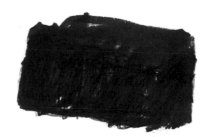

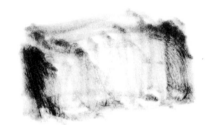

This book explains and reviews some of the significant events involved in human implantation and the establishment of the placenta in the uterus. This critical phase in human reproduction has proved to be an elusive and challenging area of research, not least because of the immunological and genetic interactions between the mother and fetus. The volume focuses on the most recent advances in our understanding of the basic mechanisms involved, with particular emphasis on cell biology and immunology. Although there are still gaps in our knowledge, the authors have succeeded in producing a timely, coherent and stimulating account of this subject. This lucid volume will benefit all those studying or undertaking research in reproductive biology and immunology, perinatal pathology, fetal medicine and obstetrics.

HUMAN IMPLANTATION
Cell Biology and Immunology

HUMAN IMPLANTATION

Cell Biology and Immunology

Y. W. LOKE AND ASHLEY KING
Research Group in Human Reproductive Immunobiology,
Department of Pathology, University of Cambridge

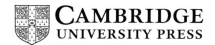

CAMBRIDGE
UNIVERSITY PRESS

Published by the Press Syndicate of the University of Cambridge
The Pitt Building, Trumpington Street, Cambridge CB2 1RP
40 West 20th Street, New York, NY 10011-4211, USA
10 Stamford Road, Oakleigh, Melbourne 3166, Australia

First published 1995

Printed in Great Britain by Biddles Ltd, Guildford & King's Lynn

A catalogue record for this book is available from the British Library

Library of Congress cataloguing in publication data
Loke, Y. W.
Human implantation : cell biology and immunology / Y. W. Loke and
Ashley King.
p.   cm.
Includes index.
ISBN 0 521 44193 5 (hc)
1. Ovum implantation. 2. Human reproduction – Immunological
aspects. I. King, Ashley. II. Title.
[DNLM: 1. Ovum Implantation – immunology. 2. Trophoblast –
immunology. 3. Maternal–Fetal Exchange. QS 645 L836h 1996]
QP275.L65 1996
612.6′3–dc20   95-21095 CIP
DNLM/DLC
for Library of Congress

ISBN 0 521 44193 5   hardback

Contents

The colour illustrations (Figs. 4.2, 7.1, 7.5 and 10.5) are between pp. 34 and 35

Acknowledgements

The idea for this book arose, either directly or indirectly, from our research interest on the immunobiology of human implantation. In an era when research funding is difficult to obtain, we are extremely fortunate that various grant-awarding bodies have supported us over the years, thereby enabling us to maintain a degree of continuity with our work. This is an opportune moment to acknowledge them. They are: the American Friends of Cambridge University; East Anglian Regional Health Authority; Sir Halley Stewart Trust; Isaac Newton Trust; Journal of Reproduction and Fertility Fellowship; Lalor Foundation (USA); Meres Senior Studentship for Medical Research, St John's College; Medical Research Council; Wellcome Trust; Special Programme of Research, Development and Research Training in Human Reproduction, World Health Organization; and Well Being (Birthright).

We would like to thank all those colleagues who generously sent us preprints. This has ensured that we have included the most recent events. All unpublished data referred to in the text are from the work of our research group which consists of the following people besides the authors: Christine Boocock, Tanya Burrows, Percy Jokhi, Lucy Gardner, Marie Mack and Eva Rainbow Hills. We are especially indebted to our two graduate students, now Drs Tanya Burrows and Percy Jokhi, for allowing us to use material from their PhD theses, especially tables and figures which, otherwise, would have taken a considerable time to reproduce. In addition, Dr Burrows' expertise in computer graphics has been invaluable in helping us generate and modify illustrations when required.

We are appreciative of the high-quality photographs produced for us by our departmental photographer, Mr Philip Starling, which now grace the pages of this book.

Our departmental librarian, Mrs Ann Nash, has spent a great deal of effort searching for, and usually managing to obtain, copies of obscure articles for our bibliography. We are most grateful to her for providing us with such unfailing service.

We would single out our secretary, Mrs Jenny Connor, who lost many evenings and weekends in a stirling effort to complete the final manuscript within a tight schedule. This was done with good humour and infinite patience. Above all, she exerted a calming influence on two increasingly demanding authors.

Finally, we assure our families that the frenetic days are over and a semblance of normality will return.

Y.W.L.
A.K.

Abbreviations

Ad	adenovirus
AFP	alpha (α) fetoprotein
ALV	avian leukosis virus
APC	antigen presenting cell
β_2m	β_2-microglobulin
BaEV	baboon endogenous virus
bp	base pair
cDNA	complementary DNA
CEA	carcinoembryonic antigen
CMV	cytomegalovirus
CNS	central nervous system
CNTF	ciliary neurotrophic factor
CRD	carbohydrate recognition domain
CSF-1	colony stimulating factor-1
CSF-1R	colony stimulating factor-1 receptor
CTL	cytotoxic T lymphocyte
cy	cytoplasmic
DAF	decay accelerating factor
EBV	Epstein–Barr virus
ECM	extracellular matrix
EGF	epidermal growth factor
EGF-R	epidermal growth factor receptor
EHS	Engelbreth–Holm–Swarm (mouse sarcoma)
ELISA	enzyme-linked immunosorbent assay
ER	estrogen receptor
EVT	extravillous trophoblast
FACS	fluorescence-activated cell sorter
FAK	focal adhesion kinase

FGF	fibroblast growth factor
FITC	fluorescein isothiocyanate
FN	fibronectin
FSH	follicle stimulating hormone
GALT	gut-associated lymphoid tissue
GALV	gibbon ape leukaemia virus
G-CSF	granulocyte colony-stimulating factor
GM-CSF	granulocyte-macrophage colony-stimulating factor
GM-CSF-R	granulocyte-macrophage colony-stimulating factor receptor
GMG	granulated metrial gland
GPI	glycosyl-phosphatidylinositol
HBV	hepatitis B virus
hCG	human chorionic gonadotrophin
HERV	human endogenous retrovirus
HGF	hepatocyte growth factor
HIV	human immunodeficiency virus
HLA	human leucocyte antigen
hPL	human placental lactogen
hsp	heat-shock protein
HTDV	human teratocarcinoma-derived virus
HTLV	human T-cell leukaemic virus
HUVEC	human umbilical vein endothelial cell
IEL	intraepithelial lymphocyte
IFN-α	interferon-α
IFN-αR	interferon-α receptor
IFN-γ	interferon-γ
IFN-γR	interferon-γ receptor
IFN-τ	trophoblast interferon
Ig	immunoglobulin
IGF	insulin-like growth factor
IGF-IR	insulin-like growth factor receptor (type I)
IGF-IIR	insulin-like growth factor receptor (type II)
IGFBP	insulin growth factor binding protein
IgSF	immunoglobulin superfamily
IL-	interleukin-
IL-1	interleukin-1
IL-2	interleukin-2
IL-1R	interleukin-1 receptor
IL-2R	interleukin-2 receptor
IRE	interferon response element

IUGR	intrauterine growth retardation
IVF	*in vitro* fertilisation
kb	kilobase
kDa	kilodalton
KDR	kinase domain-containing receptor
KGF	keratinocyte growth factor
KL	kit ligand
LAK	lymphokine-activated killer
LCA	leucocyte common antigen
Le^a	Lewis^a
Le^x	Lewis^x
LGL	large granular lymphocyte
LH	luteinising hormone
LIF	leukaemia inhibitory factor
LIF-R	leukaemia inhibitory factor receptor
LM	laminin
LTR	long terminal repeat
M-PV	Mason–Pfizer virus
MAA	melanoma-associated antigen
Mab	monoclonal antibody
MAC	membrane attack complex
MALT	mucosa-associated lymphoid tissue
MAP	mitogen-activated protein
MCP	membrane cofactor protein
MHC	Major Histocompatiblity Complex
MLR	mixed lymphocyte reaction
Mls	minor lymphocyte stimulating
MMP	metalloproteinase
MMTV	mouse mammary tumour virus
Mo-MuLV	Moloney murine leukaemia virus
mRNA	messenger ribonucleic acid
MUC-1	polymorphic epithelial mucin
MuLV	murine leukaemia virus
NCAM	neural cell adhesion molecule
NDF	neu differentiation factor
NK	natural killer
OTP-1	ovine trophoblast protein-1
Pa	pregnancy-associated antigen
PAI	plasminogen activator inhibitor
PAPP-A	pregnancy-associated plasma protein-A

PBL	peripheral blood lymphocyte
PCR	polymerase chain reaction
PDGF	platelet derived growth factor
PDGF-R	platelet derived growth factor receptor
PE	phycoerythrin
PET	pre-eclamptic toxaemia
PHA	phytohaemagglutinin
PI-PLC	phosphatidylinositol phospholipase C
PKC	protein kinase C
PLAP	placental alkaline phosphatase
pO_2	partial pressure of oxygen
PoD	post-ovulatory day
PP14	placental protein 14
PR	progesterone receptor
PSA	polysialic acid
RAG	recombination activating gene
RFLP	restriction fragment length polymorphism
RGD	arginine-glycine-aspartic acid
rh	recombinant human
RNase	ribonuclease
RT-PCR	reverse-transcriptase polymerase chain reaction
SBA	soy bean agglutinin
SCF	stem cell factor
SCID	severe combined immunodeficiency disease
SDS-PAGE	sodium dodecyl sulphate–polyacrylamide gel electrophoresis
SLE	systemic lupus erythematosus
SNRPN	small nuclear ribonucleoprotein polypeptide N
SP-1	Schwangerschafts protein-1
SSAV	simian sarcoma associated virus
SSCP	single strand conformational polymorphism
TAP	transporter associated with antigen processing
TCR	T cell receptor
TGF-α	transforming growth factor-α
TGF-β	transforming growth factor-β
TGF-βR	transforming growth factor-β receptor
TIMP	tissue inhibitor of metalloproteinase
TN	tenascin
TNF-α	tumour necrosis factor-α
TNF-R	tumour necrosis factor receptor
tPA	tissue-type plasminogen activator

VCAM	vascular cell adhesion molecule
VEGF	vascular endothelial growth factor
VT	villous trophoblast

1

Introduction

This book is devoted specifically to human implantation with passing reference to other animal species only when they shed light on the human situation. This approach is intentional because, of all mammalian physiological processes, implantation is one where the mechanisms involved differ so markedly even among closely related species as to make comparisons difficult. Viviparity is a major advance in the evolution of vertebrate reproductive strategy because it allows the fetus to develop inside the maternal uterus protected from the vagaries of the external environment. This form of reproduction is made possible by the formation of a specialised organ, the placenta, where maternal nutrients are delivered to the fetus and gaseous exchange takes place. Placentation is initiated when the blastocyst makes contact with the epithelial lining of the uterus, leading to a series of events known as implantation. Essentially, this involves fetally derived placental trophoblast cells coming into close apposition with maternal tissues. It is in this process that species variations occur, ranging from merely superficial contact such as that seen in ungulates to deep penetration like in humans. Also, in the latter type of implantation, the uterine endometrial lining is transformed during pregnancy into a specialised tissue, the decidua, whose function is not known. The proposal that it may protect the mother from excessive trophoblast invasion is attractive. The human decidua contains a variety of cell types. Elucidation of their role in influencing trophoblast behaviour is currently a major focus of research interest.

Because of this species variability, attempts to extrapolate animal data to man have largely confused the issue. It is not to say that animal studies are of no value. They are useful for the species being studied, but they should not be considered as exact replicas of human implantation. To be valid, investigations on human implantation have to be performed on our own species, and the only way that this can be achieved is to design *in vitro* assays that simulate the *in vivo* situation. A major technical difficulty had been the lack of suitable methods by which relevant cell types could be isolated with a sufficient degree of purity for valid experimentation. However, in recent years great strides have been made in this direction. Experiments using these isolated cells are now beginning to provide an insight into the cellular mechanisms involved in human implantation.

The association between trophoblast and decidual cells is highly complex and a detailed knowledge of the histology of the implantation site is required before a clear view of the overall process can be obtained. Older studies based on morphology, by either light or electron microscopy, did not provide a sufficiently precise identification of the cell types involved. However, the availability of appropriate specific antibodies directed at cell markers and their use in immunohistology have greatly increased our understanding of the topography of the human implantation site.

There are many aspects of the cell biology of human implantation that will be of interest to both basic scientists and clinical obstetricians. Trophoblast invasion of uterine tissues and eventual destruction of the arterial walls of decidual spiral arteries are essential features of human implantation. This is to ensure an adequate blood supply to the developing feto-placental unit. Such aggressive cellular behaviour is normally only associated with malignant cells, the cardinal difference being that trophoblast invasion is tightly controlled while that of cancer cells is not. At present, very little is known about what controls trophoblast migration. Based on studies in other physiological systems, binding to extracellular matrix proteins via adhesion molecules is one possible mechanism. In particular, recent advances in the understanding of the structure and function of integrins as well as the biochemistry of matrix proteins such as laminin and fibronectin, have emphasised the potential role of these receptor–ligand interactions in trophoblast migration. Besides acting as an intercellular 'glue', it is now generally accepted that matrix proteins can transduce signals into a cell via its integrin receptors, thereby providing a mechanism for a cell to respond to information from its external environment. This could be a very important way by which maternal decidua can influence the behaviour of invading trophoblast cells.

A family of molecules which is receiving increasing attention in relation to cellular growth and differentiation is the cytokines. These are proteins which dictate cellular functions by acting in an autocrine or a paracrine manner. It has been known for quite some time that many cytokines can be detected in the human placenta and the uterus, but it is comparatively recently that the actual cellular sources within these organs have been identified by techniques such as immunohistology and *in situ* hybridisation on tissue sections together with PCR, ELISA and bioassays on isolated cells. Similarly, the cells expressing cytokine receptors are also being documented. Once a complete picture is obtained regarding the sources of production and the potential responding cells, the next stage would be to design experiments to examine the effects of individual or groups of cytokines on defined cell populations isolated from the trophoblast–decidual interface.

Perhaps the most intriguing aspect of implantation is that it involves two distinct individuals – the fetus and the mother. This has genetic and immunological implications. The phenomenon of gene imprinting in which genes inherited from a paternal or maternal source have differing effects on embryonic development has led to the hypothesis that this could be an evolutionary device by which the activity of paternal genes is nullified by maternal genes. This paternal–maternal conflict may have arisen because paternal genes have evolved to enhance the growth of the embryo at whatever cost to the mother, while maternal genes are there to ensure that she survives the demands of the present pregnancy in order to breed again. Immunologically, the close admixture of cells from two antigenically disparate individuals is analogous to that seen in clinical organ transplantation. The question of why the conceptus is not rejected by the mother like an allograft has preoccupied reproductive immunologists for a long time. A solution to the problem remains tantalisingly beyond reach. Recent observations, however, have indicated that reproduction may not be governed by the laws of classical transplantation immunology, in spite of superficial resemblance of the conceptus to an organ graft. Instead, there are many aspects of reproduction which seem to involve an immune system more akin to that seen in invertebrates. This realisation has completely changed our conceptual view of the immunology of human implantation. Thus, there is need for a reappraisal of this central paradigm in reproductive immunology.

Many pathological conditions of pregnancy encountered in clinical obstetrical practice, such as miscarriage, intrauterine growth retardation and pre-eclampsia, are all due to failure of the normal controlling mechanisms on trophoblast migration, leading to insufficient invasion and vascular adaptation with the final result of poor perfusion of the feto-placental unit. Recent reports that inadequate fetal nutrition *in utero* can lead to a higher incidence of heart disease and diabetes in adult life further emphasise the importance of this process. Research into how implantation is controlled could lead eventually to the development of therapeutic regimes to alleviate some of these conditions.

This volume attempts to collate the relevant available information pertaining to the immunology and cell biology of human implantation in the hope that it will serve as a useful reference point for all those interested in this aspect of human reproduction. We would emphasise that research in this field is still very much in its infancy, so that many conclusions are necessarily speculative, either because available data are conflicting or because they cannot yet be formulated into any meaningful concept. In addition, the views expressed are entirely our own and may contrast with those held by others. Nevertheless, we believe that there is now sufficient information to permit at least a preliminary evaluation of the mechanisms that may be involved in human implantation.

2

Evolution of the maternal–fetal interaction

Evolution of placentation

Major landmarks in the phylogenetic history of vertebrates are two developments in early reptiles which eliminated reliance on open water for reproduction. These are the possession of copulatory organs by the male that can deliver sperm directly into the female's body rather than into the surrounding water (internal fertilisation), and the production of amniote eggs by the female (Postlethwait and Hopson 1992). The amniote egg contains yolk and albumen which supply nutrients to the embryo via the yolk sac, while the allantoic sac carries out gaseous exchange with the external environment across the porous egg shell as well as serving as an excretory organ by converting nitrogenous waste into relatively non-toxic uric acid (Morriss 1975). Thus, an independent viable unit is formed. This adaptation subsequently emancipated reptiles from the necessity to breed in water and allowed them to colonise the land, sea and air, making them the most successful species during the Mesozoic era – which became known as the Age of Reptiles.

The first step on the road to viviparity is taken by some reptiles retaining the egg inside the maternal oviduct where embryo–maternal exchange is carried out between the allantoic and oviductal blood streams (Sharman 1976). This is facilitated by hypertrophy of the blood vessels within the oviductal region in contact with the egg and by thinning of both the uterine epithelium and chorio-allantoic membrane, resulting in close apposition of the two blood streams. From this area, a specialised organ, the placenta, is eventually formed. Thus, some of the viviparous reptiles (e.g. the adder) already have well-developed chorio-allantoic placentae, but in none of these species does the chorion invade the uterine epithelium.

Early in the Mesozoic era, a group of reptiles, the Therapsids, diverged from the primitive reptilian stock and ultimately evolved into three groups. These are the monotremes, marsupials and eutherian mammals. The monotremes (e.g. the duck-billed platypus and spiny ant eater) remain egg-layers and are probably the most primitive of the group. The marsupials do have a placental form of reproduction, but the young is born highly immature and needs to be nurtured for a further period in the pouch where it obtains nutrients via the mammary gland (e.g. kangaroo). In marsupial placentation, different degrees of trophoblast invasion into maternal uterine tissues can be seen. For example, the placenta of the North American opossum (*Didelphis virginiana*) is only superficially apposed to the uterine epithelium, but in the four-eyed opossum (*Philander opossum*) the trophoblast is mildly invasive, penetrating the uterine epithelium and extending into the uterine stroma. The function of this process is probably to anchor the placenta so that the embryonic and uterine epithelia remain in close apposition. At first, the bilaminar amphalopleure where nutrient material secreted by maternal tissue is absorbed by the trophoblast (i.e. histiotrophic nutrition) consists of an outer layer of trophectoderm and an inner layer of yolk sac endoderm. Later in gestation, vascularised embryonic mesoderm extends between the two layers to form a trilaminar amphalopleure which is the basic structure of the marsupial yolk sac placenta. Here, the trophoblast layer develops numerous prominent microvilli which can take in maternal molecules by pinocytosis which are then transferred across to the fetal circulation (i.e. haemotrophic nutrition).

The extensive diversity of fetal membranes is a feature only of Eutheria. Essentially, the types of placentation are classified according to the number and form of the layers which intervene between fetal and maternal circulations (Table 2.1). As can be seen from the table, it is the presence or absence of certain maternal layers that is the basis for the variation. The category of syndesmochorial has since been modified because many anatomists are of the opinion that the uterine epithelium persists in certain areas of ruminant placental implantation, so that this kind of placentation is essentially epitheliochorial. However, Wooding (1992) has argued from studies in the sheep that there is fusion between fetal chorionic cells and maternal uterine epithelial cells to form a hybrid feto-maternal syncytial layer. Thus, the sheep placenta is neither epitheliochorial nor syndesmochorial. Wooding has suggested synepitheliochorial as a term that best describes this kind of ruminant placentation.

The deepest invasion is in those species with haemochorial placentation (e.g. humans) where placental trophoblast cells come into direct contact with maternal blood. The advantage of this is obvious as it establishes the most intimate association between the developing embryo and its source of nutrition from the mother. However, it must not be assumed that this form of placentation is necessarily the most advanced in evolutionary terms. As can be seen in the dendogram of mammalian evolution (Fig. 2.1), haemochorial placentation occurs in a variety of species that are unconnected in their evolutionary lineage.

Table 2.1. *Classification of different types of chorio-allantoic placentae according to the number of maternal and fetal layers present*

Type of placenta	Maternal tissues			Fetal tissues			Examples
	Endothelium	Connective tissue	Uterine epithelium	Chorion	Connective tissue	Endothelium	
Epitheliochorial	+	+	+	+	+	+	Horse, pig
Syndesmochorial	+	–	–	+	+	+	Most ruminants, e.g. sheep, cow
Endotheliochorial	+	–	–	+	+	+	Most carnivores, e.g. cat, dog
Haemochorial	–	–	–	+	+	+	Man, primates, rodents

Adapted from Amcroso (1968).

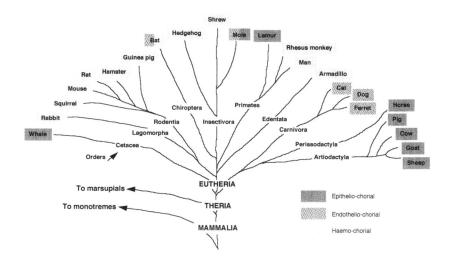

Fig. 2.1. Mammals with different types of placentation.

Therefore, a high degree of trophoblast penetration is not the ultimate end-point of a stepwise progression in placental evolution, but has developed in a species-specific manner, probably as a result of some unique requirements in their reproductive process. Because of its highly invasive nature, the disadvantage of haemochorial placentation is that it is dangerous to the mother. It is not surprising, therefore, to find there is a concomitant evolution of the uterine endometrium into a pregnancy-transformed decidua which appears to have the capacity to control the extent of trophoblast invasion.

The importance of decidua can be seen experimentally by transplanting murine blastocysts into extrauterine sites where trophoblast is observed to invade uncontrollably (Kirby 1960). In human pregnancy, implantation into areas deficient in decidua, such as a previous Caesarian section scar or in ectopic tubal pregnancy, also results in uncontrolled trophoblast invasion. Significantly, in species with epitheliochorial placentation there is no decidualisation of the endometrium. Thus, in the evolution of mammalian placentation, the development of a highly invasive trophoblast occurs concomitantly with adaptation of the uterine mucosa to resist this invasion. There is, therefore, a compromise between the nutritional benefit to the embryo and the risk of uterine rupture in the mother. Out of these observations has arisen the concept that there has been an evolutionary accommodation between fetal genes encoding for enhanced trophoblast invasion and gaining greater access to maternal nutrients and maternal genes which limit this potentially dangerous invasion (Haig 1993). This could provide a rationale for imprinting of maternal and paternal genes (Chapter 3), a phenomenon restricted to placental mammals (Moore and Haig 1991).

During the period when the placenta is evolving, a well-developed immune system is already in place. Thus, an important factor that needs to be taken into account, particularly in the highly invasive variety of placentation, is the potential immune defensive response of the mother. The process of implantation involves the intimate association of cells from two antigenically disparate organisms (embryo and mother) so some form of non-self or allogeneic immune recognition would be expected to occur. This is a problem which hampers clinical organ transplantation to-day. Both Medawar (1953) and Billingham (1964) have addressed the question of fetal allograft survival based on their studies of graft rejection. However, this analogy is becoming increasingly inappropriate because there is accumulating evidence to indicate that the human conceptus is not subjected to the laws of classical transplantation immunity. Instead, reproduction appears to involve a more primitive maternal defence system (King and Loke 1991). Indeed, there are many aspects of human reproduction which resemble the immune defence of invertebrates. For this reason, it would be illuminating to trace the development of vertebrate immunity from its invertebrate ancestry, and to see how the human maternal–fetal interaction fits into this evolutionary framework (Millar and Ratcliffe 1994). The phylogenetic relationship between the main groups in the animal kingdom is shown in Fig. 2.2. The major division into the two lineages of Protostomata and Deuterostomata based on differences in embryological development of the mouth and anus probably occurred more than 500 million years ago. As can be seen from Fig. 2.2, vertebrates are descended from the Deuterostomata lineage so that it will be among invertebrates, such as Urochordata and Echinodermata, that homologous (i.e. sharing a common ancestry) immune cells are likely to be found. While immune cells with similar structure and function to those in vertebrates may also be encountered in Protostomata invertebrates, these are probably a result of convergent evolution (i.e. analogous rather than homologous).

Evolution of cells for defence

Phagocytes are as old as life itself. The process of phagocytosis was utilised by unicellular organisms and has been retained in higher vertebrates. As pathogens became more adept at evading killing by phagocytes, other cells emerged which could eliminate infected cells or provide help by secretion of soluble products (Fig. 2.3). The first to appear were natural killer (NK)-like cells which can be traced back to invertebrates and which continue to play an important defensive

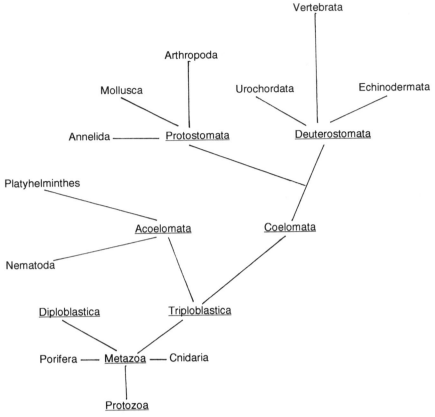

Fig. 2.2. Evolution of the animal kingdom.

role in these organisms, such as annelids and urochordates. Analogous NK-like cells can be seen also in the freshwater snail. This mollusc possesses lymphocyte-like cells which stain for several surface markers of human NK cells such as CD56, but are devoid of T cell markers such as CD3, CD4 and CD8 (Franceschi *et al*. 1991). These cells are also cytotoxic to the human NK-sensitive cell line, K562. NK cells are generally considered to be the evolutionary precursor of T cells (Janeway 1992), but when T cells actually first emerged is still a matter of dispute. T-cell-receptor-like genes are present at the earliest stages in the phylogenetic emergence of jawed vertebrates (Rast and Litman 1994). The important distinguishing feature between mammalian T cells and NK cells is the expression of a clonally distributed T cell receptor which arises by a process of genetic recombination under the influence of the recombination activation gene (RAG). This allows T cells a highly diverse and specific repertoire compared with the more broad spectrum recognition system of NK

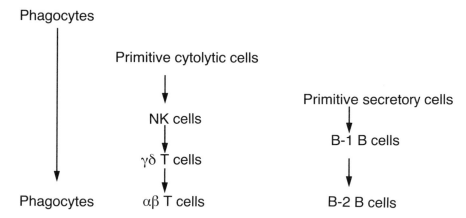

Fig. 2.3. Evolution of cells for defence.

cells. T cell effector mechanisms also require clonal expansion, and are capable of memory. Both these features are not typical of NK cells.

There are subpopulations of T cells: γδ T cells and αβ T cells. Although the phrase 'ontogeny recapitulates phylogeny' is often over-used, it is interesting that in the human fetus, NK cells are the first lymphocyte lineage to emerge followed by γδ T cells and subsequently αβ T cells. Certainly, γδ T cells are still something of an enigma with regard to target ligands and function. They often demonstrate limited receptor diversity and tissue-specific localisation. There are also subtypes of the B cell lineage: B-1 and B-2 cells. B-1 cells are the most primitive and produce low-affinity, broad specificity IgM antibodies compared with the diverse and highly specific antibodies secreted by conventional B-2 cells.

To summarise, phagocytic cells were the earliest defensive cell. The most primitive lymphocyte appears to be the NK cell. Both these cells have persisted and now comprise the so-called innate or natural immune system of vertebrates. Later, cells with clonally distributed receptors emerged (T and B cells) to provide the specific adaptive immune system. Thus, the immune system may be viewed as having been created in layers by evolution, where each new layer is more complex and sophisticated than the preceding one (Herzenberg et al. 1992). It is important to note that the preceding layers are not replaced, but have evolved either to cooperate with the subsequent layers or to develop some other function.

Anatomic compartmentalisation of the immune system

Alongside the onset of increasing sophistication and types of defensive cells, there is a concomitant development of greater complexity of the anatomic organisation of the immune cells during evolution. Phagocytes in diblastic phyla were able to wander between the two body layers separated by a primitive connective tissue, the mesoglea. In the triblastic phyla, the mesodermal layer eventually became the basis for the development of organs and a circulatory system. The simplest form is exemplified by flatworms and the ribbon worms, which have a vascular system filled with a variety of phagocytic and lymphocyte-like cells. The development of a coelom situated between the intestinal tract and the body wall is another development allowing movement of phagocytic and other cells between the two body layers. The annelids are representative of this protostome coelomate phylum and have both a well-developed coelom and a closed circulatory system allowing more complex compartmentalisation of the cellular components. In molluscs the primary body cavity has developed further into a large open vascular system, the haemocoel.

With the emergence of the chordate and vertebrate body plans in deuterostomes came the appearance of specialised organs concerned with immune defence. This allowed microenvironments to be strategically placed where cellular interactions could more easily take place. Eventually, these became the vertebrate spleen, thymus and lymph nodes (Kroemer *et al.* 1993). It should be emphasised that the defensive systems at the body surfaces were in place far earlier than any of the complex systemic immune systems (Du Pasquier 1993). These surface systems were probably populated by lymphocyte-like cells, possibly early B-1 type cells and cytotoxic cells together with phagocytic cells, and were already present in several invertebrate phyla. A similar system is conserved in vertebrates and is known as GALT or gut-associated lymphoid tissue. This can be expanded to include all mucosal surfaces by the designation MALT for mucosa-associated lymphoid tissue.

Allorecognition

Virtually all invertebrates are capable of some form of histocompatibility reactions. However, the nature of the experiments in these animals and lack of genetic information makes the data difficult to interpret. Furthermore, it can be confusing if data from the diverse groups of invertebrates are considered together. Nevertheless, despite these constraints, several general conclusions can be drawn.

In the crowded marine environment, direct cellular contact between sedentary metazoans will frequently occur. The possibility of fusion or contamination by other members of the species poses a threat, and needs to be combated. Thus, allorecognition has developed to maintain the individuality of each colony. This could be the origin of histocompatibility reactions.

In vertebrate allorecognition, cytotoxicity and rejection is the expected result. However, in some invertebrate phyla, e.g. Porifera (sponges), there are two possible outcomes when genetically different colonies meet on the sea bed. Cytotoxicity or rejection reactions may occur, but another is the production of a collagen barrier between the two apposing colonies, known as the encapsulation reaction, which is rapidly infiltrated by large granular wandering cells (Smith and Hildemann 1986; Humphreys and Reinherz 1994).

In the allorecognition systems of invertebrates, no prior sensitisation is necessary. This observation prompted Burnet (1971) to conclude that the primary mechanism must be based on 'self-recognition' with the primitive immunocytes expressing receptors which bind to the individual's own histocompatibility antigens. Any foreign cells that lack these antigens will be immediately detected without prior sensitisation. Subsequent detailed investigations on the allogeneic responses on colonial tunicates, such as *Botryllus*, have confirmed Burnet's view. Killing or rejection is observed to occur between interacting cells or tissues unless they share some alleles in common (Smith and Davidson 1992). For example, in this organism, the progeny from an AB × CD cross will be of four different types: AC, AD, BC and BD. Any two sets with a gene in common will be able to fuse with each other (e.g. AC/BC, AC/AD), whereas those with no gene in common will undergo necrosis when brought into contact (e.g. AC/BD, AD/BC), producing a barrier between the two colonies, a phenomenon known as 'colony specificity'. Thus, the recognition system in *Botryllus* detects absence of shared alleles rather than the presence of different alleles. This, in turn, implies that invertebrate immune recognition is directed inwards towards self-recognition, whereas in vertebrates the focus of the immune system is directed outwards for specific recognition of foreign molecules. It seems that some aspects of this invertebrate histocompatibility system are retained in higher vertebrates. In the phenomenon of 'hybrid resistance' described in mice, F_1 hybrids from homozygous parents are observed to reject bone marrow grafts from either one of the parents (Fig. 2.4). This again appears to be an example of recognition of the absence of a gene in common rather than the presence of a foreign gene, and is now known to be mediated by NK cells. There is accumulating evidence from many species, including humans, that NK cells tend to be cytolytic to target cells which are deficient in Major Histocompatibility Complex (MHC) class I molecules. Thus arose the concept that, while T cells recognise 'non-self', NK cells recognise 'missing self' or the absence of self (Ljunggren and Kärre 1990). Neoplastic transformation or viral infection can lead to downregulation of class I molecules, and it is possible that NK cells will provide the defence in these situations. Therefore, the phylogenetically more primitive NK cells have been designed for internal surveillance and to monitor the integrity of self, while T

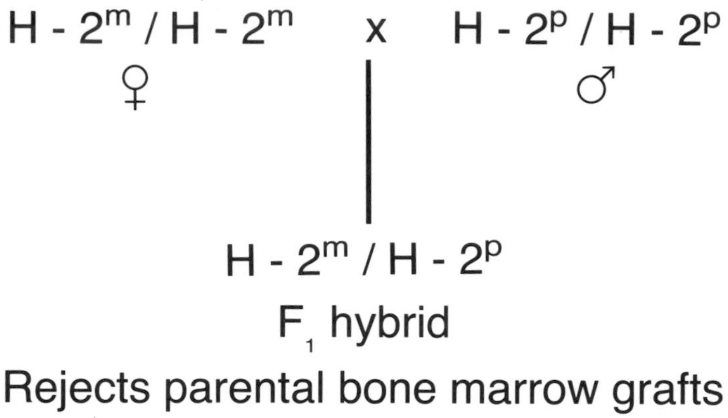

$$H - 2^m / H - 2^m \quad \text{x} \quad H - 2^p / H - 2^p$$

♀   ♂

$$H - 2^m / H - 2^p$$

F$_1$ hybrid

Rejects parental bone marrow grafts

Fig. 2.4. The phenomenon of hybrid resistance where the F$_1$ hybrids from homozygous parents reject bone marrow grafts from either one of the parents.

cells have been developed to guard against non-self external aggressors. This idea is not a new one. It was already the basic concept of Metchnikoff's work over a century ago when the early immune processes were considered to be concerned mainly with embryogenesis and only later in development used to defend the host against invading pathogens (Tauber 1994). In mammals, these disparate functions of NK cells and T cells have been retained.

Further studies on *Botryllus* have shown that while colonies sharing one but not both alleles will initially fuse, one member of the resultant chimera will eventually die and be absorbed by the other. This is known as 'colony resorption' (Weissman *et al*. 1990). Thus, there are two phenomena in *Botryllus* allorecognition: colony specificity and colony resorption. The first is the result of the recognition of shared alleles leading to the delivery of negative signals, while the second is probably caused by the presence of a foreign allele with generation of positive signals.

Although the genes involved in invertebrate histocompatibility reactions are still largely unknown, more recent work has indicated that, in *Botryllus*, there are several loci controlling the fusion/non-fusion and the resorption reactions which can be highly polymorphic and may contain as many as 100 alleles (Sima and Vetvicka 1993). Allorecognition is governed by multiple codominantly expressed alleles at a single highly polymorphic haplotype. Whether this elaborate gene system is related to the MHC genes of vertebrates is unknown (Schofield *et al*. 1982). According to Klein (1991), an ancestral MHC probably existed at the time of the emergence of vertebrates over 500 million years ago. If the *Botryllus* allorecognition histocompatibility systems have evolved prior to the protochordate/chordate split, it is possible that these systems could be the precursor of the self + foreign antigen type of immune recognition utilised by vertebrate T cell receptors.

Immunology of the maternal–fetal interaction

Many of the features of the local maternal–fetal interaction in the uterus are those associated with the primitive immune system. The defensive cells present at the feto-maternal interface in the human uterus are macrophages and NK cells which are cells of the innate system. B cells are absent and T cells sparse. Furthermore, the NK cells closely resemble the fetal NK cells which first appear in ontogeny (Chapter 7). Although uterine NK cells have been most extensively investigated in humans, equivalent NK-like cells, granulated metrial gland (GMG) cells, are present in rodents (Croy 1994). The presence of granulated lymphocytes at the feto-maternal interface in species with epitheliochorial placentation has been harder to establish. Nonetheless, by functional analysis in the pig (Croy *et al.* 1994), morphological analysis in the horse (Enders and Liu 1991) and phenotypic analysis in the sheep (Lee *et al.* 1992) it seems that granulated non-T lymphocytes are also present in these species. Their anatomic localisation is, however, different from that in mice and humans as they seem to be predominantly intraepithelial. This may reflect the fact that the feto-maternal boundary in these species is at the epithelium. The presence of abundant NK cells throughout the human decidual stroma may correlate with the deep infiltration of trophoblast. Perhaps uterine NK-like cells will invariably be found to accumulate at the actual physical feto-maternal interface as more species are examined.

The uterus is a mucosal surface and has many features of the MALT system rather than the complex structure of a lymph node (Morris *et al.* 1985). Even the presence of lymphatics in the human endometrium is disputed. In evolutionary terms, therefore, it is a relatively primitive lymphoid compartment.

Unlike the artificial situation of an organ transplant, the intermingling of cells from genetically different individuals occurs naturally during placentation. Also unlike a transplant, the mammalian conceptus is not rejected. As we have seen, a possible outcome of invertebrate allorecognition is the formation of a collagen interface. This interface provides a mutual demarcation of territorial boundaries, and can be viewed as an extension of the monitoring of self. There is no killing of either of the two organisms. The feto-maternal interface is far more analogous to this situation. It has often been viewed as a 'battlefield', and in humans there is a layer of fibrinoid material, the Nitabuch's layer (Kaufmann and Burton 1994), which may be akin to the boundary. Yet it has always been a mystery how the battle is resolved. Neither parasitism nor rejection occurs. Does delineation of this boundary depend on some form of allorecognition by the mother? If so, how might this be mediated?

Despite the original definition of NK recognition as 'non-MHC restricted', it is now generally accepted that NK cells are capable of allorecognition and that human NK cells can broadly discriminate between some MHC class I antigens (Kärre 1993; Trinchieri 1994). This may be a legacy from the time when MHC molecules interacted with other cells in the absence of T cell receptors (TCR) because it is still an open question whether MHC molecules or the TCR evolved first (Bartl *et al.* 1994). Interestingly, human extravillous trophoblast expresses class I HLA-G and maybe HLA-C also, but not the usual class I HLA-A,B like other somatic cells (Chapter 5). Perhaps these class I antigens provide the recognition molecules by which decidual NK cells detect the allogeneic nature of trophoblast (Chapter 8). This recognition can then result in the generation of either negative or positive signals analogous to the *Botryllus* colony specificity or colony resorption phenomena. However, it must not be assumed that MHC class I molecules are the only ones involved. Classical immunology defines 'self' and 'non-self' according to the MHC, but this may not be the case in primitive immune systems such as NK cells. Carbohydrate–lectin interactions are often used by cells of the innate immune system such as macrophages whereby foreign cells such as bacteria are detected and phagocytosed. Of great interest is the recent discovery that NK cells in mice, rats and humans express type II membrane glycoproteins which contain a C-type lectin-like domain (Chambers *et al.* 1993). Some of these NK receptors have been found to recognise oligosaccharide ligands which deliver stimulatory or inhibitory signals to the NK cell (Bezouska *et al.* 1994). A search for trophoblast-specific carbohydrate antigens might prove very fruitful. There is already evidence that sialylated type I blood group related carbohydrates are preferentially expressed on certain human extravillous trophoblast sub-populations (King and Loke 1988). Thus, the concept of 'self' and 'non-self' in terms of NK cells may be very different to how it is generally perceived in classical T cell immunology.

An effector mechanism frequently used by primitive defence systems is secretion of cytokines. These are highly conserved proteins as suggested by the structural homologies observed in the cytokines of different vertebrate classes. Indeed, there is evidence that cytokine-orchestrated host defences are not restricted to vertebrates but are also present in invertebrates, such as annelids, echinoderms and urochordates (Beck and Habicht 1991). Even single cell protozoa may possess cytokine-like molecules. Human IL-2 can compete effectively for receptor binding with a protozoan pheromone (Er-1) and, reciprocally, a Mab raised to Er-1 blocks the IL-2 induced proliferation of a mouse T cell line (Ortenzi *et al.* 1990).

Many cytokines are pleiotropic and function not only in host defence but also in tissue development. For example, the colony stimulating factors (CSF) play an important role in the proliferation and maturation of cells, particularly during haemopoiesis. Cytokines produced by NK cells in the bone marrow, either constitutively or upon activation, are important mediators of this process (Trinchieri 1989). It is interesting to note that decidual NK cells also produce colony stimulating factors, among other cytokines (Chapter 10), so the possibility arises that during evolution trophoblast has managed to utilise certain aspects of the maternal cytokine response to sustain its own development. These cytokines will provide either positive or negative signals to ensure the correct degree of trophoblast migration within the uterine environment in the same way as haemopoiesis is controlled in the bone marrow.

The overall conclusion from this chapter is that the mammalian placenta, unlike other organs, exhibits a wide range of structural and functional characteristics based on the degree of interaction between fetal and maternal tissues so that major differences can be found even among closely related species. This is due to the fact that different species have evolved different means to achieve the same end, which is to obtain the optimal method for embryonic nourishment *in utero* as a necessary prerequisite for the development of viviparity. Studies on animal placentation, therefore, cannot be readily extrapolated to humans, and this constraint should be appreciated in the interpretation of experimental data. Furthermore, the relationship between the implanted placenta and the uterus is governed by a primitive defence system whose mechanism of self and non-self recognition and the reaction invoked are not the same as for the classical adaptive immune response. Thus, although the human placenta is genetically foreign to the mother, the characteristics of its interaction with the uterus are more akin to those observed between unrelated primitive invertebrates than between mammalian allograft and host as seen in contemporary transplantation immunology. Experimental studies of human implantation, therefore, should be designed within this evolutionary framework.

3

Decidualisation

Morphology

The closely coordinated events which take place in the transformation of endometrium to decidua affect all the cell types present in the uterine mucosa. Morphologically the most obvious changes are seen in the stromal cells and epithelial glandular cells (Maslar 1988), together with infiltration by large numbers of bone marrow derived cells (King *et al*. 1991). The development of a secretory endometrium capable of supporting implantation and pregnancy is achieved when the uterus is exposed to an appropriate sequence of estrogen and progesterone. After menstruation, under the influence of estrogen, there is rapid proliferation of both epithelial and stromal cells (proliferative phase). Following ovulation, when progesterone levels start to rise, proliferation in the glands and stroma will cease and differentiation begins (secretory or luteal phase). The appearance of basal subnuclear vacuoles in the glandular epithelium 24–48 hours after the luteinising hormone (LH) surge is the first histological evidence that ovulation has occurred and the secretory phase commenced. Secretory activity in glands is maximal on the 5th to 7th post-ovulatory day (POD) when large amounts of mucin, glycogen and glycoprotein are seen in the gland lumina. Stromal cell differentiation begins later (POD 9–10) when the cells around spiral arteries and beneath the uterine epithelium become plump and glycogen rich, an appearance known as pre-decidual change. This spontaneous decidualisation of the endometrial stroma is initiated in the normal menstrual cycle and will occur even in the absence of pregnancy, a situation that differs from that in other species such as rats, mice, guinea pigs and rabbits in which the decidual reaction only begins at implantation.

This decidualised tissue eventually breaks down with bleeding at the end of the cycle at menstruation (Finn 1994). If pregnancy occurs, these decidual changes in the stroma become much more extensive and three layers of decidua can now be discerned. The upper layer, the decidua compacta, contains decidualised stroma with attenuated non-secretory glands. Beneath this the decidua spongiosa is composed of dilated secretory glands separated by a narrow rim of non-decidualised stroma. The basal layer remains undifferentiated, and it is from this layer that regeneration occurs after menstruation or parturition.

After implantation, three anatomical decidual regions in the uterus are apparent. The decidua basalis lies beneath the developing placenta, and is the maternal tissue infiltrated by extravillous trophoblast cells. Overlying the embryo is the decidua capsularis. This will eventually fuse with the decidua parietalis which lines the uterus away from the implantation site. Fusion of the decidua capsularis with the decidua parietalis in the fourth month involves degeneration of the uterine surface epithelium and obliteration of the uterine cavity. The amniochorion formed from regression of the capsular villi therefore comes into contact with maternal decidua parietalis and an additional point of cell contact is formed between fetal and maternal tissues.

Estrogen and progesterone receptor expression

Estrogen and progesterone are essential for the preparation of the endometrium and the maintenance of pregnancy after implantation. The cellular distribution of estrogen receptors (ER) and progesterone receptors (PR) in the endometrium has been assessed by immunohistology of both frozen and paraffin sections (Garcia *et al.* 1988; Lessey *et al.* 1988; Press *et al.* 1988; Snijders *et al.* 1992; Bergqvist *et al.* 1993; Critchley *et al.* 1993; Amso *et al.* 1994). A summary of the findings in these reports is given (Fig. 3.1). Although there are some minor discrepancies there is general agreement that both glandular and stromal cell expression of ER increases until around the time of ovulation and then gradually declines to become undetectable by the mid-luteal phase. Staining for PR increases during the proliferative phase to become maximal at the time of ovulation and in the early secretory phase. PR expression in glands then rapidly declines, but is maintained in the stroma throughout the luteal phase although at slightly lower levels. There is some variation in both the number of cells staining positively and the intensity of staining. Several of these immunohistochemical studies have devised quantitative methods which take these variables into account.

In pregnancy the nuclei of decidual glandular epithelial cells persist in showing no staining for either ER or PR (Perrot-Applanat *et al.* 1994). Nuclear staining for PR is found in stromal cells and in endothelial and medial cells of the spiral arteries (Wang *et al.* 1992). It should be noted that in all these immunohistological studies, the proportion of stromal cells staining is quite low (25–50%). It is generally

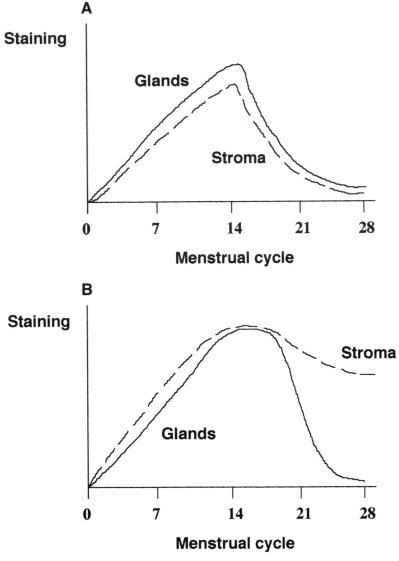

Fig. 3.1. The expression of the estrogen receptor (**A**) and progesterone receptor (**B**) in endometrial glands and stroma throughout the menstrual cycle.

assumed that ER and PR expression in the stroma is localised to stromal cells themselves, but there has been no study directly analysing hormone receptor expression by the other stromal populations such as uterine lymphocytes and macrophages, and this is an important omission. Furthermore, although cells of the placental villi, including villous trophoblast, are reportedly negative for both ER and PR, the expression of these receptors on extravillous trophoblast populations has not been extensively analysed (Perrot-Applanat *et al*. 1994; Shi *et al*. 1993a, b). There are reports suggesting differential expression of PR between decidua capsularis and parietalis, but these are difficult to interpret as it is not clear how the different decidual regions were identified (Wu *et al*. 1993).

Two distinct isoforms of the human progesterone receptor have been identified: PR-A and PR-B. The PR-B isoform contains an N-terminal fragment of 164 amino acids which is absent from the PR-A isoform. Both forms can arise either by alternate initiation of transcription from the same mRNA or by transcription from alternate promoters within the same gene (Conneely *et al*. 1987; Kastner *et al*. 1990). The expression levels of PR-A and PR-B can, therefore, differ from each other in target tissues. PR-A has been shown to function both as a repressor of PR-B transcriptional activity and as an activator (Vegeto *et al*. 1993). Alterations in the relative concentration of the two PR isoforms in the cells of the endometrium are likely to have widespread phenotypic and functional effects.

Functions of decidua

The most obvious function of the uterine lining is to provide a fertile soil for the nourishment of the developing fetus throughout gestation. However, nidation can and does occur in ectopic sites in man, with fetal development occurring successfully until term (albeit rarely), indicating that an adequate supply of nutrients to the feto-placental unit can be derived from other tissues besides decidua (Ombelet *et al*. 1988). The more usual outcome of an ectopic gestation is potentially fatal haemorrhage resulting from trophoblast invasion into maternal vessels. In addition, even if pregnancies proceed into the third trimester surgical removal of placental tissue is generally required.

Decidualisation is a feature unique to those species which exhibit invasive haemochorial placentation. Furthermore, the degree of trophoblast invasion into the uterus in different species is closely correlated with the extent of decidualisation. Both trophoblast invasion and decidual change are most pronounced in humans. This might reflect the relatively long period of intrauterine existence required for human development, which in turn depends on a very good fetal blood supply. It has been suggested that the morphological changes of decidualisation in the uterus are there to facilitate implantation and trophoblast migration (Ramsey *et al*. 1976). However, it can be argued that the opposite is the case, and that trophoblast is inherently programmed to invade into any tissue and decidua provides the necessary restraining influence to control against over-invasion.

In tubal pregnancy, trophoblast invasion from the cytotrophoblast shell into maternal stroma and vessels occurs as in intrauterine pregnancies. Foci of decidualisation can be present in tubal pregnancies, but no true decidua is seen. In the absence of decidua the pattern of trophoblast invasion is different (unpublished). Trophoblast cells migrating into the Fallopian tube tend to retain the morphology of cohesive rounded cells unlike the isolated elongated cells moving through the uterine decidual stroma. Furthermore, in tubal pregnancies, the terminal stage of extravillous trophoblast differentiation, the placental bed giant cell, is rarely seen. These morphological observations suggest that the important role of decidua is to control trophoblast migration, perhaps by converting the inherently invasive trophoblast from motile mononuclear cells to static giant cells. Observations of ectopic implantation in mice led Kirby to the same conclusion many years ago: 'The full invasive proclivities of trophoblast are not realised during normal pregnancy' and 'the presence of decidual tissue curtails the invasiveness of trophoblast' (Kirby 1970; Billington 1971).

To summarise, invasiveness by trophoblast is essential to provide an adequate maternal blood supply, but regulation of this invasion requires interaction with decidua. How do the various cell types present in decidua fulfil this role? The contributions of surface and glandular epithelium, stromal cells, and blood vessels will be considered in this chapter. The leucocytic populations are discussed separately in Chapters 7 and 8.

Surface epithelium

The initial contact between the blastocyst and the uterus is by adhesion of the embryonic trophectoderm to the uterine surface epithelium. The surface epithelium differs from the epithelium lining the endometrial glands in several respects. The surface cells do not undergo the cyclical secretory changes of the glands. In addition, ciliated cells are present so that morphologically the surface epithelium resembles more the lining of the Fallopian tube rather than the underlying glands. These differences are important when interpreting *in vitro* experiments using uterine epithelium, even if the cultured cells show appropriate polarity. Successful isolation of human surface, as opposed to glandular, epithelium has not yet been achieved.

As Denker has pointed out, epithelial surfaces are normally repellent and do not normally adhere to other cells via the apical plasma membrane (Denker 1990). At the time of implantation, the epithelium has been considered to become 'receptive' under the influence of steroid hormones. Although this period of receptivity or 'window of implantation' has been well characterised in rodents, there is much less data on the period when implantation can occur in humans and it is only by inference that such a 'window' is said to be present (Rogers

1993). In other species it would appear that the uterine epithelium does play a central role in receptivity as, if it is removed, implantation occurs independently of hormonal control (Cowell 1969). However, as other species do not show the same degree of decidual change before implantation the relative contributions of surface epithelium and underlying stroma to receptivity in humans are not known. Human blastocysts will readily adhere to other adult tissues, notably the Fallopian tube, which do not undergo hormonally regulated cyclical changes. This has led to the idea that unlike other sites the uterus is normally 'hostile' to implantation and only becomes receptive under the correct hormonal stimulus. The state of embryonic development is also important although the amount of uterine–embryonic assynchrony which can be tolerated in humans appears quite considerable. The human implantation window has been estimated to be at least 7 days (Rogers 1993).

It has been difficult to identify any definitive phenotypic or morphological changes in the human surface epithelium around the day of implantation which would support the presence of a window of receptivity in humans. The glycoprotein coat at the apical cell surface is principally composed of heavily glycosylated mucin-type glycoproteins. Ultrastructural changes have been observed such as loss of microvilli, alteration in tight junctions and modifications of the glycocalyx (Murphy *et al.* 1992). The possibility that apical surface membrane glycoproteins may be responsible for the adhesiveness of the uterus at the time of implantation has received much attention but, so far, few conclusions can be drawn. Many studies have looked for changes in glycoconjugates in several species with such techniques as lectin binding, but the data in humans are still rather inconclusive (Aplin 1989, 1991a; Mazur *et al.* 1989). SBA-binding lectins are observed to be present on proliferative phase surface epithelium, but absent from glands in the same sections, but this was the only lectin out of 22 tested to show any qualitative difference between the surface and glandular epithelium (Lee and Damjanov 1985).

Blood group related carbohydrate antigens such as those of the Lewis system have been shown to be important in adherence of microorganisms to mucosal surfaces (Borén and Falk 1994) and, therefore, might also be important in blastocyst attachment, especially as an estrogen-dependent specific H-type-1 determinant may have a role in attachment of mouse blastocysts (Lindenberg *et al.* 1990; White and Kimber 1994). Determinants of the A, B, H and Lewis-related blood group antigens are carbohydrate structures carried on both glycoproteins and glycolipids (Feizi 1985). They are found particularly on erythrocytes, epithelial cells and in secretions. The antigenic specificities are determined by only small differences in the sugar composition and linkages between residues of the oligosaccharides. Their structures are based on backbone

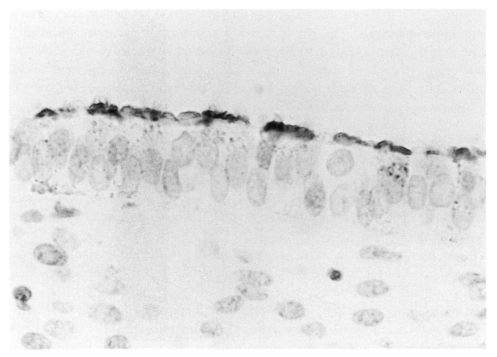

Fig. 3.2. The surface epithelium of proliferative phase endometrium showing intense staining of the apical surface and cilia with a monoclonal antibody to Le^a. (Obj × 100)

sequences (types 1–4) to which are sequentially added monosaccharides such as L-fucose, *N*-acetyl-D-galactosamine, D-galactose or sialic acid to produce the various blood group specificities. Several independent genes control the synthesis of the different glycosyl transferases responsible for the addition of the different monosaccharides.

The expression of blood group antigens in human endometrium has been studied by immunohistology, revealing a complex expression of carbohydrate antigens related both to the ABO, secretor and Lewis genetic status of the individual as well as to hormonal status and epithelial cell type (surface or glandular) (Inoue *et al.* 1987, 1990; Ravn *et al.* 1992a, b, 1993, 1994a, b). It would be surprising if blastocyst attachment to surface epithelium were to be related to ABO, secretor or Lewis genes. The most interesting antigens for reproductive biologists are likely to be those which are expressed in all women independently of genetic status. These include Le^a, Le^x, sialyl-T and the type 2 chain precursor. Le^a is of particular interest as it is found on the apical surface of luminal epithelium staining the ciliated cells, with expression being most intense in the proliferative phase (Fig. 3.2). This antigen is found only on the luminal epithelium and is not observed when the epithelium is invaginated to form glands (Fig. 3.3). This is a further example of the phenotypic difference

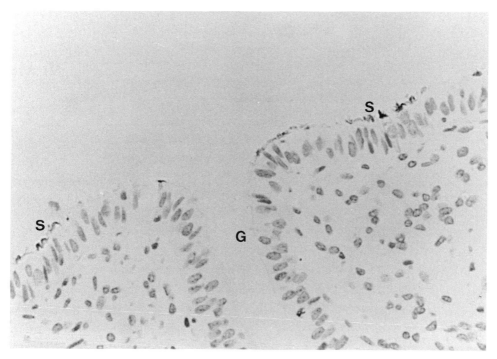

Fig. 3.3. Proliferative phase endometrial glands (G) show no expression of Le^a. The apical surface (S) becomes positive for Le^a at the neck of the glands. (Obj × 40)

between the two surfaces. A drawback of all the studies published to date is that they have studied normal endometrium in relation to changes in blood group antigens found in endometrial adenocarcinomas. The surface epithelium is generally only mentioned in passing and the biopsies are not dated very accurately. Studies of ubiquitously expressed blood group antigens in surface epithelium using precisely timed biopsies from normal and infertile women are clearly needed.

Production of lactosaminoglycans, such as keratan sulphate, is increased in glands during the secretory phase (Graham *et al.* 1994). Keratan sulphate is associated with a mucin-type secretory glycoprotein, MUC-1, also known as polymorphic epithelial mucin. The core protein of MUC-1 is localised at the apical cell surface of both glandular and luminal epithelium (Hey *et al.* 1994). Production of MUC-1 increases markedly in the secretory phase. The functional significance of these hormonally regulated glycans is at present unknown, although in mice glycosaminoglycans such as hyaluronic acid facilitate attachment and spreading of blastocysts *in vitro* (Carson *et al.* 1990).

Integrins are another group of adhesion molecules which are important in cell–cell interactions (Chapter 9). There is speculation that integrins could participate in the molecular events at implantation as there are both menstrual cycle and epithelial cell-specific patterns of expression of particular integrins (Lessey 1994). The α_1 and α_4 integrin subunits are found on glandular epithelium during the luteal phase (α_1 on days 15–28; α_4 on days 14–24). Sub-unit β_3 only appears on day 19 and expression continues into pregnancy. There is therefore co-expression of α_1, α_4 and β_3 from day 20 to day 24, the time of implantation. As β_1 and α_v integrin subunits are expressed constitutively by uterine epithelium, the possible heterodimers expressed during the period of implantation are $\alpha_v\beta_3$, $\alpha_v\beta_1$, $\alpha_4\beta_1$ and $\alpha_1\beta_1$ (Lessey *et al.* 1992, 1994a). Clinically, β_3 has been found to be absent during days 20–23 in luteal phase insufficiency and in certain patients with endometriosis (Lessey *et al.* 1992, 1994b). Integrin $\alpha_v\beta_3$ binds ligands via the RGD sequence and can engage in cell–cell interaction when both cells bind to a bridging molecule containing RGD binding sites. Integrin $\alpha_4\beta_1$ binds fibronectin (including oncofetal fibronectin) as well as VCAM, a member of the Ig superfamily. The main problem in the interpretation of these studies is that none of the three cycle-related epithelial integrin subunits are exposed on the surface luminal epithelium but are confined to glands. Furthermore, in contrast to expression in glands, the β_3 subunit appears only on day 24 on the luminal surface, a period after implantation should have occurred. Thus, it is hard to envisage how these integrins can play a role in blastocyst attachment unless the blastocyst always adheres initially to the mouth of a gland. Nevertheless, further studies along these lines should be pursued because matrix proteins, such as laminin and fibronectin, are secreted by mouse and human embryos which also express a variety of integrins (Turpeenniemi-Hujanen *et al.* 1992; Damsky *et al.* 1993; Campbell *et al.* 1995). In addition, preliminary data in mice suggest that activation of the blastocyst itself can determine the state of receptivity of the uterus and this activation might involve integrins (Paria *et al.* 1993).

Cytokines may also play a role in blastocyst implantation, notably IL-1 and LIF. IL-1α and IL-1β are secreted by pre-implantation mouse embryos, with correlation of high levels of secretion with successful implantation after *in vitro* fertilisation (Zolti *et al.* 1991; Sheth *et al.* 1991). Implantation can be blocked by intraperitoneal administration of soluble IL-1 receptor antagonist in mice (Simón *et al.* 1994a). In humans the type 1 IL-1R is present on glandular epithelium with maximal expression in the luteal phase (Simón *et al.* 1994b). Furthermore, other cytokines which are important in implantation may also act indirectly via activation of the IL-1R as IL-1 has a regulatory effect on both CSF-1 and LIF. LIF has an essential role in murine implantation events as shown by failure of normal embryos to implant in LIF knock-out mice (Stewart *et al.* 1992) (Chapter 10).

It can be seen that trophoblast–epithelial interactions are likely to involve a sequential cascade of events similar to those occurring when leucocytes leave the circulation by rolling, attachment and migration. These events are initiated by selectin–carbohydrate interactions followed by adhesion mediated by integrins and members of the Ig superfamily. Cytokines also play a role. At present there are only scattered observations that similar adhesion molecules might play a role in human blastocyst attachment. Finally, although it is generally assumed that the initial attachment is by trophectoderm, studies in the baboon, macaque and marmoset indicate that the primitive syncytium has already formed by the time the blastocyst is moving through the surface epithelium (Enders 1993). Adherence to the epithelium may signal this differentiation from trophectoderm to syncytium although syncytial trophoblast has been seen in blastocysts obtained from baboons by uterine flushing (Enders *et al.* 1989). As yet, there is no information on the expression of adhesion molecules on primitive human syncytium, and almost nothing is known of the molecular signals occurring during the initial period of nidation (<14 days) in humans.

Glands

Remarkably, little is known about the products of uterine glands and their functions. Secretion is maximal during the first 2–3 weeks, and thereafter the glandular epithelium becomes attenuated in the decidua compacta, although secretion continues in the underlying decidua spongiosa. It has been assumed that products from glands provide nutrients for the early embryo before tapping of the maternal blood vessels occurs. Certainly, in species where implantation is superficial (e.g. sheep/pigs/horses), and in which the embryo undergoes extensive development while remaining free in the uterine cavity, 'uterine milk' does serve this function (Maslar 1988). However, it has not been easy to find any evidence in support of the nutritional value to the embryo of human uterine fluid, which may essentially be a filtrate of plasma. Only about 1% of 'endometrial' proteins are different from those in plasma as analysed by two-dimensional gel electrophoresis (MacLaughlin *et al.* 1986). This is surprising in view of the obvious abundant secretions from glands. Large amounts of glycogen, mucins and glycoproteins are secreted into the lumina of the glands, and these include blood group related glycoproteins some of which (sialyl-Tn and sialyl-Le[a]) show cyclical changes. Other mucins such as MUC-1 are also found in secretions (Hey *et al.* 1994). Maybe this material is retained in the lumina or absorbed by the epithelial cell surface. Furthermore, after hatching of the blastocyst from the zona pellucida the embryo rapidly attaches and buries itself in the endometrium to become completely embedded. The primitive syncytium can be seen occluding glands in specimens from the Carnegie collection and glandular secretions may influence trophoblast behaviour in the first 14 days. However, once the cytotrophoblast shell has formed and invasion by trophoblast into the decidual stroma has begun, little contact occurs between glands and their secretions and extravillous trophoblast.

The most abundant glandular protein is PP14, which is a major decidual protein product (Seppälä *et al.* 1994). It was not thought to be produced in any abundance outside the reproductive tract (Chard and Olajide 1994). However, this view needs to be modified in view of the recent finding that PP14 is expressed in cells of the megakaryocytic and erythroid lineages, which may share a common precursor cell (Furmanski 1994; Kämäräinen *et al.* 1994). PP14 is synthesised and secreted by uterine glandular epithelium and the concentrations are high throughout the first trimester (Waites and Bell 1989). In non-pregnant endometrium, levels are low in the proliferative phase apart from in basal glands. During the secretory phase, around the time of implantation, PP14 becomes detectable and levels increase until 10 days post-ovulation when all glands are strongly stained (Seppälä *et al.* 1988). PP14 is a member of the β-lactoglobulin family, and its functions are unknown although there have been suggestions that PP14 may modulate NK activity (Seppälä *et al.* 1994). Indeed, many proteins secreted during early pregnancy from either maternal or placental tissues, such as human placental lactogen (hPL), Schwangerschafts protein-1 (SP-1), pregnancy-associated plasma protein-A (PAPP-A) and placental alkaline phosphatase (PLAP) have no established functions in spite of a considerable amount of research (Chard 1993). Successful pregnancies have been recorded where one of these substances, e.g. hPL, is absent (Simon *et al.* 1986).

Expression of both class I and class II HLA antigens has been analysed in human uterine glandular epithelium. The results for expression of HLA-DR by glands are conflicting. While there seems to be fairly uniform staining of the surface epithelium, the expression in glands is variable with some reports describing expression mainly in the basal glands (Morris *et al.* 1985; Tabibzadeh *et al.* 1986; Marshall and Jones 1988). HLA-DP and HLA-DQ are not expressed (Tabibzadeh and Satyaswaroop 1988). In pregnancy, only occasional patchy staining of glands is seen throughout gestation (Bulmer and Johnson 1985; Bulmer *et al.* 1986). HLA class II expression can be induced *in vitro* in cultured uterine epithelial cells by IFN-γ, raising the possibility that cytokines secreted by peri-glandular lymphocytes and basal aggregates may be responsible for the class II expression *in vivo* (Tabibzadeh *et al.* 1986). The functional significance of surface epithelial HLA class II expression is unknown. However, epithelia at other surface locations such as the skin and intestine are either constitutively or inductively positive for HLA class II molecules, making a functional role in antigen presentation likely (Nickoloff *et al.* 1993).

HLA class I antigens demonstrable by immunohistology using W6/32, a Mab directed to a monomorphic determinant of the β_2m–class I heavy chain complex, are expressed by glands in non-pregnant endometrium. The precise localisation of these class I heavy chains was investigated using an immunogold technique. Class I molecules were found to be solely on the basolateral membrane and not on the apical surface (Van Eijkeren *et al.* 1991). This polarised expression of class I molecules to the basolateral surface where T cells and NK cells are likely to come into contact with the epithelial cell does make sense functionally. Class I HLA expression in uterine glands is lost during early pregnancy in both decidua basalis and parietalis (Johnson and Bulmer 1984). By term W6/32 reactivity has returned in the attenuated glands of the decidua compacta, but is still negative in glands retaining an obvious columnar lining (Bulmer *et al.* 1986). At present, the relevance of these observations to pregnancy is not known.

Stromal cells

The transformation of the endometrial stromal cells from small densely packed cells to large polygonal cells with an open vesicular nucleus provides one of the most characteristic hallmarks of decidualisation. Despite this dramatic morphological change, the function of decidual stromal cells remains a mystery, and in particular it is not clear how they contribute to the control of trophoblast development and invasion.

Decidualisation of endometrial stromal cells occurs under the influence of ovarian steroid hormones. Decidualised stromal cells produce a variety of growth factors (e.g. FGF and EGF) (Chapter 10), and several extracellular matrix (ECM) proteins including laminin and fibronectin (Chapter 9). The importance of decidual ECM proteins is discussed in Chapter 9. However, the main protein products are prolactin, insulin-like growth factor binding protein-1 (IGFBP-1) and renin, none of which are produced in non-decidualised endometrium. Prolactin secretion is increased following stimulation by several factors such as steroid hormones, EGF, FGF, IGF-I, and the free alpha form of hCG, and is inhibited by IL-1, TNF-α and endothelin (Huang *et al.* 1987; Thrailkill *et al.* 1988; Blithe *et al.* 1991; Chao *et al.* 1993; Handwerger *et al.* 1993). Factors regulating production of pituitary prolactin such as bromocriptine have no influence on the secretion of decidual prolactin (Handwerger *et al.* 1992). IGFBP-1 is similarly secreted under the influence of progesterone, EGF and insulin (Seppälä *et al.* 1994).

As for decidual glandular products, it has been hard to find any biological role for the major decidual stromal products of prolactin, renin and IGFBP-1.

Prolactin is not secreted into the maternal or fetal blood streams, but high levels are found in the decidua and amniotic cavity, and it has been suggested that prolactin may regulate amniotic fluid volume and ion content as it affects water and ion transport in lower vertebrates (Handwerger and Brar 1992). There is an intriguing possibility that prolactin may influence the recruitment and retention of decidual NK cells and macrophages. The prolactin receptor belongs to the same family of cytokine receptors as IL-2βR (Sato and Miyajima 1994). Prolactin has been considered an evolutionary precursor of IL-2, and there is evidence that prolactin is necessary for lymphocyte proliferation in response to IL-2 (Clevenger *et al*. 1991). However, we have not been able to induce proliferation of decidual lymphocytes with soluble prolactin *in vitro*, but perhaps it needs to be membrane bound (unpublished). Also, a preliminary analysis of the distribution of the prolactin receptor by immunohistology and flow cytometry shows that receptor expression is mainly on decidual macrophages, and only a small subset of CD56$^+$ cells are reactive (unpublished). Thus, prolactin may be involved more with the functions of decidual macrophages than with decidual NK cells.

IGFBPs are proteins which are found in many tissues. They specifically bind IGF-I and IGF-II, and their effects have been thought to modify IGF functions (Seppälä *et al*. 1994). At the implantation site, extravillous trophoblast expresses IGF-IR, IGF-I and IGF-II mRNA, and it has been proposed that decidual IGFBP-1 might regulate trophoblast growth by inhibiting IGF-I. However, IGFBP-1 also contains an RGD integrin recognition sequence which can bind to the $\alpha_5\beta_1$ integrin (fibronectin receptor) (Jones *et al*. 1993). This $\alpha_5\beta_1$ receptor is expressed by extravillous trophoblast as it moves off the columns (Chapter 9). Since IGFBP-1 binds to cell surfaces and can cause an increase in cell migration in cells expressing $\alpha_5\beta_1$, this IGFBP-1/$\alpha_5\beta_1$ interaction may contribute to the coordinated migration of trophoblast, thus illustrating the complex interaction between growth factors, matrix and surface receptors which could occur during implantation.

Blood vessels

The intervillous space of the placenta is supplied with blood from decidual spiral arteries. These arise as radial branches from the uterine arcuate arteries and supply the stratum functionale. Their growth and structure are modified by ovarian hormones. Basal arteries, which also arise from the radial arteries, supply the stratum basalis. These arteries are unaffected by hormonal stimuli. After menstruation, the spiral arteries extend only into the stratum basale, but during the proliferative phase under the influence of estrogen the arteries thicken, lengthen and become progressively coiled. Unlike the endometrial glandular and stromal cellular elements, endothelial cell proliferation continues into the luteal phase and during the early weeks of pregnancy (Kaiserman-Abramof and Padykula 1989). Angiogenesis occurring in the adult in a physiological rather than a pathological situation such as a bone fracture has been considered exceptional (Findlay 1986). However, this angiogenesis in the uterine mucosa may not be exactly analogous to that seen in pathological situations such as a healing wound, bone repair and tumour cell growth. In these circumstances, the new capillaries sprout from pre-existing microvasculature, mainly capillaries and venules, rather than from larger arterioles or arteries surrounded by a media of smooth muscle. The lengthening, thickening and coiling of the spiral arteries throughout the menstrual cycle appears to be a different process involving growth of a pre-existing artery together with its media (Goodger and Rogers 1994). Vascular sprouts are not observed and there are no associated inflammatory changes such as are seen in wound or early scar tissue, showing that repair of the endometrium is not like repair of other adult tissues but is more like that seen in repair of fetal tissue. Angiogenesis or new blood vessel growth may therefore be something of a misnomer for the development of the endometrial spiral arteries during each menstrual cycle.

Several factors stimulating and inhibiting angiogenesis have been identified in the endometrium and decidua, but it is not yet known how these factors operate to produce the tightly controlled hormonally-regulated development of spiral arteries (Klagsbrun and D'Amore 1991). FGF and VEGF, both heparin binding growth factors, together with other angiogenic factors such as EGF/TGF-α are produced in the uterine mucosa (Chapter 10), but so far there are no functional studies using endometrial or decidual endothelial cells. The successful isolation of decidual endothelial cells for *in vitro* studies opens the way for future investigation (Chapter 5). In intact vascular explants where both endothelial cells and other cells of the arterial wall are present, VEGF, PDGF and IGF-I all stimulated angiogenesis (Nicosia *et al.* 1994).

4

Human trophoblast development

Early trophoblast development

The formation of the human placenta begins at the time the blastocyst penetrates the maternal endometrium to become rapidly embedded in the uterine stroma. A brief description of the anatomy of the implantation process and the development of trophoblast populations is given in this chapter. Particular emphasis is given to the placental cells which penetrate into maternal tissues, as events regulating correct trophoblast migration are the subject of this volume. More detailed descriptions on other aspects of the placenta can be found elsewhere (Boyd and Hamilton 1970; Kaufmann and Burton 1994; Pijnenborg 1994).

The first element to differentiate in the morula is the trophectoderm. As the morula is converted into a blastocyst, trophectoderm cells form a layer encircling the blastocyst with the inner cell mass at one pole. The blastocyst inserts itself between the epithelial cells of the uterine mucosa on the 6th–7th day after ovulation. This process has never been visualised in humans, but in the macaque monkey trophectoderm has already differentiated into a syncytial mass at the site of attachment (Boyd and Hamilton 1970). Indeed, formation of the primitive syncytium from trophectoderm may be induced by contact with the surface epithelium. Syncytial trophoblast formation is not thought to occur in pre-implantation human blastocysts. By the 8th day, trophoblast has differentiated into an outer multinucleated syncytiotrophoblast (primitive syncytium) and an inner layer of primitive mononuclear cytotrophoblast. The syncytial mass penetrates between epithelial cells and rapidly expands into the underlying stroma, but this expansion must result from differentiation of underlying cytotrophoblast cells as mitoses are never seen in the syncytium. By the 9th day, vacuoles or lacunae appear in the syncytium and these rapidly enlarge and fuse to communicate with each other. The establishment of a potential uteroplacental circulation occurs when maternal venous capillaries are eroded by the syncytium so that blood can seep into the lacuna system. The lacunae will eventually

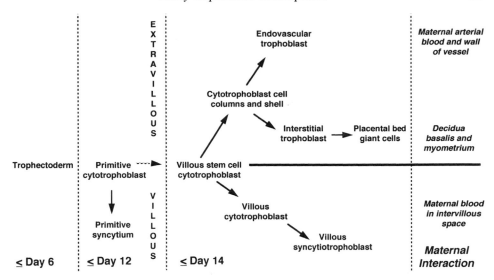

Fig. 4.1. Trophoblast differentiation at the implantation site.

become the intervillous space of the definitive placenta. By 12–13 days after fertilisation, the blastocyst is completely embedded in the decidual stroma and the uterine surface epithelium has grown over the overlying defect. It is remarkable that this early stage of implantation is accompanied by so little tissue necrosis or inflammatory reaction in the mucosa.

After this initial phase of nidation, trophoblast differentiation may be considered to occur along two main pathways – villous and extravillous (Fig. 4.1). It is useful to consider these two main differentiation pathways separately as both the function of these two main trophoblast subsets and the type of maternal cells with which they come into contact are different. Villous trophoblast ultimately covers all the chorionic villi of the definitive placenta and is concerned with transport of oxygen and nutrients from mother to child. The villi are bathed in blood and hence contact is only with maternal cells present in the circulation. In contrast, extravillous trophoblast migrates deep into the uterine mucosa as far as the myometrium and encounters many maternal cell types as it infiltrates through uterine tissues (Fig. 4.2, opposite p. 34).

Villous trophoblast

The earliest sign of villous development is the appearance of buds of cytotrophoblast protruding into the primitive syncytium in the second week of gestation. These primary villi are soon converted into secondary villi by the penetration of the solid cytotrophoblast buds by mesenchymal cells and then into tertiary villi when the mesenchymal core is supplied by embryonic blood vessels. The embryonic vessels link with vessels in the mesoderm of the chorionic plate, and ultimately with vessels in the fetus so that by the fourth week the feto-placental circulation is established. The mesodermal core of the chorionic villi is derived from cells of the inner cell mass which originate from the caudal margin of the embryonic disc (Crane and Cheung 1988). That the villous mesenchyme may provide the essential stimulus for trophoblast growth is suggested by studies in the development of the equine chorionic girdle (Stewart *et al.* 1995). In this species, the girdle arises by proliferation of trophoblast cells in a discrete region of the chorion, indicating a locally produced mitogenic signal. This trophoblast proliferation overlies an area of allantoic mesoderm which is demonstrated to express hepatocyte growth factor (HGF) while the overlying trophoblast expresses the relevant receptor, the proto-oncogene c-*met*. Since allantoic mesoderm is adjacent to proliferating trophoblast in all eutherian mammals, this could be a conserved mechanism involved in trophoblast development. Recently, mutant mice have been generated with targeted disruption of the HGF gene (Uehara *et al.* 1995; Schmidt *et al.* 1995). These mice die *in utero* with disruption of the labyrinthine trophoblast which further confirms the importance of this cytokine in influencing normal placental development.

During the second and third months of pregnancy, rapid extension and branching of the villi result in the villous tree characteristic of the mature placenta. Initially, the villi are covered by primitive syncytium which subsequently becomes the villous syncytiotrophoblast. In the first 3 months there is an obvious two-layered trophoblast covering of the villi. The inner cytotrophoblast cells sit on a basement membrane covered by the outer syncytiotrophoblast layer (Fig. 4.3). It is this syncytiotrophoblast which lines the entire intervillous space and thus comes into contact with maternal blood in a manner similar to endothelial cells. In the first trimester, the core of the villus contains loose mesenchymal cells, embryonic blood vessels and fetal macrophages (Hofbauer cells). Hofbauer cells appear very early in gestation (by the third week) and increase in number throughout the first trimester (Fig. 4.3). As gestation proceeds, the villi become smaller, the cytotrophoblast layer appears less prominent as the cells become widely separated and the syncytiotrophoblast becomes more irregular and narrow with clustering of the nuclei. The stroma contains the same elements, but the fetal capillaries become much more prominent and come to lie directly under the basement membrane at the periphery of the villus. By the last few weeks of gestation, thinned areas of syncytiotrophoblast form only a narrow rim over the fetal capillaries to become vasculosyncytial membranes, which are specialised zones for the facilitation of

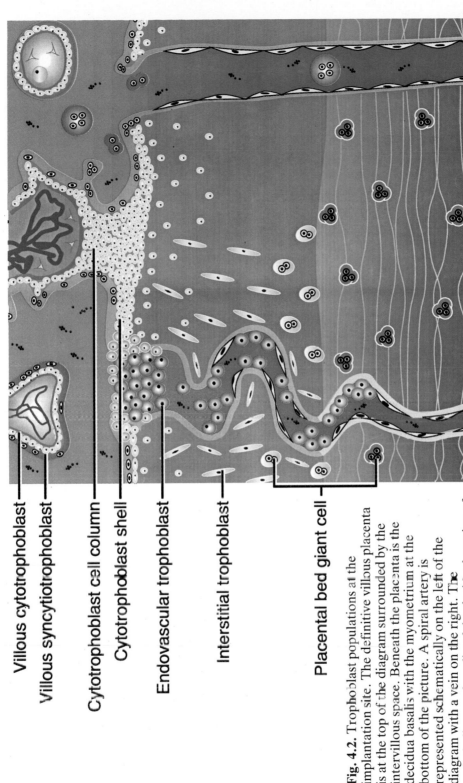

Villous cytotrophoblast

Villous syncytiotrophoblast

Cytotrophoblast cell column

Cytotrophoblast shell

Endovascular trophoblast

Interstitial trophoblast

Placental bed giant cell

Fig. 4.2. Trophoblast populations at the implantation site. The definitive villous placenta is at the top of the diagram surrounded by the intervillous space. Beneath the placenta is the decidua basalis with the myometrium at the bottom of the picture. A spiral artery is represented schematically on the left of the diagram with a vein on the right. The endothelium and media of the decidual portion of the spiral artery are replaced by trophoblast and fibrinoid material as a result of infiltration by endovascular and interstitial trophoblast. Placental bed giant cells are present in the myometrium. Syncytial sprouts originating from the villous syncytiotrophoblast are deported via uterine veins to the lungs.

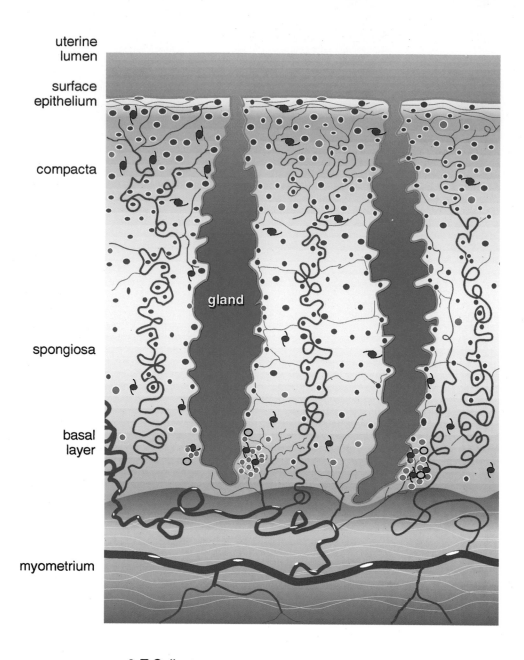

uterine
lumen

surface
epithelium

compacta

gland

spongiosa

basal
layer

myometrium

● T Cells
● CD56+ LGL
⟨ Macrophages
○ B Cells

Fig. 7.1. The distribution and relative proportion of leucocytes in the decidua.

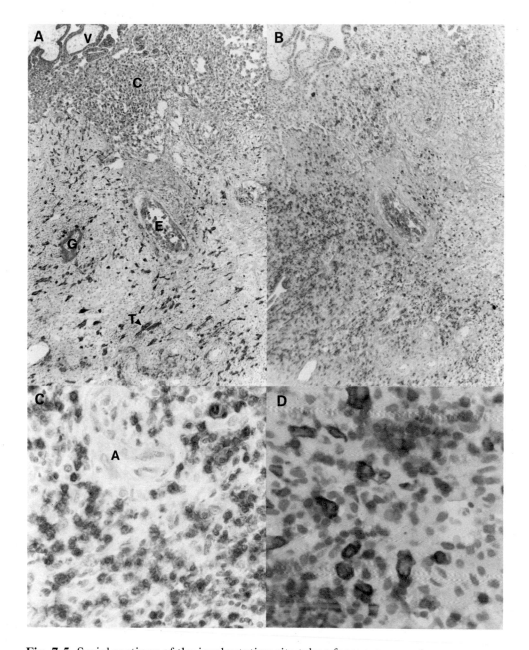

Fig. 7.5. Serial sections of the implantation site taken from a pregnant hysterectomy of 7 weeks gestation. **A.** Trophoblast cells are identified by staining with anti cytokeratin. The thick cytotrophoblast shell (C) is formed from fusion of cell columns migrating off anchoring villi (V). From this shell interstitial trophoblast (T) can be seen streaming into the decidua basalis. The media of the artery in the centre of the picture is destroyed and the lumen partially filled by endovascular trophoblast (E). One gland (G) is present in this section. (Obj × 4). **B.** The distribution of CD56$^+$ NK cells is shown in a serial section. Large numbers of NK cells are present in the decidua in areas infiltrated by interstitial trophoblast. The endovascular trophoblast and scattered cells in the overlying cytotrophoblast shell are also CD56 (NCAM)- positive. (Obj × 4) **C.** A high-power photograph of the same section shown in **B**. The dense infiltration of CD56$^+$ cells in areas of trophoblast invasion and around an artery (A) is obvious. (Obj × 40) **D.** A similar section of the implantation site double stained for CD56$^+$ NK cells (red) and for cytokeratin$^+$ trophoblast cells (brown) to show the close intermingling of the two cell types.

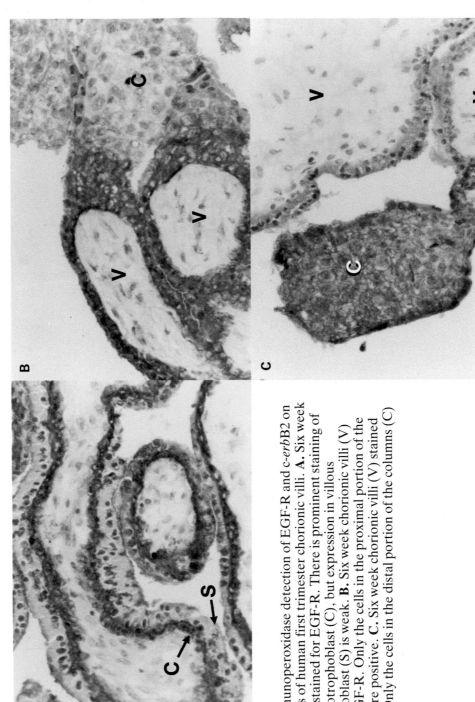

Fig. 10.5. Immunoperoxidase detection of EGF-R and *c-erb*B2 on frozen sections of human first trimester chorionic villi. **A.** Six week chorionic villi stained for EGF-R. There is prominent staining of the villous cytotrophoblast (C), but expression in villous syncytiotrophoblast (S) is weak. **B.** Six week chorionic villi (V) stained for EGF-R. Only the cells in the proximal portion of the columns (C) are positive. **C.** Six week chorionic villi (V) stained for *c-erb*B2. Only the cells in the distal portion of the columns (C) are positive.

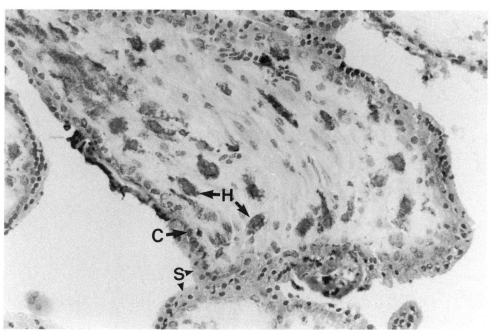

Fig. 4.3 A section of a first trimester placental villus stained with an antibody to CD68 which is a marker for macrophages. Hofbauer cells are clearly visible (H). The villus is covered by a double layer of villous cytotrophoblast (C) and syncytiotrophoblast (S). (Obj × 25)

gas transfer across the placenta. As a result of the prominent capillaries, Hofbauer cells and mesenchymal cells appear less numerous.

Extravillous trophoblast

Interstitial trophoblast

After the second week, the budding cytotrophoblast which will ultimately form the villous tree breaks through the primitive syncytium. At the tips of these early villi, cytotrophoblast cells remain as a solid core known as the cytotrophoblast cell columns which fix the villi to the decidua (Fig. 4.4). These are known as anchoring villi. The cytotrophoblast cell columns spread laterally and fuse with neighbouring columns to form a cytotrophoblast shell which encircles the entire embryonic sac. During the first 8–10 weeks, remnants of primitive syncytium are seen close to the anchoring villi and the cytotrophoblast shell. Invading trophoblast cells arise from this cytotrophoblast shell. Once the shell has come into physical contact with decidua, isolated interstitial trophoblast cells stream into the uterine mucosa (Fig. 4.4). The morphology of these cells changes as

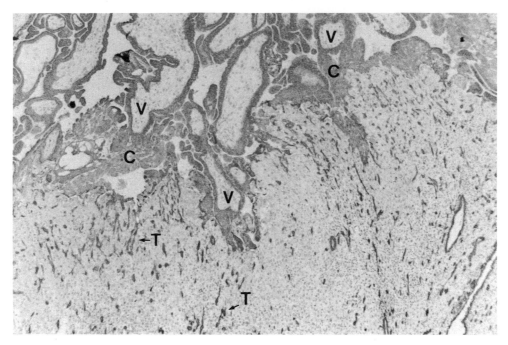

Fig. 4.4. A frozen section taken from the implantation site at 7 weeks gestation. Trophoblast is identified with an anti-cytokeratin antibody. Cytotrophoblast cell columns (C) extend from the anchoring villi (V) to attach the placenta to the decidua. From these columns isolated interstitial trophoblast cells (T) are streaming into the decidua basalis. (Obj × 4)

soon as they lose contact with the cytotrophoblast shell where they appear as rounded uniform cohesive cells. After invasion into decidua has occurred, the interstitial trophoblast cells become isolated fusiform pleomorphic cells. The nuclear morphology also changes from open nuclei with prominent nucleoli in the columns to hyperchromatic pleomorphic nuclei with an irregular nuclear membrane.

On the maternal side of the cytotrophoblast shell in the region of the original primitive syncytium, two irregular narrow strips of fibrinoid necrosis appear known as Rohr's layer and Nitabuch's layer. Apart from these small foci of necrosis at the placental–decidual junction, the migration of trophoblast into maternal tissues is remarkable for the lack of tissue destruction or inflammatory response. The invading interstitial trophoblast cells apparently move towards the decidual spiral arteries as trophoblast is always concentrated around the arteries with a much sparser number of invading cells in the intervening areas (Fig. 4.5). Around the arteries the trophoblast cells appear larger and rounder than when moving through decidua. In addition, these interstitial trophoblast cells seem to have a specific and remarkable effect on the spiral arteries. Arteries in the decidua

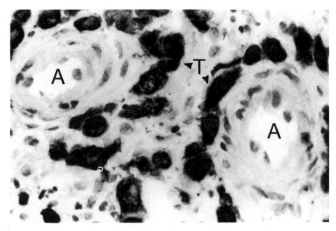

Fig. 4.5. A section of the implantation site at 7 weeks gestation stained with an anti-cytokeratin antibody. Two spiral arteries (A) are surrounded by interstitial trophoblast cells (T). The endothelium and media are intact. (Obj × 40, H & E)

basalis which are surrounded by trophoblast show endothelial swelling and a characteristic destruction of the muscular media which is replaced with 'fibrinoid' material. This disruption of vessel walls is not found in decidual vessels away from the implantation site. By 8 weeks of pregnancy interstitial trophoblast has extensively colonised the full thickness of the uterine mucosa to reach the decidual–myometrial border. As the cells move deeper into the decidua, the trophoblast cells become multinucleated and more rounded (Fig. 4.6). These trophoblast cells are known as placental bed giant cells, and they can be regarded as the terminally differentiated sessile end-point of the extravillous pathway. It is not known if they arise by fusion or endoreduplication. During the second trimester, there is further invasion into the inner myometrium. Destruction of the musculo-elastic tissue of the intramyometrial segments of the spiral arteries occurs with similar fibrinoid change of the media. However, in the myometrium the interstitial trophoblast does not appear to show the same preference for perivascular regions. Diffuse infiltration of the inner myometrium by trophoblast is seen and most of the trophoblast cells here have the morphology of placental bed giant cells.

Endovascular trophoblast

The cytotrophoblast shell formed from the cell columns of the anchoring villi provides almost a continuous and complete rim around the developing villous tree and gestational sac during the first trimester. This shell provides the origin not only for the interstitial trophoblast invading into decidual tissue, but also for endovascular trophoblast. Where the shell comes to lie over the openings of the

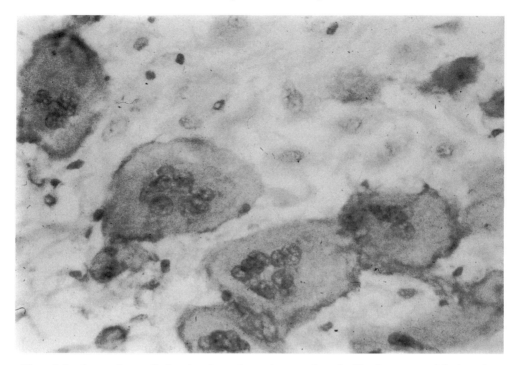

Fig. 4.6. A section of the implantation site at the decidual–myometrial junction. Multinucleated placental bed giant cells are clearly seen. (Obj × 40, H&E)

maternal spiral arteries, the trophoblast cells form a plug seemingly occluding the lumen. From these plug-like areas of the shell, trophoblast moves in a retrograde manner down the spiral arteries 'like wax dripping down a candle' (Ramsey and Donner 1980). The cells in these plugs and in the lumina of the arteries remain rounded and loosely cohesive (Fig. 4.7), unlike interstitial trophoblast. Extension of endovascular trophoblast continues into the arteries throughout the first trimester. In portions of the arteries furthest from the intervillous space, vessels may be only partially lined by trophoblast with residual endothelial cells frequently seen. In the second trimester intramyometrial arterial segments also come to be lined partly by endothelial cells overlying the fibrinoid material and partly by trophoblast. It is important to note that endovascular trophoblast is only seen in vessels which have already been surrounded by interstitial trophoblast and undergone medial disruption. Eventually, trophoblast cells become incorporated into the fibrinoid material in the wall, although the relative contribution of endovascular trophoblast and interstitial trophoblast to this process is uncertain, and indeed may differ in the different segments of the vessel.

Interestingly, the walls of the decidual veins are not similarly invaded by trophoblast. However, these decidual veins are the channels by which syncytial

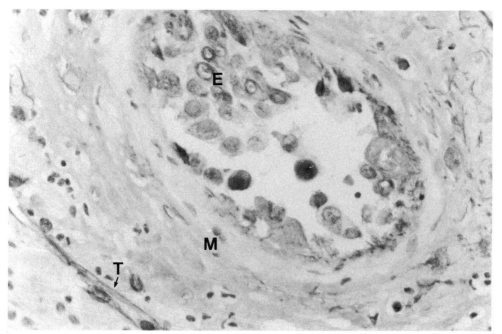

Fig. 4.7. A section of a spiral artery in the implantation site at 7 weeks gestation stained with an anti-cytokeratin antibody. There is degeneration of the smooth muscle of the arterial media (M). The lumen of the artery is partially filled by a loose plug of endovascular trophoblast cells (E) which are attached to the wall of the vessel. Interstitial trophoblast cells (T) are present in the perivascular region. (Obj × 40)

knots, detached from chorionic villi into the intervillous space, are deported into the maternal circulation to be trapped in the blood vessels of the lungs where they are eventually lysed. Some investigators, such as Hawes *et al.* (1994), believe that these syncytiotrophoblast cells can traverse the pulmonary capillary bed to appear in the peripheral blood of pregnant women. This, of course, has very important potential clinical applications because these cells, when isolated from maternal blood, could be a very useful source of fetal genetic material for pre-natal diagnosis. There is still some residual doubt that all multinucleated cells detected in maternal peripheral blood are necessarily of fetal origin (Adinolfi 1992). Maternal cells, such as megakaryocytes, are also multinuclear. This point needs to be settled unequivocally before this technique can be heralded as a non-invasive method to obtain cells for pre-natal diagnosis.

Immunohistology of trophoblast sub-populations in early pregnancy

It is clear that a heterogeneous population of fetally derived trophoblast comes into close contact with a variety of maternal tissues in the implantation site.

Pijnenborg *et al.* (1981), in their extensive histological studies, have commented on the difficulty in recognising trophoblast cells in the placental bed using morphological criteria alone. 'Like songs in love, they much describe, they nothing prove' (from Matthew Prior 1687–1729). The availability of polyclonal and monoclonal antibodies reactive with trophoblast cell products or antigens has now made it possible to identify trophoblast cells with a greater degree of confidence (Loke and Butterworth 1987). Much can be learnt about the *in vivo* situation by examining the distribution of these molecules on trophoblast sub-populations in sections of the placenta and implantation site throughout gestation. This knowledge is also an essential prerequisite to *in vitro* studies both in characterising primary cultures of trophoblast and in indicating the direction functional studies should take.

Although the technique is relatively simple, there are obvious problems in obtaining the relevant areas of placental bed in humans, particularly the deciduo-myometrial junction. There are also difficulties in orientating and interpreting placental bed biopsies (Pijnenborg 1994). Thus, the rare pregnant hysterectomy specimens are very precious material. Furthermore, many antigens do not survive the harsh treatment associated with the process of tissue embedding in paraffin. This means that frozen sections have to be used, which immediately precludes retrospective studies with archival material from histopathological laboratories.

Great care has to be taken in the interpretation of data. It must be remembered that localisation of a protein does not necessarily mean production by that cell. This is most pertinent when analysing villous syncytiotrophoblast, which is capable of a remarkable absorptive and pinocytic capacity. This layer is also notorious for non-specific binding to antibodies in immunohistology and careful controls are necessary. Ideally, immunohistological studies should be performed in conjunction with *in situ* hybridisation with appropriate probes to localise the relevant mRNA in the cell. For example, Hoshina *et al.* (1982) detected mRNA for hCG and hPL in human syncytiotrophoblast thereby confirming that the protein equivalents localised to the cytoplasm of these cells by immunohistology are likely to be synthesised by the cells. Interestingly, in a recent study using an oligo-dT probe for total mRNA, we were surprised to find relatively little mRNA in syncytiotrophoblast relative to cytotrophoblast because the former has always been thought to be the major source of many placental proteins (unpublished). From this observation, we would conclude that most of the placental proteins detected in syncytiotrophoblast are probably initially transcribed in the villous cytotrophoblast and are then stored in the overlying syncytial layer. It has always been a puzzle how a multinuclear cell like syncytiotrophoblast can synchronise its transcriptional activity. The finding of mRNA, of course, does not guarantee that the protein is made. This is well illustrated in HLA class I expression where villous cytotrophoblast has mRNA but does not express the antigen, whereas syncytiotrophoblast is mRNA$^-$ and protein$^-$ and extravillous trophoblast is mRNA$^+$ and protein$^+$ (Hunt *et al.* 1990). Thus, while immunohistology has divided trophoblast into two populations on the basis of class I antigen expression, detection of class I mRNA by *in situ* hybridisation has expanded this into three populations (Chapter 6).

Many phenotypic differences are evident among the trophoblast sub-populations, particularly between villous and extravillous trophoblast. For example, it can be seen that while multinuclear cell formation is the terminal differentiated state of both villous and extravillous developmental pathways, the two end products are not identical. While many placental proteins are detected in syncytiotrophoblast, placental bed giant cells are largely unproductive (Table 4.1). This suggests that these hormones are synthesised predominantly for transfer to the maternal systemic circulation via the intervillous space. In addition, syncytiotrophoblast is HLA class I$^-$ (W6/32$^-$) and placental bed giant cells are class I$^+$ (W6/32$^+$), indicating that the immunology of the trophoblast–maternal blood interface is likely to be different from the trophoblast–uterine interface.

There are other markers that distinguish between villous and extravillous cytotrophoblast, such as BC-1 (Loke *et al.* 1992b), cytokine receptors EGF-R and c-*erb*B2 (Jokhi *et al.* 1994a) and integrins $\alpha_6\beta_4$ and $\alpha_5\beta_1$ (Burrows *et al.* 1993a). Interestingly, endovascular trophoblast is the only population which expresses NCAM (Burrows *et al.* 1994). These molecules will be discussed in more detail in later chapters. There are presently no reliable markers that can differentiate between the various interstitial trophoblast populations as they move through the placental bed towards the spiral arteries or into the myometrium where they become giant cells. Perhaps Mabs reactive with different sets of intracellular keratin filaments could prove useful in this regard. Many keratins are expressed in epithelial cells as specific heterodimers in a differentiation-specific fashion *in vivo* (Coulombe 1993). The differentiation sequence of skin keratinocytes has been followed in this way (Fuchs 1993). Certainly, the interstitial trophoblast directly encircling the spiral arteries has a curious distribution of cytokeratin filaments reminiscent of the 'star-like structures' described in carcinoma cells treated with antimitotic drugs (Fig. 4.8) (Knapp *et al.* 1983). These structures may be preventing collapse of the cell.

Finally, proliferation is observed only in villous cytotrophoblast and at the base of the cytotrophoblast cell columns by the presence of mitotic figures and staining for the proliferation marker Ki-67 (Bulmer *et al.* 1988a). No proliferation is seen in the rest of the extravillous trophoblast populations so that proliferation is not an appropriate end-point to measure when assessing this trophoblast population *in vitro*.

Table 4.1. *Production of placental proteins by trophoblast populations*

Product	Villous cytotrophoblast	Villous syncytiotrophoblast	Columns and shell	Interstitial trophoblast	Endovascular trophoblast	Placental bed giant cells
hCG	–	+	–	–	–	–
hPL	–	+	–	±	+	–
SP1	–	+	–	–	–	–
PLAP	–	+	–	–	–	–

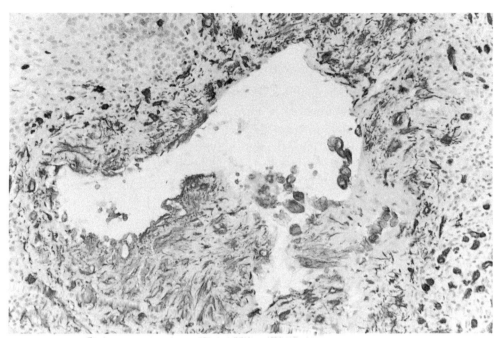

Fig. 4.8. A spiral artery in the decidua basalis at 10 weeks gestation stained with an anti-cytokeratin antibody. The smooth muscle media and the endothelium are replaced by trophoblast cells. The cytokeratin staining pattern of the trophoblast cells in the arterial wall shows a disruption of the normal pattern of keratin filaments resulting in a 'star-like' appearance. (Obj × 25)

Second and third trimesters

As pregnancy proceeds, there is a shift in the distribution of changes in the placental bed. Vessels are initially invaded in the centre, but then invasion spreads outwards to occur in all implantation site arteries. In the second half of pregnancy, there is no further trophoblast penetration of the myometrium although vascular transformation by trophoblast appears to continue throughout gestation (Pijnenborg 1994). For the first 2 months of gestation, villi cover the entire surface of the chorionic sac. As the conceptus expands, the villi beneath the decidua capsularis degenerate, leaving a layer of trophoblast and mesenchyme known as the chorion laeve. By the end of the fourth month further expansion leads to atrophy of the decidua capsularis. The chorion laeve fuses with the decidua parietalis with obliteration of the uterine lumen and regression of the uterine surface epithelium. In the latter half of gestation there is, therefore, another point of contact between maternal and fetal cells at this chorio-decidual junction. Transport of substances and even maternal cells in the event of infection may occur across this barrier from the decidua into the amniotic cavity.

Functions of trophoblast sub-populations

Villous trophoblast

The main function of the complex villous tree which eventually forms the definitive placenta is the transfer of nutrients and other substances including immunoglobulins and oxygen from the maternal to the fetal circulation. The villous syncytiotrophoblast is also the major source of placental proteins produced during pregnancy. There is considerable functional reserve in the placenta and up to 40% of the villous population can be lost without compromising physiological function.

Extravillous trophoblast

'The integrity of the conceptus in man must depend directly upon the provision and maintenance of an adequate supply of maternal blood to the intervillous space' (Brosens *et al.* 1967). To provide the blood supply necessary for the growing conceptus, the invasion of trophoblast into the spiral arteries is essential. Vascular adaptation by extravillous trophoblast (known as physiological change) is a remarkable phenomenon whereby non-neoplastic cells invade and destroy an artery. The result is a large sac-like vessel incapable of responding to vasoactive stimuli.

The different extravillous populations exhibit different functional characteristics in relation to the spiral arteries, although both are ultimately concerned in the regulation of the placental blood supply. It is obvious that the function of the migrating interstitial trophoblast is primarily to mediate the destruction of the arterial wall. It has been described as 'priming' the vessel (Pijnenborg *et al.* 1983). These cells must therefore be allowed to move around the arteries in both decidua and the inner myometrium by 16 weeks. Placental bed giant cells are found in the deeper part of the decidua and in the myometrium and have been described as 'effete' and 'passive' (Robertson 1987). If morphological studies can be any guide these cells would appear to have lost invasive capacity and the potential for medial destruction. Transformation from invasive trophoblast to inert placental bed giant cells is, therefore, an important feature of placentation and reflects correct trophoblast differentiation.

In contrast, the endovascular plugs which are in continuity with the cytotrophoblast shell have a different function in the first trimester. They are thought to prevent arterial blood from entering the intervillous space at high pressure in the first weeks of pregnancy (Hustin 1992). The plugs are only loosely cohesive and can act like valves, allowing seepage of serum through to the intervillous space until early in the second trimester when the haemochorial placenta becomes properly established and the plugs disappear. Thus, endovascular trophoblast plugs act as both valves and sieves to prevent pressure damage to the fragile early gestational sac. After 12 weeks gestation, endovascular trophoblast is seen lining the spiral arteries where it has replaced the endothelium to become incorporated into the vessel wall. Thus, endovascular trophoblast prevents blood reaching the early embryo at high pressure in early gestation and later contributes to the lining of the arteries supplying the intervillous space.

Abnormal trophoblast invasion

There is no animal model which can be used to study trophoblast invasion into the human uterus as no other species shows a similar degree or pattern of invasion. Insight into the normal process has, however, come from the histopathological study of abnormal pregnancies. Abnormalities of trophoblast invasion do occur, both over-invasion to a deeper level as in placenta percreta, and under-invasion which occurs in pre-eclampsia and other conditions (Robertson 1987) (Chapter 11). Limitation of trophoblast invasion is therefore the main feature of defective placentation and the failure to develop a normal uteroplacental blood supply. Normal fetal growth and development must therefore ultimately depend on how trophoblast invasion is controlled (King and Loke 1994).

Effects of genomic imprinting on trophoblast development

The term genomic imprinting refers to the phenomenon whereby genes have differential expression depending on the parental source from which they are inherited. The parental gene that is silent is said to be imprinted. The existence of genomic imprinting in mammals was first observed in the aberrant development of murine embryos after experimental induction of parthenogenesis (Barton *et al.* 1984; McGrath and Solter 1984). Creation of gynogenomes (both sets of haploid chromosomes are derived from the mother) by replacement of the male pronuclei with female pronuclei after fertilisation leads to the development of relatively normal sized embryos with poor development of extraembryonic membranes and the placenta. These conceptuses remain viable until the early somite stage, and then undergo involution. In contrast, androgenomes (paternally derived chromosomes) created by transplantation of male pronuclei into ova in which the female pronuclei have been removed result in conceptuses with severely stunted embryos, but with normally developed extraembryonic trophoblast tissues. These experiments led to

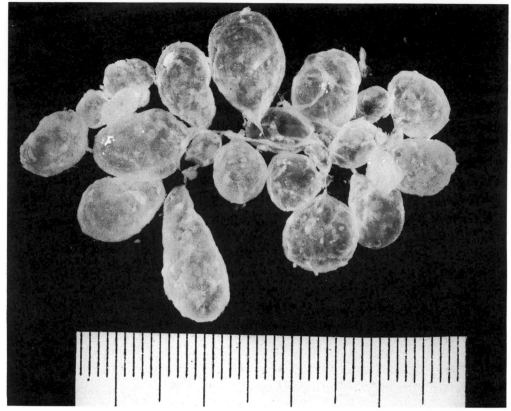

Fig. 4.9. Hydatidiform molar villi photographed under water. The translucent distended terminal villi are attached to slender stem villi giving the appearance of a bunch of grapes.

the conclusion that, while both parental genomes are essential for murine embryonic development, their contributions are not equivalent. The paternally transmitted genome appears to provide the necessary genetic information for trophoblast growth whereas the maternally transmitted genome is associated with the development of the embryo itself. Because of this, mammals are not capable of parthenogenetic reproduction. Two reviews on genomic imprinting during placental development (De-Groot and Hochberg 1993) and in human pathology (Tycko 1994) have recently been published.

The classic human example of genomic imprinting is complete hydatidiform mole. The essential features of these tumours are a pregnancy without an associated fetus, grape-like distension of chorionic villi together with excessive placental tissue and trophoblast proliferation (Fig. 4.9). Genetic analyses of these tumours revealed that they contain two paternally derived sets of haploid chromosomes (diploid androgenomes) (Lawler and Fisher 1993). The

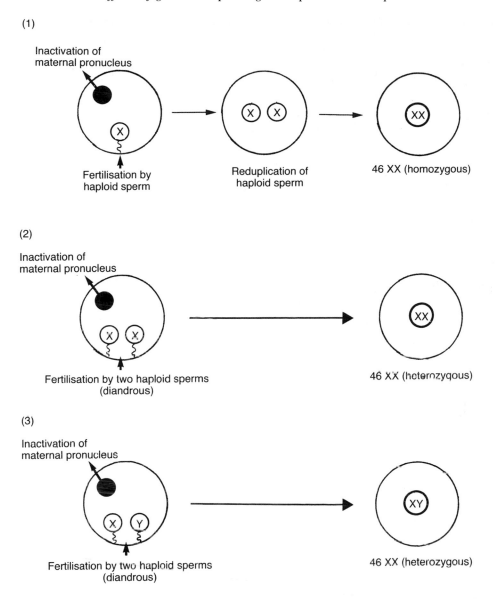

Fig. 4.10. Mechanisms of androgenetic fertilisation in complete hydatidiform moles.

characteristics of complete hydatidiform moles, therefore, are consistent with that of maternal imprinting (i.e. only paternal genes are expressed). Several mechanisms are possible for the production of these tumours (Fig. 4.10). The main distinguishing features between these are whether the condition is caused by fertilisation by one haploid sperm with eventual reduplication or by two haploid sperms, because the resultant mole will be either homozygous or heterozygous. Among the heterozygous variety the mole can either be XX or XY depending on the sex chromosomes carried by the sperms. YY combinations are non-viable.

It is interesting to compare the situation in a related condition known as a partial mole. As its name implies, only part of the placenta is involved in molar transformation, unlike complete hydatidiform mole, and there is an associated embryo although it may die *in utero*. Partial moles are triploid (Szulman and Surti 1978), and genetic analyses have shown they contain one set of maternal chromosomes plus two sets of paternal chromosomes (diandrous triploid) (Lawler *et al.* 1979). Digynous triploid pregnancies, in contrast, are characterised by small underdeveloped placentae. The origin of triploidy could be by the same mechanism as for the production of complete hydatidiform mole except for the retention of the maternal set of chromosomes. Thus, in a partial mole, the paternal contribution is two-thirds of the genome compared with 100% in complete mole. These findings further confirm the role of genomic imprinting in placental development and trophoblast growth.

The reverse situation demonstrating paternal imprinting can be seen in ovarian teratomas. These tumours arise by reduplication of the complement of maternal chromosomes in an unfertilised oocyte. They are, thus, gynogenomes (Linder *et al.* 1975). These tumours contain embryonic tissues from all three germ layers, but no extraembryonic elements including trophoblast. Ovarian teratomas are generally benign. In contrast, trophoblast cells from complete hydatidiform moles are prone to malignant change, with the risk of developing into choriocarcinoma calculated to be 1000 times greater than after normal pregnancy (Bagshawe and Lawler 1982). This indicates that androgenetic trophoblast is more inclined to undergo malignant change than normal trophoblast which, in turn, implies that paternal genes may play a role in this transformation. Homozygous and heterozygous complete moles are equally susceptible to becoming choriocarcinomas (Lawler and Fisher 1993) so it is not a question of the inheritance of some recessive alleles due to homozygosity. Perhaps mutations are more frequent in the paternal genome. For example, new germ line mutations in retinoblastoma are usually of paternal origin (Ejima *et al.* 1988). Alternatively, the loss of suppressor genes on maternally derived chromosomes could influence malignant change in complete moles, which may explain the relative rarity of choriocarcinomas following partial moles. In Wilms' tumour, preferential loss of maternal alleles and retention of paternal alleles for chromosome markers on 11p, where the Wilms' tumour suppressor gene (WT1) is located, has been observed (Schroeder *et al.* 1987; Pal *et al.* 1990).

From the evidence discussed, it could be concluded that the paternal genome provides some genetic information vital for the growth of trophoblast while the maternal genome acts in an inhibitory way (Hall 1990). In the context of mammalian reproduction, this has been viewed as a parental tug-of-war where the paternal genes, by having a positive effect on the growth of the placenta, give the fetus a greater chance of survival while the maternal genes, by limiting the growth of the placenta, will reduce the nutritional burden of each pregnancy and thus promote the mother's chances of a successive pregnancy (Moore and Haig 1991; Haig 1993). That this kind of imprinting has evolved in vertebrates only in placental mammals, where the embryo is nourished directly from maternal tissue, and is not present in oviparous species, where the amount of yolk laid down in the egg is already determined before fertilisation, is in support of such a hypothesis.

Recently, Varmusa and Mann (1994) proposed a more provocative idea to explain why genomic imprinting has evolved in mammals. They view imprinting as a mechanism by which female mammals are protected from the potential danger of developing trophoblast disease from parthenogenetically activated ovarian teratomas. As discussed earlier, ovarian teratomas are usually benign and lack extraembryonic tissue including trophoblast, and it is this tissue which has a predilection for malignant change. Indeed, most testicular germ line tumours contain abundant extraembryonic tissues including yolk sac elements and trophoblast which frequently develop into malignant tumours in the same way as complete hydatidiform moles. Genomic imprinting could certainly explain this difference in behaviour between ovarian and testicular germ cell tumours (Porter and Gilkes 1993). However, it is a major conceptual leap from a proposal that the benign nature of ovarian teratomas is a consequence of imprinting to one which states that this is the evolutionary rationale for the existence of imprinting. That nature has not deemed it worthwhile to protect the males of the species in a similar way is rather disappointing! A further difficulty about this 'ovarian time bomb' hypothesis is its failure to explain the imprinting of other genes which have no obvious links with trophoblast growth – apart from invoking the idea that these are innocent bystanders which happen to be caught up in the imprinting process.

Only some genes are imprinted and the effects of imprinted genes may be developmentally complex. Even closely linked genes may be differentially affected by the imprinting mechanism. In humans four genes are known to be imprinted, H19, IGF-II, WT1 and SNRPN (Jinno *et al.* 1994). At present, it is not known what imprinted gene(s) are important for trophoblast development or for implantation (Goshen *et al.* 1994).

The gene encoding insulin-like growth factor II (IGF-II) is maternally imprinted (Giannoukakis *et al.* 1993). Studies in mice that carry a targeted disruption of the IGF-II gene have shown that transmission of this mutation through the male germ line results in progenies that are growth deficient, whereas transmission of the disrupted gene through the maternal germ line gives rise to offspring which are phenotypically normal (DeChiara *et al.* 1991). This observation can be interpreted as due either to a direct effect on the embryo or to an indirect consequence of impaired placental function. Immunohistological studies on human placentae have shown that those trophoblast cells with mitotic activity express receptors for IGF (Chapter 10), so the paternally expressed gene encoding this growth factor could be one important element in trophoblast development. Interestingly, the receptor for IGF-II is reciprocally imprinted in mice, with exclusive maternal expression. Since the receptor plays a significant role in controlling the action of the polypeptide, this may be an example of maternal genes having evolved to counter the effects of paternal genes in reproduction. This is supported by the observation that mutant mice with disruption of this receptor gene are approximately 30% larger than normal mice at birth and generally do not survive (Wang *et al.* 1994). Either maternal inheritance or homozygosity of the inactivated allele leads to similar results, indicating that maternal expression of this receptor is essential for embryonic growth regulation. However, the significance of these murine observations in relation to human reproduction is unclear because the type I and II receptors for IGF-II are not imprinted in humans (Ogawa *et al.* 1993). This lack of conservation between mouse and human suggests that the physiological role of this growth factor may differ between these two species, and that imprinting of certain genes are species specific.

The H19 gene is paternally imprinted (Zhang and Tycko 1992). Its function is unclear because, although it expresses abundant RNA, it does not appear to code for any protein product (Brannan *et al.* 1990). H19 is expressed by normal trophoblast (Rachmilewitz *et al.* 1992) as well as by trophoblast derived from complete moles (Mutter *et al.* 1993), placental site trophoblast tumours and choriocarcinomas (Ariel *et al.* 1994). Since complete moles are androgenetic, it would appear that the parental source of certain imprinted genes can sometimes be reversed. It remains to be determined what the functional implication of this relaxation of imprinting is in relation to molar trophoblast development. Loss of imprinting of IGF-II and H19 is also commonly associated with choriocarcinomas (Hashimoto *et al.* 1995). Intriguingly, relaxation of imprinting has been detected in human cancers (Rainer *et al.* 1993).

Recently, maternal monoallelic expression of the Wilms' tumour suppressor gene WT1 was demonstrated in five of nine human placentae while this gene was biallelically expressed in the kidney (Jinno *et al.* 1994). This suggests that imprinting of WT1 may occur in a tissue-specific manner. Furthermore, because monoallelic expression of WT1 was not found in all placentae examined, the possibility also arises that imprinting for this gene may be genetically polymorphic within the human population. This makes it difficult to formulate a hypothesis for a role of this gene in placental development.

The fourth human gene which has been shown to be imprinted is the gene called small nuclear ribonucleoprotein polypeptide N (SNRPN) (Reed and Leff 1994). In both mouse and man, only the paternally inherited allele is expressed, with monoallelic expression demonstrable in human brain and heart. A defect in paternal chromosome 15q12 is associated with the human neuroendocrine disorder Prader-Willi syndrome. To date, there is no evidence that imprinting of this gene affects the reproductive process.

A recent report that the murine *Mash2* gene is paternally imprinted is interesting (Guillemot *et al.* 1995). This gene encodes a transcription factor required for the development of trophoblast progenitors and homozygous mutants die from placental failure. This finding, therefore, is in contrast to the generally accepted view that paternal genes alone are important for trophectoderm development.

In the context of possible maternal 'recognition' of trophoblast, a crucial question would be whether MHC genes are imprinted in the placenta. Both maternally and paternally inherited MHC class I antigens are expressed by cells of the invasive equine trophoblast so that, in this species, expression of these genes does not appear to be affected by genomic imprinting (Donaldson *et al.* 1994). Similar findings have been reported for the mouse where RNA extracted from whole placentae as well as from separated spongio- and labyrinthine trophoblast shows no evidence of imprinting for MHC class I H-2K or H-2D expression (Drezen *et al.* 1994). In contrast, the classical class I antigen (RT1.A) and the non-polymorphic pregnancy associated antigen (Pa) of the rat are imprinted in the placenta with preferential expression of the paternal allele (Kanbour Shakir *et al.* 1993). If this imprinting does have a biological function for the rat, then it is further evidence for the disparate evolutionary pathways taken by even closely related species during placental development (Chapter 2). From these observations in animals, it seems unlikely that imprinting of MHC class I genes would be a general phenomenon involved in maternal–fetal recognition. No data are available for MHC imprinting in the human placenta. Since the monomorphic rat Pa locus is imprinted, the question arises whether the relatively invariant HLA-G molecule may be similarly imprinted in human trophoblast. Using a specific antibody against HLA-G, we have recently observed that this antigen is expressed by androgenetic complete hydatidiform mole (Chumbley *et al.* 1994a), indicating that the paternally derived allele is not suppressed, but whether there is co-expression of the maternal HLA-G allele is unknown.

While studies on androgenetic hydatidiform moles have focussed attention on the positive effects of paternally expressed genes on trophoblast growth, it must not be forgotten that normal trophoblast development is likely to be subjected to the opposing influence of maternally expressed genes. The X chromosome may be especially important in this regard. The paternal X chromosome is preferentially inactivated in normal murine trophectoderm (Takagi and Sasaki 1975; West *et al.* 1977) and in human trophoblast (Harrison 1989) whereas X inactivation is random in somatic tissues, affecting the paternal and maternal X chromosome equally (Lyon 1993). Since the male trophoblast has a single maternal X and female trophoblast has the paternal X preferentially inactivated, this could be a device whereby some X-linked genes important for trophoblast development could behave as though they were paternally imprinted. However, duplication of the maternal X is detrimental to early mouse embryogenesis and prevents differentiation of the trophectoderm (Takagi 1991). Differential methylation of CpG sites in the promoter region of the *Xist* gene in sperm and oocyte of mice has recently been reported (Ariel *et al.* 1995; Zuccotti and Monk 1995). This difference in gametic methylation could provide a mechanism whereby the paternal X chromosome is marked for preferential inactivation in the trophectoderm. The gene encoding tissue inhibitor of metalloproteinases (TIMP) which may control trophoblast degradation of extracellular matrix and hence trophoblast invasion (Chapter 9) is X-linked. It would be tempting to suggest that the expression of this gene is a further example of how the mother can exert a balancing influence on trophoblast invasiveness.

Thus, in the search for imprinted genes that affect placentation, it is important to identify those which have a positive and those with a negative influence on trophoblast development. Success in this venture would greatly enhance our understanding of how human implantation is controlled, especially in those pathological conditions such as pre-eclampsia where the interaction between a paternal and maternal genetic element is a tantalising feature of its aetiology (Chapter 11). The concept of imprinting as a mechanism designed to control maternal–fetal interaction during the evolution of the placental form of reproduction is an attractive one.

Retrovirus expression and trophoblast development

Biology of retroviruses

Retroviruses are RNA enveloped animal viruses which contain a single-stranded RNA genome and an RNA-dependent DNA polymerase to transcribe the viral RNA into a double-stranded insertion element for integration into host DNA (Hellman *et al.* 1979; Coffin 1990). Genetic mapping studies have identified three genes in the retroviral genome. In order from the 5′ to 3′ end, these are: (1) a *gag* gene which codes for viral structural core proteins, (2) a *pol* gene which codes for reverse transcriptase, (3) an *env* gene which codes for the major envelope proteins. Flanking these are the 5′ and 3′ long terminal repeat (LTR) regions which contain sequences essential for viral expression. The inserted retroviral genome is known as the *provirus*, which can be expressed with the production of viral particles. These viral particles can be classified morpohologically into four types (A, B, C and D) that can be transmitted horizontally like other viruses (exogenous transmission). However, an important characteristic of retroviruses is that they can remain unexpressed in the host cell, and be transmitted vertically in the genome through the germ line (endogenous transmission).

Because of this ability of retroviruses to integrate into host DNA to become part of the host genome, most animal species have accumulated large numbers of integrated retroviral sequences (Larsson *et al.* 1989). It has been estimated that as much as 0.05% of the total mouse genome is composed of retroviral-related sequences. Similarly, retroviral sequences have also been identified in the human genome, usually by low-stringency nucleic acid hybridisation with DNA probes from evolutionary conserved animal retrovirus genes. From 0.1% to 0.6% of the human genome consists of endogenous retroviral sequences, with the proviral element present in copy numbers between 1 and 1000 per haploid genome. These human endogenous retroviruses are collectively given the designation HERV and followed by a one-letter amino acid code indicated by the tRNA specific primer binding sequence. Thus, if the amino acid is lysine, then the virus is called HERV-K.

Nearly all the HERVs so far described appear to be defective. For example, HERV-H sequences do not contain long open reading frames in their structural genes that can code for intact viral proteins (Mager and Freeman 1987). Similarly, O'Connell *et al.* (1984) described an apparently full length human endogenous proviral clone ERV-3 (now classified as HERV-R because of its arginine), located as single copy loci per haploid genome in chromosome 7, which has retained the typical LTR-*gag-pol-env*-LTR gene order of a type C retrovirus, but the presence of terminator codons in the open reading frames of both its *gag* p30 sequence and its *pol* gene suggests that it probably cannot function as an infectious virus. However, the LTRs do contain normal transcription regulatory sequences in spite of 8.8% divergence between the 5′- and 3′-LTR with differences in the number of nucleotides as well as nucleotide substitutions (O'Connell and Cohen 1984). These functional LTRs could direct the expression of at least some viral genes, although complete viral particles cannot be made. For example, the *env* glycoprotein gene of HERV-R has been shown to be capable of encoding a polypeptide product and antibody generated against this envelope protein reacts against several normal human tissues (Cohen *et al.* 1985). Since retroviruses have probably been inserted into the vertebrate germ line in the distant evolutionary past, the virus genes could have evolved within the eukaryotic chromosomal environment into essential elements which encode important cellular products for the normal function of the host cell (Repaske *et al.* 1985). Alternatively, functional retroviral LTRs may promote the expression of flanking host genes. The best example of this was first described in chicken B cell lymphomas induced by avian leukosis virus (ALV), where transcription of the cellular proto-oncogene *myc* was upregulated through the integration of a provirus in its vicinity. AVL integrates preferentially just upstream of the c-*myc* coding region where its 3'-LTR is juxtaposed to the c-*myc* gene. The transcriptional influences from the proximal LTR will lead to elevated production of c-*myc* protein (Torry and Cooper 1991). This insertional activation of cellular oncogenes without structurally altering the host gene is now recognised as one of the major mechanisms of retroviral oncogenesis (Kung *et al.* 1991).

Unlike other HERVs, HERV-K, which was originally characterised by the partial homology of its polymerase gene to corresponding sequences in mouse mammary tumour virus (MMTV), has sequences that contain the open reading frames for all structural retroviral genes (Ono 1986). Therefore, HERV-K appears to possess all the characteristics of an intact endogenous human retrovirus (Lower *et al.* 1993). Supporting evidence is now available that HERV-K could indeed code for the human teratocarcinoma-derived retrovirus (HTDV) in that an antiserum raised against recombinant *gag* protein of HERV-K is observed to react specifically against HTDV particles in immunoelectronmicroscopy. In Western blots, this same antiserum recognises a protein of 30 kDa which is presumably the major core protein of HTDV particles (Boller *et al.* 1993).

Selective expression in the placenta

Retroviral mRNA

The reason why placental biologists are interested in endogenous retroviruses is that many of these viruses appear to be selectively expressed in the placenta (Johnson *et al.* 1990). Kato *et al.* (1987) have demonstrated that three polyadenylated RNAs of 9, 7.3 and 3.5 kb long of HERV-R are abundant in first trimester and term human chorionic villi, representing 0.03–0.05% of the total mRNA for this tissue. In contrast, associated embryos had relatively little of these transcripts. All three RNAs were spliced mRNAs that lacked 5.9 kb of proviral sequences, including the *gag* gene and most of the *pol* gene. Recent *in situ* hybridisation studies by Boyd *et al.* (1993), who probed with ERV-3 (HERV-R) envelope DNA generated by PCR amplification of genomic ERV-3 sequences, confirm that the syncytiotrophoblast layer of term placentae is the major site of expression. Northern blot of term trophoblast cells in culture revealed a 3.5 kb transcript detectable after 96 hours of culture. The 7.3 kb or the 9 kb transcripts described by Kato *et al.* (1987) were not detected, indicating that these mRNAs may be expressed by other non-trophoblast elements of the placenta. Because no significant bands were detected before 96 hours of culture, the authors concluded that cytotrophoblast probably did not express any retroviral message until it has differentiated into syncytiotrophoblast *in vitro*. This is supported by the finding that βhCG production by the cells paralleled the level of expression of transcripts. This hormone is a syncytiotrophoblast product. It would be interesting to perform similar experiments with first trimester chorionic villi where cytotrophoblast cells are more abundant, and also on extravillous trophoblast at the implantation site, to ensure that other trophoblast populations are not involved.

Interestingly, Kato *et al.* (1988) did not find ERV-3 mRNA expression in choriocarcinoma cell lines and in one case of invasive hydatidiform mole, although in general other tumour cell lines had levels of transcripts 10–60% higher than in normal placenta. This is not due to deletion of the locus because the ERV-3 genome is present and unaltered in the DNA of the choriocarcinoma cells. Also, trace levels of ERV-3 mRNA can sometimes be found, which indicates that the cells have not completely lost their ability to process the primary transcripts. Thus, it was concluded that, in choriocarcinomas, the ERV-3 gene may be abnormally transcribed, and that a gene product encoded by ERV-3 could act as a tumour suppressor gene in trophoblast. There is a precedence for this in that the retinoblastoma susceptibility locus is also abnormally transcribed in retinoblastomas. The possibility that ERV-3 may encode a protein with a physiological function is intriguing. In evolutionary terms, ERV-3 is a very old insertion and was present in the primate germ line before the divergence of apes and Old World monkeys about 30 million years ago. Furthermore, unlike the majority of the other known HERVs, ERV-3 is a single copy element which is inserted into a common integration site in all primates studied. It would be difficult to imagine that this retrovirus had persisted in the genome for so long if it did not have a role to play in the host cell.

Retroviral proteins

There are now many studies demonstrating the presence of retroviral-encoded proteins in the placenta. J. Nelson *et al.* (1978) examined 100 normal human placental extracts for RNA-directed DNA polymerase activity and found this in 80 of the specimens studied. This activity banded at a density of 1.15–1.17 g/ml in sucrose and examination of material within this band revealed numerous retrovirus-like particles 100–150 nm in size with central electron-dense cores and double-membraned envelopes. It was concluded that the enzyme might be associated with these particles. Prior to this, similar enzymes with virus-like particles have been detected only in human malignant tissues so this was the first demonstration in a normal human tissue. Subsequently, the same authors found a specific inhibitor of the enzyme they originally described in placental extracts and believed that interference by this inhibitor could be the reason why the enzyme itself is not detected more frequently (Nelson *et al.* 1981). The chemical nature of the inhibitor was not established. Sedimentation behaviour in glycerol gradients suggests that it is not lipoprotein and immunodiffusion tests for IgG and IgM proved negative. The authors observed very high levels of this inhibitor in placental extracts from a woman with a history of several spontaneous abortions. While it is tempting to postulate that aberrant regulation of reverse transcriptase activity by inhibitor could upset placental development, this is just one sample. Although not specifically stated, this placenta was presumably obtained from a subsequently normal pregnancy so it is difficult to explain why the high inhibitor levels had not affected this pregnancy also.

Besides reverse transcriptase, other viral-associated proteins have been detected in placenta by many investigators and by a variety of immunological assays. Using indirect immunofluorescence and goat antisera against the p30 core protein of the simian sarcoma associated virus (SSAV)/gibbon ape leukaemia virus (GALV) primate retrovirus group, Maeda *et al.* (1983) localised a cross-reactive antigen at the basal aspect of the syncytiotrophoblast near the underlying basement membrane from all ten full-term human placentae examined. This is the location where C-type particles are seen by electronmicroscopy. Subsequently, this placental protein was shown to be also 30 kDa in size by electrophoresis and immunoblotting (Jerabek *et al.* 1984). This similarity in molecular weight and antigenicity supports the conclusion that the placental protein is indeed encoded by the endogenous retrovirus-related p30 *gag* gene segment.

Similar results have been obtained with antibodies against other retroviral antigens. Suni *et al.* (1984a) used a monoclonal antibody specific for the p19 protein of the human T cell leukaemic virus (HTLV), which is one of the major antigenic polypeptides of this virus. The antibody was found to stain syncytiotrophoblast of normal placentae, hydatidiform moles and choriocarcinomas. Other embryonic or adult tissues were not stained. Immunoblotting of proteins from JAR choriocarcinoma cell line with this antibody detected a single protein band of 28 kDa. A rabbit antiserum generated against a synthetic 11 amino acid polypeptide which has partial sequence homology with the murine leukaemia virus (MuLV) and baboon endogenous virus (BaEV) p30 protein was found to react with the trophoblast layer of first trimester chorionic villi and also with hydatidiform mole and choriocarcinoma tissues, but not with other fetal or adult tissues (Suni *et al.*

1984b). Immunoblotting detected a 75 kDa protein from first trimester placenta, and from three different choriocarcinoma cell lines. The authors felt that, in studies such as these, polyclonal antibodies capable of reacting against several epitopes of a peptide sequence could be preferable to monoclonal antibodies directed at a single epitope because there is less chance of the former giving false cross-reactivities due to molecular mimicry between two proteins. Thus, they are inclined to believe that their antibody is recognising the gene products of a human endogenous retroviral sequence which may be selectively expressed in syncytiotrophoblast.

In Rhesus monkeys, Stromberg and Huot (1981) screened for the expression of a C-type viral p26 antigen by radioimmunoassay and found this protein to be present in 16 of 16 placentae, but not in a variety of fetal tissues tested, including heart, lung, spleen, liver, kidney, intestine, skeletal muscle, testis and thymus. Interestingly, the level of expression of p26 is very much higher in the portion of placenta in direct apposition to decidua compared with the portion facing away, which seems to imply that endogenous retroviral products could play a role in placental–uterine interaction.

Additional evidence from a different approach has shown that a rabbit antibody generated against purified human syncytiotrophoblast plasma membrane (Whyte and Loke 1979) mediated complement-dependent cytotoxicity against cells infected with the Mason-Pfizer virus (M-PV) or BaEV (Thiry *et al.* 1981), indicating there may be shared antigenic determinants on the cell membrane of syncytiotrophoblast and retroviral infected cells. Prior absorption of the antiserum with virus or viral glycoproteins partially neutralised the cytotoxicity of the antiserum, which supports the idea that the shared antigens are viral coded. All these viral-encoded trophoblast proteins described may be immunogenic to the mother. Both sensitised lymphocytes and specific antibodies against retroviral-related antigens have been demonstrated (Hirsch *et al.* 1978; Thiry *et al.* 1978). Whether this maternal immune response is important for reproduction or is merely a by-product is unclear.

Retroviral particles

In addition to proteins, the presence of actual retroviral particles in the placenta of a variety of mammalian species has long been documented (Parem 1979; Kalter 1983). These include humans and eight species of non-human primates as well as mice, guinea pigs and rabbits. The earliest reports are electronmicroscopic demonstration of C-type viral particles (Kalter *et al.* 1973; Benveniste *et al.* 1974; Dalton *et al.* 1974; Vernon *et al.* 1974; Feldman 1975; Kalter *et al.* 1975; Seman *et al.* 1975; Imamura *et al.* 1976; Dirksen and Levy 1977). There is general agreement that these viruses are normally located on the convoluted plasma membrane at the basal border of the syncytiotrophoblast in apposition with either the underlying villous cytotrophoblast or basement membrane. Occasionally, C-type particles have also been seen budding from cytotrophoblast. Viral particles have never been observed at the brush border of the syncytiotrophoblast in contact with maternal blood in the intervillous space. Among human placentae surveyed, positive sightings of C-type particles ranging from 36.7% to 80% of specimens examined have been reported. This is a significantly higher success rate than for other human tissues, indicating that the placenta is especially permissive for retroviral replication (Chandra *et al.* 1970).

In addition to the usual locations of viral particles reported in the vicinity of syncytiotrophoblast, Feldman (1975) has observed particles among cells of the cytotrophoblast columns in the region of the basal plate in Rhesus monkeys. This finding, of course, is of great relevance to the theme of the present volume because it shows that the extravillous trophoblast population also expresses viral particles. However, although these particles resemble C-type particles in their formation by budding from the plasma membrane and the presence of a central nucleoid, they are much smaller in size ($\approx$30 nm compared with 100 nm for C-type particles) and differ in their internal structure.

In the most recent study, Lyden *et al.* (1994) analysed retroviral particles isolated from human first trimester and term chorionic villi. These particles display reverse transcriptase activity and have a buoyant density of 1.17 g/ml on sucrose which is consistent with type C retroviruses. They have a diameter of around 120 nm, are membrane-bound and contain capsid particles within an internal matrix structure. A Mab generated against these particles was subsequently observed to stain cytoplasmic structures within syncytiotrophoblast (Mwenda *et al.* 1994).

From the preceding survey, it can be concluded that retroviral genetic information is expressed preferentially in the human placenta. The cumulative evidence is convincing and is summarised as follows: (1) Retroviral transcripts are more abundant in chorionic villous tissue than in associated embryos. (2) Placental extracts contain retroviral reverse transcriptase. (3) Antisera raised against various retroviral-related proteins react against placental proteins. (4) The reverse is also the case in that antisera raised against trophoblast membrane antigens recognise shared determinants on retroviral-infected cells. (5) Pregnant women show cell mediated and humoral immunity against retroviral proteins, indicating that these proteins are immunogenic *in vivo*. (6) Even complete viral particles may be expressed since C-type particles are frequently observed in human placentae.

Retroviral activation and possible functions

Why retroviruses are especially transcriptionally active in the placenta is not known. The two most likely factors are hormonal and immunological (Hellman *et al.* 1979). Estrogen (17β-estradiol) but not progesterone induced the production of retroviral proteins and RNA-directed DNA polymerase in the uteri of ovariectomised mice (Hellman and Fowler 1971; Fowler *et al.* 1972). In normal mice, the levels of retroviral p30 protein in the uterus are also highest during the follicular (estrogen) phase of the estrous cycle. Retrovirus activation has also been observed in situations of immunological activity such as graft-versus-host reaction, allograft rejection and *in vitro* mixed lymphocyte reactions. The implantation site represents the interface between tissues from two dissimilar individuals, so that their mutual recognition of each other could, in some way, trigger retroviral expression in the placenta as well as the uterus.

Perhaps an even more important question is the role these retroviral products may play in placental development. Although no definitive functions have so far been attributed to them, it would be surprising if at least some of these sequences had not acquired biological importance in the host cells since they have been part of the vertebrate genome for millions of years. That proviral LTR can promote the expression of cellular genes has already been alluded to earlier in relation to AVL and c-*myc*. Indeed, this proto-oncogene is upregulated in the developing human placenta with the 2.4 kb transcript of c-*myc* exhibiting a stage-specific appearance, varying 20- to 30-fold over the period of gestation (Pfeifer-Ohlsson *et al.* 1984). The peak of expression was at 4–5 weeks gestation, when the *myc* transcripts comprised 0.05% by weight of total placental mRNA, and then declined by the end of the first trimester. *In situ* hybridisation revealed highest expression of *myc* transcripts among cells of the cytotrophoblast shell where most [³H]thymidine incorporation was also found, leading to the conclusion that the pattern of *myc* expression is correlated with the proliferating cytotrophoblast population. A later report on the immunohistological localisation of the c-*myc* product in human chorionic villi also recorded similar findings (Maruo and Mochizuki 1987). The human placenta is known to express a number of proto-oncogenes besides c-*myc*, such as c-*fms*, c-*sis*, c-*fos*, c-*erb-B* (Adamson 1987). Perhaps the expression of some of these others may also be influenced by viral encoded promoters.

The promoter of the gene encoding the calcium-binding protein, oncomodulin, is thought to be a retroviral LTR in the rat (Banville and Boie 1989). The function of this protein is unknown. It is expressed by villous and extravillous cytotrophoblast cells in the human placenta and also by various tumours (Brewer and McManus 1987). Because of this pattern of distribution, oncomodulin has been included in the group of oncodevelopmental proteins such as alpha fetoprotein (AFP), placental alkaline phosphatase (PLAP), human chorionic gonadotrophin (hCG) and carcinoembryonic antigen (CEA).

More examples of the potential role of retroviral LTR in host gene expression are appearing in the literature, such as the expression of the human phospholipase

A2 gene in teratocarcinoma cells (Feuchter-Murthy *et al.* 1993) and the transcriptional control of immunoglobulin genes during B cell differentiation in the mouse (Hummell *et al.* 1993). Therefore, it would not be too improbable that the expression of some placental genes could also be controlled by proviral LTR sequences.

So far there is no definite assignment of a retroviral encoded protein to a specific placental function. It is tempting to suggest that the fusion of villous cytotrophoblast to form the overlying layer of syncytiotrophoblast could be mediated by some retroviral fusion protein since retroviruses are frequent inducers of syncytium formation (Owens *et al.* 1990). This hypothesis may also apply to placental bed giant cells at the implantation site, although it is not known whether the multinuclear characteristic of these cells is a result of endoreduplication rather than cell fusion.

Of relevance to the immunological relationship between the placenta and the uterus is the observation that a transmembrane envelope protein (p15E) encoded by the murine and feline retrovirus has immunosuppressive properties as demonstrated by its ability to inhibit lymphocyte blastogenic response to mitogens and alloantigens *in vitro* and to block macrophage accumulation at inflammatory sites in mice *in vivo* (Copeland *et al.* 1983; Lindeskog *et al.* 1993). A region of p15E has been conserved among murine and feline retroviruses and a homologous region is also found in a human endogenous retrovirus. A synthetic peptide (CKS-17) of this conserved region was found to inhibit alloantigen stimulation of murine and human lymphocytes whereas four other peptides representing different regions of the virus proteins were inactive, suggesting that the immunosuppressive portion of retroviral transmembrane envelope protein p15E may reside in a conserved sequence (Cianciolo *et al.* 1985). Of particular significance in the context of extravillous trophoblast is the demonstration that p15E also abrogates peripheral blood natural killer (NK) cell cytolytic function (Harris *et al.* 1987) because analogous effector cells at the implantation site are thought to be pivotal in the control of trophoblast migration (Chapter 8). In a ^{51}Cr-release cytotoxic assay against the prototype NK target K562, the peptide (CKS-17) was observed to suppress this activity at concentrations as low as 1.5 mM. This suppression was reversible, indicating that CKS-17 was not toxic to the NK cells themselves but somehow interferes with the lytic phase of NK cytolysis.

The recent experiments of Kim *et al.* (1994) also point to retroviruses having an influence on target cell susceptibility to NK lysis. Transfection of BL6-8 (H-2K^{b-}, H-2D^{b+}) and BL6-2 (H-2K^{b-}, H-2D^{b-}) melanoma clones with H-2K^b or H-2K^d gene resulted in a stable increase in their sensitivity to lysis by NK cells. This transfection was associated with a variety of phenotypic changes in the melanoma cells including the downregulation of the melanoma-associated antigen (MAA) and loss of endogenous A- and C-type retrovirus production. Transfection with other MHC genes, H-2D^d or H-2L^d, had no effect on the phenotype of these melanoma cells or on their susceptibility to NK lysis. The authors postulated an interaction between the H-2K gene and the endogenous retroviruses which could lead to the elimination of viral-induced resistance. Two possible mechanisms may be considered: (1) These retroviruses may contain a gene that regulates target cell resistance against NK effectors, perhaps by the production of some viral-encoded protein, such as p15E. (2) These retroviruses direct inhibitory signals to some cellular genes that control NK susceptibility and these cellular genes become expressed once retroviral production is suppressed by the H-2K gene. As discussed in Chapter 8, the influence of MHC class I molecules on susceptibility to NK cells is highly complex with different genes exhibiting different effects. The present finding of divergent behaviour of H-2K and H-2D genes on the susceptibility of melanoma cells to NK cytolysis confirms the complexity of the relationship.

Viral modulation of host cell MHC expression is a well-known phenomenon found among both DNA and RNA viral groups (Maudsley and Pound 1991; Rinaldo 1994). A variety of mechanisms have been observed, such as effects on transcription factors for MHC genes used by Ad12 and HBV or blocking transport of MHC antigens to the cell surface by Ad2 and CMV. Retroviruses are most likely to exert their influence by acting on the transcription of MHC genes. Howcroft *et al.* (1993) observed that an HIV-1 construct which expresses all viral gene products except *gag* and *pol* transfected into HeLa cells reduced the level of MHC class I surface expression 12-fold. That this is mediated by viral repression of promoter activity is shown by co-transfecting HeLa cells with the 86 amino acid (two-exon) HIV Tat protein, a viral-encoded regulatory protein that transactivates HIV LTR-directed gene expression, together with a class I promoter construct and observing markedly decreased activity of the latter. Since human trophoblast cells are devoid of MHC class I antigens, the implications for some form of retroviral control is clear. However, the situation in human trophoblast is complicated by the fact that villous cytotrophoblast does express class I mRNA although there is no protein product (Chapter 6), so the controlling step here is post-transcriptional.

Besides affecting the host cell's own expression of class I antigen, endogenous retroviruses may also encode their own transplantation antigen. Colombo *et al.* (1987) described a non-H-2 histocompatibility antigen (designated as H-43) in mice which appears to be encoded by sequences of the Mo-MuLV endogenous retrovirus. This antigen is able to stimulate skin graft rejection and cytotoxic effector T cell generation in strains where this retrovirus is not expressed. The encoding of the murine minor lymphocyte stimulating (Mls) antigens by endogenous proviruses of MMTV is another example of this phenomenon (Coffin 1992). These antigens can stimulate T cell proliferation in mixed lymphocyte cultures between mice that are otherwise matched at the MHC. Interestingly, these Mls antigens can act as superantigens (Coffin 1992) that stimulate an inordinately large proportion of the T cell population by binding to the Vβ region of the T cell receptor (Scherer *et al.* 1993). The functional consequences of T cell interaction with superantigens are varied, ranging from stimulation and the production of cytokines to anergy and unresponsiveness (Goodglick and Braun 1994). Because of the unusual characteristics of superantigens compared with conventional antigens, it would be of great interest to reproductive biologists if they were to be expressed by trophoblast cells at the implantation site.

Analysis of extensive nucleotide sequence information from a variety of viruses has identified the presence of numerous viral open reading frames that encode for proteins with homology to cytokines and cytokine receptors (Spriggs 1994). Trophoblast expresses many such proteins and receptors. It would further enhance their importance in trophoblast development if endogenous retroviruses also encode similar molecules.

In conclusion, it will be appreciated that endogenous retroviruses are potentially capable of playing an important role in placental development. Further data are required to determine how this is implemented. Meanwhile, attention may be drawn to the similarity between a normal trophoblast cell and a cancer or transformed cell in their ability to invade solid tissues and blood vessels, their production of analogous 'oncoplacental' proteins and their shared surface membrane profile (Loke 1978).

5

Isolation and characterisation of cells from the early pregnant uterus

The various methods for isolating and culturing human trophoblast have been reviewed (Loke 1983). There are basically three approaches: organ culture, explant culture and monolayer culture.

Organ culture of trophoblast

Organ culture is a technique whereby a small piece of tissue is maintained in a viable functional state *in vitro* over a period of time (Fell 1976). Unlike an explant culture, no outgrowth of cells occurs from the primary piece of tissue. The normal architecture is not disrupted and would, therefore, permit a study of the different cellular components in their proper relationship to each other. This type of culture technique is frequently employed to study biosynthesis by chorionic villous trophoblast. Radiolabelled protein precursors are introduced to the culture medium and autoradiographed tissue sections of the pieces of tissue are subsequently examined by either light or electron microscopy to localise the site of protein synthesis (D. Nelson *et al.* 1978a, b).

Organ culture can also be used to evaluate the effect of oxygen concentration on different trophoblast populations. Fox (1970) observed that, within 24 hours of culture in 6% O_2, the syncytiotrophoblast layer of chorionic villi showed signs of degeneration and necrosis. In contrast, not only were there no visible degenerative changes in the underlying cytotrophoblast cells, they actually appeared to be increasing in numbers, so that by the 10th day of culture the syncytiotrophoblast layer had disappeared from many villi, which became covered by a surface mantle consisting entirely of cytotrophoblast cells. These *in vitro* observations may reflect similar changes occurring in trophoblast under hypoxic conditions *in vivo*. For example, in toxaemia of pregnancy, the increased number of cytotrophoblast cells described in the placenta could be due to ischaemia.

63

The reverse situation also applies in that syncytiotrophoblast in organ culture is equally susceptible to hyperoxic conditions (Ishimara 1971). Indeed, trophoblast *in vivo* during the early stages of pregnancy appears to survive best in a relatively low O_2 environment. Rodesch *et al.* (1992) measured the partial pressures of oxygen (pO_2) in placental and endometrial tissues *in vivo* during the first trimester of pregnancy using a polarographic oxygen electrode and found pO_2 values of 17.9 ± 6.9 mmHg in placental tissues and 39.6 ± 12.3 mmHg in endometrial tissue between 8 and 10 weeks gestational age. The low pO_2 in the early villous placenta may be related to the presence of the trophoblast plugs over the mouths of decidual spiral arteries which serve to prevent too much blood flowing into the intervillous space (Chapter 4). A pO_2 value of 17.9 mmHg is roughly equivalent to 2–3% O_2. The usual gas mixture used for trophoblast culture is 95% air. This contains about 20% O_2 which could, therefore, be much too high for the *in vitro* cultivation of first trimester trophoblast.

Explant culture of trophoblast

Explants are grown from tissue fragments of about 1–2 mm^3 in size. They differ from organ cultures in that cellular outgrowths extend from the primary explant into the surrounding area of the culture dish. If the ultimate aim is to obtain outgrowths of trophoblast then the tissue employed as the starting point must be chosen from those chorionic villi which contain cells capable of giving rise to trophoblast. Based on observations of the number of mitotic figures, staining for Ki-67 in histological sections and the incorporation of radiolabelled DNA precursors using autoradiography, it is generally agreed that cells at the base of the cytotrophoblast columns are likely to be the optimum source of trophoblast cells which are capable of proliferation. These columns are present mainly in the first trimester and not at term so early gestation material is a necessary prerequisite for such cultures. Yagel *et al.* (1989a) and Genbacev *et al.* (1992, 1993) have obtained trophoblast outgrowths by this method. It appears that only trophoblast cells have the ability to migrate out of the explants because the tissue has not been disrupted by enzymes, so this technique can positively select for trophoblast.

In addition, this would be an appropriate model to investigate differentiation and migration of trophoblast from the cell columns. Several relevant findings were made. Signs of proliferation, such as expression of Ki-67, were seen in the cells of the outgrowth nearest the primary explant, but were no longer evident as the cells migrated away from the explant. This is analogous to the situation *in vivo* where proliferative activity is observed mainly in the cells of the columns nearest the villous core, indicating that certain factors derived from the villous mesenchyme or underlying basement membrane are required (Chapter 4). Only explants from first trimester chorionic villi gave rise to trophoblast outgrowths. Those from the second trimester did not. This provides support for the hypothesis that trophoblast has an intrinsic differentiation programme which switches off invasive behaviour after a certain stage of gestation (Aplin 1991b). A substrate of Matrigel or rat tail collagen type I supplemented by decidual extract appears to be the optimal condition for induction of trophoblast outgrowth from explants. Subsequent identification of the actual matrix protein and the factors derived from decidua which influence this process is awaited with great interest.

Monolayer culture of trophoblast

For most types of experiments designed to investigate trophoblast behaviour, it is desirable to obtain large numbers of these cells with a high degree of viability and homogeneity. For this, monolayer cultures of trophoblast cells are required. Theide (1960) was the first to attempt this method by using enzymic digestion of chorionic villi to release isolated cells which were then seeded in culture to produce the monolayers. It was immediately obvious that a variety of cell types were released by this procedure and the subsequent culture contained mixed cell populations (Loke 1983). For this reason, a great deal of effort has been devoted to developing isolation techniques which will select for trophoblast. This has not been easy because of the composite nature of the human placenta (Loke and Hussa 1987). It was not until the latter part of the 1980s that significant technical advances were made in the methodologies for human trophoblast isolation (Loke 1990). Currently, there are four main approaches to human trophoblast cell isolation. They are: (1) outgrowth from explants, (2) density gradient separation, (3) immunological separation and (4) receptor–ligand interaction. Most investigators will agree that, if available, first trimester placental tissue is to be preferred as starting material to that obtained at term delivery because the early part of pregnancy is when major events in implantation take place. Furthermore, extravillous trophoblast is only abundant in young placentae and this is the population which is required for *in vitro* immunological and invasion studies.

Outgrowth from explants

Yagel and his colleagues (1989a) reported that pure, long-term trophoblast cultures can be established by allowing cells to grow out from small pieces of explants of chorionic villous tissue (see Explant Culture). By this method, viable trophoblast cells can be maintained for as long as 8 months in culture and up to 13 passages. The authors believe that, because no enzymic disaggregation has been used, there is less chance of non-trophoblast cells being released to contaminate the cultures. The surprising thing is that the trophoblast cells obtained proliferate so readily. The experience of most investigators is that trophoblast does not behave in this way in culture. However, some cytotrophoblast cells, particularly those situated at the proximal end of the cytotrophoblast columns, are capable of proliferative activity *in vivo* as evidenced by the presence of mitotic figures as well as their expression of the transferrin receptor and the proliferation marker, Ki-67 (Bulmer *et al.* 1988a). Perhaps these are the progenitor cells from which trophoblast which grows outwards from explants are derived.

Density gradient separation

Apart from outgrowth of trophoblast from explants, all other trophoblast isolation procedures are initiated by enzymic disaggregation of cells from chorionic villi and subsequent enhancement or purification. Kliman and his colleagues (1986) are of the opinion that the density of dissociated trophoblast cells from term placentae is sufficiently different from that of other placental cells to be separable by centrifugation over a Percoll gradient. They reported that a homogeneous population of trophoblast cells can be recovered within the density band of 1.048–1.062 g/ml. When plated out in culture, many of these trophoblast cells are transformed into multinucleated syncytiotrophoblast which synthesises placental proteins and hormones such as SP-1, hCG and hPL. However, not all who try this method are equally successful. For example, Bierings *et al.* (1988), using an identical protocol, reported that up to 40% of the cells obtained from the 1.048–1.062 g/ml density band were CD14[+] and DR[+], both of which are macrophage markers, and none stained for hCG, hPL or SP-1. From our own experience, we would concur that macrophages (presumably villous Hofbauer cells) are the major population of contaminating cells from disaggregated chorionic villi (Butterworth and Loke 1985) and we are therefore not surprised with Bierings' findings. Furthermore, we have been unsuccessful in adapting this method for the isolation of trophoblast cells from first trimester placentae.

Immunological separation

In recent years, many monoclonal antibodies (Mabs) have been generated towards human trophoblast specific or restricted molecules so these reagents have opened up new approaches towards trophoblast isolation. After incubation with an appropriate Mab, trophoblast cells can then be pulled out from a mixed cell population by a variety of methods.

Contractor and Soorana (1988) have used a 'panning' technique whereby cells labelled with an anti-trophoblast Mab are incubated on culture dishes coated with an anti-mouse IgG. However, the reported yield of trophoblast is only in the region of 50–60%, which is not sufficiently pure for most kinds of studies. Sorting of antibody-coated cells by flow cytometry should be more discriminating and, indeed, Caulfield *et al.* (1992) have reported the isolation of trophoblast cells with greater than 95% purity using the anti-trophoblast Mab, NDOG2

Even this degree of homogeneity may be insufficient if trophoblast cells are to be used in experiments such as searching for transcripts by amplification of trophoblast mRNA using the polymerase chain reaction (PCR) because 5% of contaminants will render any PCR data invalid. On the basis of an observation that Mabs against EGF-R and c-*erb*B2 surface proteins can be used to discriminate between villous and extravillous trophoblast respectively (Jokhi *et al.* 1994a), flow cytometry has been used to obtain highly purified preparations of these two trophoblast populations to screen for cytokine mRNA expression by reverse transcriptase (RT)-PCR (King *et al.* 1995). Fig. 5.1 shows cells dissociated from chorionic villi of two placentae of 7 weeks and 14 weeks gestational age double stained either for EGF-R and for the macrophage marker CD14 or for c-*erb*B2 and CD14. The fluorescence gate R2 was used to select EGF-R$^+$ or c-*erb*B2$^+$ cells while placental macrophages were excluded using gate R3. The purity of villous and extravillous trophoblast cells obtained was found to be in excess of 99.5%. It is interesting to note that considerably more macrophages are present at 13 weeks than at 7 weeks so this should be borne in mind when selecting tissue to isolate trophoblast. Also, relatively fewer c-*erb*B2$^+$ cells are present at 13 weeks than at 7 weeks indicating a reduction in cytotrophoblast cell columns and therefore extravillous trophoblast cells from the older placenta. To our knowledge, this is the first report of an isolation method whereby villous and extravillous trophoblast can be obtained separately from the same placental sample. This should permit valid comparison between the two populations. The major disadvantages of sorting trophoblast cells by flow cytometry are that this method is labour intensive, time-consuming and only small numbers of cells are obtained.

Trophoblast cells do not express many antigens present on other somatic cells so negative selection procedures have also been tried. Morrish *et al.* (1991) removed contaminating fibroblasts using a Mab against CD9 which should theoretically prevent long-term cultures of trophoblast from being overgrown by these cells. Yui *et al.* (1994) have improved on this technique by removing the cells reactive with CD9 through a goat anti-mouse immunoglobulin column, resulting in a 95% yield

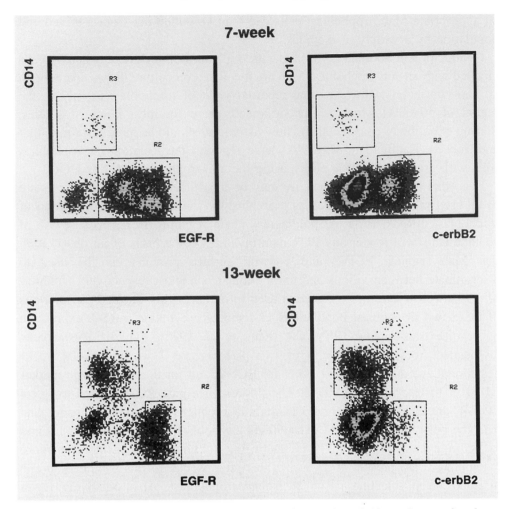

Fig. 5.1. Cells dissociated from chorionic villi of 7 week and 13 week gestational age double stained either for EGF-R and the macrophage marker CD14 or for c-*erb*B2 and CD14. The fluorescence gate R2 was used to select EGF-R$^+$ or c-*erb*B2$^+$ cells while placental macrophages were excluded using gate R3. The purity of villous (EGF-R$^+$) and extravillous (c-*erb*B2$^+$) trophoblast cells obtained was in excess of 99.5%.

of trophoblast cells. These cells can then be cultured for at least 2 weeks with almost no contamination by fibroblasts. Douglas and King (1989) removed all non-trophoblast cells by reacting them with a pan anti-class I Mab. The obvious constraint with both these protocols is that all extravillous trophoblast will also be lost because this sub-population, unlike villous trophoblast, does express both CD9 (unpublished) and a class I-like molecule which will be reactive with a monomorphic class I antibody. A way round this conundrum is to use a Mab directed against a class I antigen (such as 4E against HLA-B) which is not expressed by villous or extravillous trophoblast. Shorter and his colleagues (1990) reported the isolation of trophoblast to 97% homogeneity from term amniochorion using this technique. However, Shorter *et al.* (1993) subsequently showed that Mab 4E stains some trophoblast cells of first trimester cell islands, so this antibody also is not ideal for isolating early gestation trophoblast.

Douglas and King (1989) used an alternative method for selection of labelled cells. Immunomagnetic beads coated with anti-mouse immunoglobulin, rather than the cell sorter, were used to pull out non-trophoblast class I$^+$ contaminating populations. The advantage of immunomagnetic beads is that the procedure is quick and there is no need for sophisticated equipment. However, this method is particularly suitable for negative rather than positive selection because it can be difficult to remove attached beads from the cells. It would not matter if these cells are the ones to be discarded; otherwise the beads can adversely influence any subsequent functional studies.

Receptor–ligand interaction

Receptor–ligand interaction is the method which is used routinely in our laboratory. The rationale of the technique is based on the observation in other culture systems that epithelial cells (of which trophoblast is an example) require a substrate of extracellular matrix for adhesion. From this, we described a method using extracellular matrix coated culture flasks (Loke and Burland 1988). Subsequently, the component in extracellular matrix responsible for trophoblast adhesion was identified to be the protein laminin (Loke *et al.* 1989b), and this is now used to coat either culture dishes or magnetic beads (Loke *et al.* 1989a). Since these earlier studies, various modifications have been made. By trial and error, it has been established that the optimum time for enzymic disaggregation of trophoblast is exactly 9 minutes. This is just enough to dissociate the cytotrophoblast cell columns (Fig. 5.2). Any longer will disrupt the mesenchymal core, thereby releasing unwanted contaminants. After removal of red cells and debris by centrifugation over Lymphoprep, the cells at the interface are left to settle for 1 hour at 37 °C in a plastic culture dish. During this time, contaminating macrophages will readily adhere to the plastic while trophoblast will not, after which the non-adherent trophoblast cells are transferred to laminin-coated culture dishes. We regularly obtain trophoblast cells in excess of 80–90% homogeneity and these are the cells we use for all *in vitro* experiments. To characterise these isolated trophoblast cells, a panel of Mabs as shown in Table 5.1 is currently used to stain cytospin smears or for analysis by flow cytometry.

The trophoblast cells isolated by this technique are observed to be 18B/A5$^+$, PKK1$^+$, HMFG-2$^-$, W6/32$^+$, 71.1$^-$ and BC-1$^+$. They therefore have the phenotype

Table 5.1. *Monoclonal antibodies used to identify isolated extravillous trophoblast cells*

1.	18B/A5 is generated in our own laboratory and stains both villous and extravillous cytotrophoblast, but not villous syncytiotrophoblast (Loke and Day 1984)
2.	PKK1 (Labsystems) stains cytokeratin microfilaments in villous and extravillous trophoblast (Loke and Butterworth 1987)
3.	HMFG-2 (Unipath) stains uterine glandular epithelial cells but not trophoblast, and therefore controls against contamination by the former
4.	W6/32 (Sera-Lab) is directed at a monomorphic determinant of the HLA-A,B,C molecule which is expressed by extravillous trophoblast but not by villous trophoblast
5.	71.1 is generated in rat against horse endometrial cup cells by Prof. Doug Antczak at Cornell University (Antczak *et al* 1987). We have observed that this Mab stains human villous cytotrophoblast but not extravillous trophoblast
6.	BC-1 identifies an antigen expressed on the surface membrane of human extravillous trophoblast (Loke et al. 1992b)

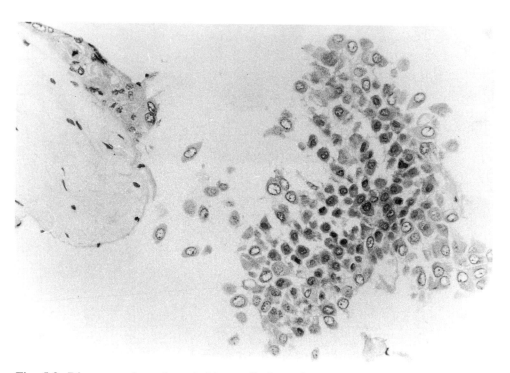

Fig. 5.2. Disaggregation of trophoblast cells from first trimester chorionic villi after 9 minutes of enzyme treatment.

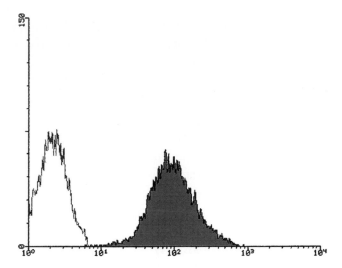

Fig. 5.3. Flow cytometric analysis of cells isolated by adherence to laminin and stained with Mab BC-1 reactive against extravillous trophoblast. This confirms the purity of the trophoblast cells obtained with 98% of the cells staining positively.

of extravillous trophoblast and should be appropriate cells to use for investigations on the implantation process. The homogeneity of the trophoblast cells obtained is shown in the FACS analysis of isolated cells stained with Mab BC-1 (Fig. 5.3). Fisher *et al.* (1989) have used a similar method to isolate extravillous trophoblast.

A wide variety of experiments relevant to implantation have been performed using monolayer cultures of trophoblast cells. They have been used for invasion assays, adhesion to matrix proteins, response to cytokines and as targets for lysis by decidual effector cells. All these will be described in detail in subsequent chapters under the appropriate headings. Experiments such as these require only short-term cultures to generate a sufficient number of cells. Long-term cultures, however, have proved more difficult to achieve. Apart from the explant-derived cells described by Yagel *et al.* (1989a), most investigators are agreed that isolated trophoblast, even from the first trimester of gestation, cannot be readily propagated in culture. It is not clear why this should be so. It is possible that the necessary stimulatory factors are not present or that the prevailing culture conditions are driving the cells immediately towards terminal differentiation. Alternatively, the number of mitotically active trophoblast stem cells isolated may be too small to support viable growth.

To circumvent this problem, Chou (1978a, b) succeeded in transforming trophoblast cells with the temperature-sensitive mutant, tsA255, of the SV40 virus. This has the distinct advantage that the transformed phenotype can be maintained continuously as cell lines at the permissive temperature (33 °C) and yet will revert to normal cell behaviour at the non-permissive temperature (40 °C). Several cell lines were established. One of these, SPA 255-26, has recently been characterised and found to have many properties of first trimester invasive trophoblast, such as a similar profile of adhesion molecule expression and the ability to invade Matrigel substrates (Logan *et al.* 1992). Graham *et al.* (1993) have also produced trophoblast cells with extended life-spans by transfecting these cells with the gene encoding SV40 large T antigen. The transfected cells appear to have similar phenotypic characteristics to the parental trophoblast cells, except that the transfected cells secrete hCG. These cells could prove useful for investigation of the implantation process if it is accepted that they truly represent normal invasive trophoblast cells in their behaviour. However, by virtue of their immortality alone, it is questionable whether transformed cells can ever be considered as identical to normal cells, especially if they are to be used for functional studies.

Monolayer cultures have frequently been used to study trophoblast differentiation in response to various stimuli. Multinucleated cells can be found in trophoblast monolayer cultures and these have been used as a marker representing terminal differentiation of cytotrophoblast cells into syncytiotrophoblast. We, however, believe that the multinucleated cells found in culture, at least with our system, have characteristics of placental bed giant cells rather than syncytiotrophoblast in being MHC class I$^+$ but hCG$^-$ and hPL$^-$, so that the cells are differentiating along the extravillous and not the villous pathway (Loke 1988; Loke and Burland 1988). This distinction is important because the extravillous differentiation route is the one which is directly relevant to the study of implantation. The confusing aspect about multinucleated trophoblast cells in culture is the continued presence of syncytial sprouts derived from the original enzymic digest of chorionic villi. These, of course, have all the characteristics of syncytiotrophoblast (MHC class I$^-$, hCG$^+$, hPL$^+$) and can remain among the cultured cells for a considerable period of time. The gradual distintegration of these cells may be responsible for the placental hormones detected in supernatant fluid of trophoblast cultures. This could explain why a graph constructed for trophoblast secretion in culture is frequently in the form of a bell-shaped curve in spite of continued viability of the cells. Assaying for trophoblast products, such as hCG, in culture supernatants, therefore, is not a valid measure of *in vitro* extravillous trophoblast differentiation. Indeed, the major difficulty in studies of extravillous trophoblast differentiation *in vitro* is the lack of a marker that can follow the developmental sequence of this trophoblast sub-population from its origin in the cell columns through its migration within decidua until its final transformation into placental bed giant cells (Chapter 4). Until such markers become available, it will be difficult to reach meaningful conclusions.

Endometrial and decidual explants

In order to preserve the three-dimensional structure, explants of endometrial (Kliman *et al.* 1990; Bersinger *et al.* 1993) or decidual tissue (Vicovac *et al.* 1993, 1995) have been used as *in vitro* models to study trophoblast invasion. Usual tissue culture conditions, either with or without a collagen gel support for the explant, appear to maintain good viability as shown by ultrastructural morphology or protein synthesis.

Isolation of cells from decidua

The decidua is composed of a mixture of cell types and isolation of purified cell populations is necessary to identify which cells are involved in interaction with trophoblast. In general, dispersal of the tissue by mechanical or enzymic means is followed by some sort of selective procedure to purify the cell population of interest. Techniques to isolate all the main decidual cell components have now been described. For successful cell isolation, the quality of the primary tissue digest is crucial. Poor quality digests have often been the stumbling block in separation of specific cell types from a heterogeneous starting population. After the cells have been isolated, it is essential that they are adequately characterised. This is usually performed by immunostaining of cytospins or culture chamber slides/dishes or by immunofluorescence and flow cytometry. Markers that can be used to identify the various decidual cell types are summarised in Table 5.2. It must be remembered that *in vitro* studies are always an approximation to the *in vivo* situation and the dissociation of cells from their surrounding matrix and neighbouring cells can produce artefactual results.

The separation of the decidual fragments into decidua basalis, compacta or spongiosa is the first step in cell isolation (Chapter 3). Decidua spongiosa is easily recognisable by its bright red appearance and, as the name implies, sponge-like consistency. These fragments are used for the isolation of decidual glands as there is only sparse stroma present. Decidua compacta has a smooth firm grey appearance, and after washing the fragments become paler and pinker. Decidua compacta is used to isolate bone marrow derived cells and stromal cells. Endothelial cells may be isolated from both decidua compacta and spongiosa. The presence of extravillous trophoblast (EVT) in the decidua basalis means these fragments are excluded from decidual cell isolation procedures, but they

Table 5.2. *Markers used to identify isolated cells from the decidua*

Decidual cells	Markers
Stromal cells	EGF-R
	PDGF-Rα and β
Epithelial cells (surface and glands)	Cytokeratin
	HMFG-2
Endothelial cells	QBEND/40
	Factor VIII
	Ulex europaeus
Vascular smooth muscle cells	PDGF-Rβ
Leucocytes	CD45(LCA)
NK cells	CD56
T cells	CD3
Macrophages	CD14, HLA-DR

are vital for *in vivo* studies of the implantation process by immunohistology and *in situ* hybridisation. Decidua basalis can be recognised with some practice. The fragments are more irregular and haemorrhagic than decidua compacta and often yellowish flecks of necrosis (Nitabuch's layer) are visible. If decidua basalis is required, the tissue fragment should always be routinely processed for histological analysis and immunostaining for cytokeratin to confirm the presence of EVT.

Stromal cells

Stromal cells grow easily in culture and their adherence to plastic means they are easily obtained. Smooth grey pieces of decidua compacta contain abundant stromal cells and only a few attenuated glands, and these should be used for stromal cell isolation. Dissociation of the cells is achieved using enzymes such as collagenase or trypsin. The few glandular elements present may be removed by sieving out epithelial clumps with an appropriately sized sieve, by allowing stromal cells to attach to plastic and removing non-adherent epithelial cells after a short period of incubation (20 minutes) or by differential sedimentation at unit gravity (Liu and Tseng 1979; Kirk and Irwin 1980; Cherny and Findlay 1990; Kariya *et al.* 1994). Stromal cells grow readily in a variety of media, and the addition of hormones such as medroxyprogesterone acetate retains the decidualised characteristics of stromal cells (prolactin, IGFBP-1 and fibronectin secretion) (Irwin *et al.* 1989; Tabarelli *et al.* 1992). Stromal cells can be positively identified by using immunochemical markers such as vimentin (+) and cytokeratin (−) to determine the degree of epithelial cell contamination. However, the most notable contaminants will be decidual macrophages (which are also vimentin⁺), but these are identifiable by CD14. These macrophages, being non-proliferative, will eventually be lost after two or three passages, but persist in the first 10 days of culture. We have noted by immunohistology that decidual stromal cells specifically stain for PDGF-Rα and EGF-R and this could be useful in checking stromal cell purity (Jokhi 1994).

Epithelial cells

To date, human glandular epithelial cells have not been isolated separately from the uterine surface epithelium. In any *in vitro* studies of blastocyst–uterine epithelial interaction this should be borne in mind as morphologically and phenotypically these glandular and surface epithelial cells are different (Chapter 3). Ideally, uterine epithelial cells should adhere, become confluent and polarise. This has been achieved in several species (including humans) by isolating glands and culturing on a permeable culture surface plated with extracellular matrix proteins so that the cells are perfused from all sides (Schatz *et al.* 1990; Glasser *et al.* 1991). Isolation of human decidual glands in a non-polarised state is relatively easy (Satyaswaroop *et al.* 1979; Osteen *et al.* 1989, 1994). Fragments of decidua spongiosa rather than decidua compacta are dispersed enzymically. The glands remain as clumps which can be separated by sieving and these will adhere onto plastic. Epithelial cells are cytokeratin⁺, HMFG-2⁺, vimentin⁻, unlike trophoblast which is HMFG 2⁻. In culture, they have a characteristic 'crazy-paving' or 'jigsaw puzzle' appearance (Fig. 5.4).

Endothelial cells

The isolation of endothelial cells is becoming increasingly important both for *in vitro* functional studies of uterine mucosal angiogenesis and for studying how endovascular trophoblast interacts with endothelial cells. Although human umbilical vein endothelial cells (HUVEC) are easy to obtain they are of limited value in the study of the tissue-specific microvasculature (Scott and Bicknell 1993). After mincing the decidual tissue and incubating the fragments with proteolytic enzymes, a cell suspension is obtained which will contain small numbers of endothelial cells. A further purification procedure is always required before plating, otherwise stromal cells will rapidly overgrow the culture. We have incubated mixed decidual cell isolates with magnetic beads coated with an antibody to thrombomodulin (QBEND/40) (Drake and Loke 1991). An enzyme digest method

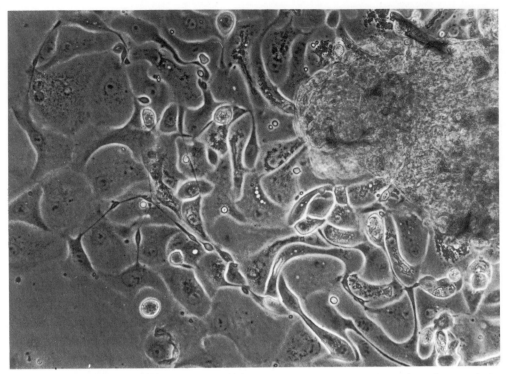

Fig. 5.4. Decidual glandular epithelial cells in culture showing the characteristic 'crazy-paving' or 'jigsaw puzzle' appearance. Phase contrast. (Obj × 20)

was used which released endothelial cells in aggregates, as endothelial cells survive better in culture if plated as small groups of cells. Endothelial cells were plated onto a gelatin or fibronectin substrate and to survive and proliferate required supplements such as endothelial cell growth supplement, heparin and high serum concentration (~50%). They are characterised by their morphological appearance which is of a 'cobble-stone' monolayer (Fig. 5.5), staining positive for von Willebrand factor antigen and with QBEND/40 Mab. Endothelial cells from first trimester decidua have been isolated by other groups. In one study, sensitivity to trypsin was used to eliminate less adherent fibroblasts (Lindenbaum *et al.* 1991). Term decidual endothelial cells have also been obtained using *Ulex*-coated magnetic beads. In this method the endothelial cells were preferentially maintained in culture with human pregnancy sera (Gallery *et al.* 1991).

Vascular smooth muscle cells

The smooth muscle media of the spiral arteries plays a crucial role in human implantation. The characteristic 'fibrinoid necrosis' of media seen in arteries

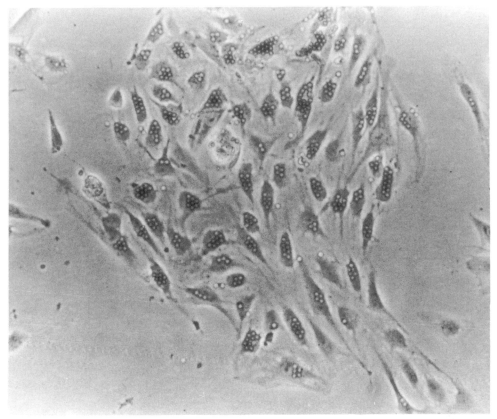

Fig. 5.5. Decidual vascular endothelial cells in culture showing the characteristic 'cobble-stone' appearance. The antibody-coated magnetic beads used for the separation procedure are still present. Phase contrast. (Obj × 20)

surrounded by interstitial trophoblast suggests trophoblast secretes media-specific proteases (Chapter 4). This phenomenon has not been studied *in vitro*, but would ideally require purified decidual vascular smooth muscle cells. We have noted that these stain for the β chain of the PDGF receptor, along with decidual stromal cells. This staining pattern could be utilised to isolate arterial media cells using a combination of cytokine receptors (EGF-R⁺ PDG-Rβ⁺ for stromal cells and EGF-R⁻ PDGF-Rβ⁺ for smooth muscle cells) and separation by either magnetic beads or flow cytometry.

Leucocytes

The bone marrow derived cells comprise a significant proportion of decidual cells (~30%). The main populations are NK cells (large granular lymphocytes) (70%), macrophages (~20%) and T cells (~10%) (Chapter 7). *In vivo* B cells, plasma cells, mast cells and eosinophils are present in negligible numbers. Leucocytes can most easily be obtained by disaggregating minced fragments of decidua compacta with enzymes such as trypsin or collagenase. After sieving to remove clumps, and layering onto Lymphoprep, the mixed cell isolates are plated into tissue culture flasks. Macrophages, stromal cells and glandular cells will all adhere after overnight incubation and the non-adherent lymphocytes can be removed. These contain >95% CD45$^+$ or leucocyte common antigen (LCA)$^+$ cells of which ~80% are CD56$^+$ NK cells on analysis by flow cytometry. The disadvantage of this method is that the use of enzymes may alter surface phenotype and function (Ritson and Bulmer 1987a). This becomes important when analysing phenotypic characteristics such as cytokine receptors. The other problem is that large numbers of stromal cells are obtained and, if these form a monolayer during the overnight culture, significant numbers of lymphocytes will attach to the stromal cells (Chapter 7). This problem can be overcome by using a flask with a large surface area.

Alternatively, we also use a mechanical method for obtaining a single cell suspension by pressing decidual tissue through a metal sieve with a particular pore size (53 μm) using a rubber bung. Larger cells in the tissues do not survive this procedure. These dead cells can then be removed by layering onto Lymphoprep. This is a very simple and rapid method and ~1 × 10^7 cells may be obtained in just 1 hour from a single sample. The cells are mainly lymphocytes with a few macrophages and other cells as contaminants. This mechanical method is the ideal way to isolate cells rapidly for functional studies as no enzymes are used, and a prolonged period of culture to allow non-lymphocytes to adhere is not required. Isolation of decidual leucocyte sub-populations requires selective procedures.

NK cells (CD56$^+$ cells)

Decidual lymphocyte preparations isolated either with enzymes or mechanically contain predominantly CD56$^+$ cells (80–90%). For many *in vitro* studies such a degree of purity is sufficient. The main contaminant cell population is T cells, and it may be necessary to remove these under certain circumstances. Immunological techniques such as panning, magnetic beads or complement-mediated lysis can be used. We have found the simplest method is panning over anti-CD3 coated flasks. After this procedure, together with overnight adherence to plastic to remove macrophages, NK cells with a purity of 96% can be obtained (Fig. 5.6). CD56$^+$ CD3$^-$ CD14$^-$ cells prepared in this way are ideal for several types of study such as cytokine production and Western blotting. However, preparations of CD56$^+$ cells of more than 99% purity are needed when techniques such as reverse transcriptase polymerase chain reaction (RT-PCR) are performed. These can be

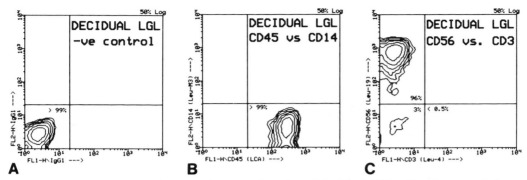

Fig. 5.6. Flow cytometric determination of purity of decidual NK cells after overnight adherence to plastic to deplete macrophages and immunodepletion of T cells by panning over anti-CD3 coated flasks. **A.** Negative control. **B.** Depleted cells double stained with CD14-PE and CD45-FITC showing virtually no macrophages remaining. **C.** Depleted cells double stained with CD56-PE and CD3-FITC showing 96% CD56+ NK cells with minimal contamination by CD3 T cells.

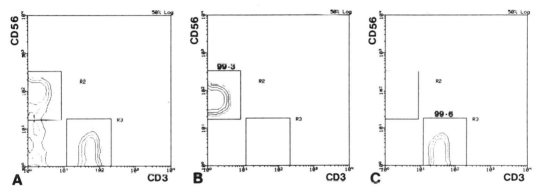

Fig. 5.7. Dual fluorescence flow cytometric analysis of decidual leucocytes before and after cell sorting. **A.** Unsorted cells double stained with anti-CD56-PE and anti-CD3-FITC Mabs. Gates R2 and R3 were used to select for CD56+ NK cells and CD3+ T cells respectively. **B.** Sorted CD56+ CD3− NK cells (99.3%). **C.** Sorted CD3+ CD56− T cells (99.6%).

obtained by immunofluorescence and sorting by flow cytometry (Fig. 5.7) (Jokhi *et al.* 1994d). The morphology of the sorted cells is shown in Fig. 5.8. The disadvantages of this method are that relatively small numbers of cells are acquired and it is necessary to have access to a cell sorter.

T cells (CD3+cells)

There are only small numbers of T cells in decidual tissue and few *in vitro* studies have been performed with purified decidual T cells. However, they can be positively isolated by panning techniques and we have looked at cytokine

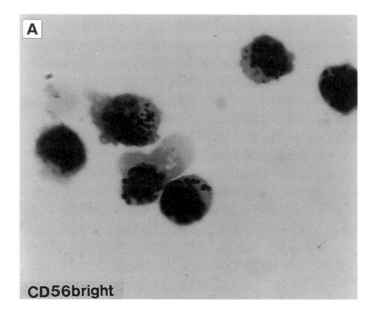

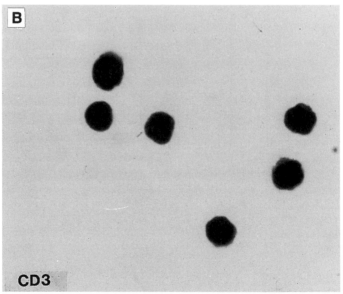

Fig. 5.8. Cytospin smears of sorted CD56$^{bright+}$ (**A**) and CD3$^+$ (**B**) decidual cells stained with Giemsa. Numerous leucocytes with typical large granular lymphocyte morphology are seen in CD56$^+$ smears. The CD3$^+$ cells appear to be small agranular lymphocytes.

production in these preparations (Jokhi 1994). Highly purified T cell preparations can also be obtained by cell sorting (Jokhi *et al.* 1994d).

Macrophages

As decidual macrophages are adherent cells, it is impossible to purify them by adherence to plastic from the more plentiful stromal cells and some positive selection is required. The initial cell digests should be obtained enzymically as rather few macrophages survive the mechanical sieving procedure. After spinning on Lymphoprep the best method is positively to select macrophages using CD14-coated or HLA-DR-coated magnetic beads. CD14 labelling and cell sorting by flow cytometry can also be performed for highly pure preparations (Vince *et al.* 1990). So far, few phenotypic or functional studies on isolated decidual macrophages have been performed.

6

Trophoblast expression of Major Histocompatibility Complex class I antigens

General aspects

Major Histocompatibility Complex (MHC) class I antigens are expressed on the surface of most nucleated cells and serve as important recognition molecules concerned with vertebrate immune responses. In humans, these antigens are also known as human leucocyte antigens (HLA). They are made up of a trimeric complex comprising a transmembrane class I heavy chain whose extracellular domains form a stable association with β_2-microglobulin (β_2m) and a short peptide of approximately eight or nine amino acids. The peptide-binding site of the HLA class I molecule has six pockets: A to F. Pockets A and F at the ends of the binding site are highly conserved between different class I alleles and may serve to anchor the ends of the peptide in the binding site. The other pockets (B,C,D,E) are highly polymorphic and may determine peptide-binding specificity, because site-specific mutagenesis of residues within the allele-specific pockets is observed to alter the repertoire of peptides bound (Barber and Parham 1993).

Trophoblast does not express HLA class II antigens but some sub-populations express class I antigens. Immunostaining with antibodies (e.g. W6/32) against the class I molecule has divided human trophoblast into two distinct populations: villous trophoblast (cytotrophoblast and syncytiotrophoblast) in contact with maternal blood in the intervillous space is class I negative (Fig. 6.1A) whereas extravillous trophoblast invading uterine decidua is class I positive (Fig. 6.1B) (Loke and King 1991). *In situ* hybridisation studies with appropriate cDNA probes for class I mRNA have, in fact, defined three trophoblast populations because villous cytotrophoblast which expresses no class I proteins has demonstrable class I message (Fig. 6.2), suggesting the presence of post-transcriptional regulation of this antigen (Hunt *et al.* 1990). This is summarised in Table 6.1. It appears that this dichotomy between mRNA and protein expression by trophoblast is also observed for MHC class II antigens. Giacomini *et al.* (1994) have reported that first trimester cytotrophoblast cells

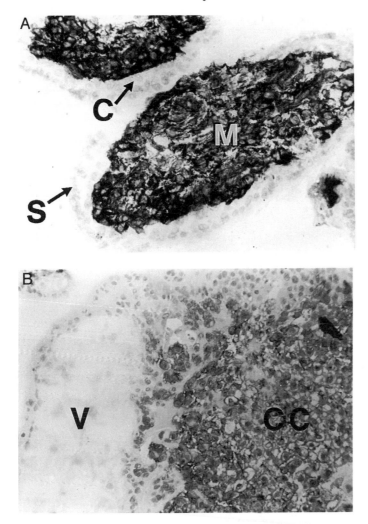

Fig. 6.1. **A.** First trimester placental villi labelled with a Mab, W6/32, which is directed against the monomorphic part of the class I HLA molecule. The villous mesenchymal core (M) is strongly stained whereas both villous cytotrophoblast (C) and syncytiotrophoblast (S) are negative. (Obj × 40) **B.** First trimester placental villus (V) labelled with Mab W6/32 showing strong staining of trophoblast cells of the cell column (CC). (Obj × 25)

showed moderate to strong expression of HLA-DRα, -DRβ and class II associated invariant chain transcripts but not the antigens.

Thus, there are two feto-maternal interfaces in human reproduction and these differ immunologically. While the maternal systemic immune response encounters a trophoblast population which is immunologically neutral, the local uterine response can potentially be stimulated by the HLA class I⁺ extravillous trophoblast migrating into decidua.

Table 6.1 *Differential expression of HLA class I antigen by human trophoblast populations*

	mRNA	Protein
Villous syncytiotrophoblast	–	–
Villous cytotrophoblast	+	–
Extravillous trophoblast	+	+

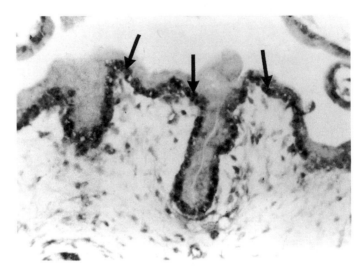

Fig. 6.2. Villous cytotrophoblast cells (arrows) in first trimester chorionic villi contain class I mRNA identified by the class I HLA heavy chain probe pWTCA11 using *in situ* hybridisation. (Obj × 40)

Because of the immunological implications, there is much interest in elucidating the nature and function of this extravillous trophoblast HLA class I antigen. The trophoblast class I molecule is uncharacteristic in many respects compared with similar antigens expressed on other somatic cells (Loke and King 1991): (1) Immunostaining revealed that while the trophoblast HLA class I antigen is reactive with certain antibodies (e.g. W6/32), other antibodies, particularly those directed at the polymorphic domains of the molecule, are unreactive. (2) Immunoprecipitation with W6/32 and SDS-PAGE identified the heavy chain of the trophoblast molecule to be somewhat smaller in molecular mass (39 kDa) than that of the class I antigen on somatic cells (45 kDa). (3) Flow cyometric analysis of isolated trophoblast cells stained with W6/32 showed the surface density of the antigen to be relatively low.

Presently, six class I loci are recognised in humans which have expressed products: three classical loci (HLA-A,B,C) and three non-classical loci

(HLA-E,F,G) (Geraghty 1993). The functions of the classical class I antigens are well established in immunology, but those of the non-classical antigens are not known. These latter usually encode oligo- or monomorphic proteins which are expressed in lower amounts on the cell surface and often in a tissue-specific fashion. The MHC class I region of chromosome 6 appears to contain many more genes than can be accounted for by these recognised loci. Some of these may well be pseudogenes, but it is possible that additional functional loci will continue to be found. A recent new gene is the non-classical locus described by Bahram *et al.* (1994) which is referred to as HLA-X until it is properly assigned (Klein and O'hUigin 1994).

It is now established that the unusual trophoblast antigen is a product of the non-classical class I locus, HLA-G. The cumulative evidence which has led to this conclusion is as follows:-

(1) Screening a series of cDNA libraries from the BeWo choriocarcinoma cell line, Ellis and colleagues (1990) obtained a nucleotide sequence which had a high homology with HLA-G (HLA-6.0 as it was originally known). Using the PCR for amplification, these investigators demonstrated that similar sequences can be found in normal term chorionic plate trophoblast cDNA.

(2) Kovats and colleagues (1990) generated HLA-G transfectants in an HLA-negative parental cell line and observed that immunoprecipitation of metabolically labelled proteins with W6/32 from these transfectants and from normal first trimester extravillous trophoblast exhibited an array of molecules with similar molecular masses (37–39 kDa) and isoelectric points (4.5–5.5 pI) on two-dimensional gels.

(3) Subsequently, Yelavarthi *et al.* (1991) demonstrated the presence of HLA-G mRNA in placental and extraplacental membrane cells by *in situ* hybridisation using an antisense probe derived from HLA-6.0 of Koller *et al.* (1984). We ourselves have constructed an HLA-G locus-specific oligonucleotide based on computer comparison of the published sequences of HLA-G and several HLA-A,B,C,E and Γ clones, and have confirmed the presence of HLA-G mRNA in all first trimester extravillous trophoblast populations using Northern blotting and *in situ* hybridisation (Chumbley *et al.* 1993).

(4) Recently, we have succeeded in generating an antibody specific to HLA-G by immunising HLA-A2/β_2m double transgenic mice with HLA-G transfected into mouse Ltk⁻ cells. This antibody has now confirmed that the class I protein expressed by trophoblast is HLA-G (Chumbley *et al.* 1994a).

HLA-G gene

The HLA-G gene is located within the MHC on chromosome 6p 21.3 and has been mapped to a position 110–220 kb telomeric to the HLA-A gene (Schmidt and Orr 1991, 1993). Like the classical genes, the gene encoding HLA-G consists of eight exons. Exon 1 encodes a leader peptide which is excised before presentation of the molecule on the cell surface. The second, third and fourth exons encode for the α1, α2 and α3 domains of the protein respectively. Exon 5 encodes the transmembrane region while exons 6 and 7 encode the cytoplasmic tail and exon 8 encodes the 3′ untranslated region. A characteristic feature of the HLA-G gene, which sets it apart from the other classical HLA genes, is the presence of a truncated cytoplasmic tail due to a termination codon at the beginning of exon 6 (Geraghty *et al.* 1987). This results in the expression of a protein with a smaller molecular mass of 39–40 kDa and may have implications for function. Initial analysis of the nucleotide (and hence the inferred amino acid) sequences of HLA-G clones from different cell lines with disparate HLA haplotypes revealed a remarkably high degree of homology (Pook *et al.* 1991). This lack of polymorphism could be a feature of an MHC gene in functional decline, but it has also been argued that this state has arisen as a result of strong evolutionary pressures, such as that required for reproduction where allorecognition may need to be kept to a minimum.

More recent work has indicated that some variability could exist in HLA-G at the genetic level. Tamaki *et al.* (1993) have isolated a genomic HLA-G clone from a Japanese placenta which they named 7.0E. The predicted amino acid sequence of this HLA-G clone is found to be identical to those of the two genomic clones, G6.0 (Geraghty *et al.* 1987) and Ice 6.23-5.4H (Pook *et al.* 1991), and two cDNA clones, BeWo G7 (Ellis *et al.* 1990) and ASR53 (Shukla *et al.* 1990). These alleles have recently been assigned as G*01011 (G6.0 and ASR53), G*01012 (BeWo G7) and G*0102 (Ice 6.23-6.4H) (Bodmer *et al.* 1994). However, a 14 bp insertion (between positions 3741 and 3742) in the 3′ untranslated region was characteristic of the Japanese clone 7.0E and BeWo G7 but not of the other clones. Analysis of PCR/ single strand conformational polymorphism (SSCP) of DNA fragments (containing the sequence position 3741) of the HLA-G locus from 45 cell lines established that HLA-G could be classified into two alleles, depending on the absence or presence of the 14 bp stretch. Harrison *et al.* (1993) have also reported variations of 14 bp in exon 8 of HLA-G.

Similarly, Alizadeh *et al.* (1993) have detected four allelic polymorphisms in the 3′ region of the HLA-G gene using an HLA-G-specific probe and analysis by RFLP after digestion with seven restriction enzymes. Allelic frequencies of the subjects tested were calculated to be: allele 1, 40%; allele 2, 36%; allele 3, 22%; and allele 4, 2%. All these reports detect polymorphism in the 3′ untranslated region. What functional implications such variations may have is unclear, but they could affect synthesis of the protein (e.g. mRNA stability). Morales *et al.* (1993) have described three allelic forms of HLA-G DNA, using the sequence of HLA 6.0 described by Geraghty *et al.* (1987) as reference.

However, all these variations either show silent mutations or result in conservative amino acid substitutions. Therefore, the overall conclusion from all the above studies is that, although the HLA-G locus appears to exhibit a degree of polymorphism, the variability is limited and of such a nature that it is not likely to affect unduly the sequence of the expressed protein. Another non-classical class I, HLA-E, also shows a remarkably high level of allelic sequence conservation. Geraghty *et al.* (1992) examined the sequence of cDNA from nine diverse individuals for HLA-E polymorphism and found only two base substitutions in exons 2 and 3; one of these is at a replacement site and the other is silent. That HLA-E alleles have accumulated only two nucleotide substitutions at a time when hundreds of new HLA-A,B alleles were fixed in the population argues that the different HLA loci are subjected to variable evolutionary pressures. A similar argument could be put forward for HLA-G.

In contrast to the above analyses, which are mainly on caucasoid individuals, van der Ven and Ober (1994) have recently presented evidence of many distinctive alleles in the African-American population. Using PCR-amplified exons in small overlapping fragments which can detect >95% of nucleotide substitutions, these investigators reported two sequence variations in exon 2 (α1 domain) and 24 variations in exon 3 (α2 domain) that resulted in amino acid substitutions in 45 healthy individuals examined. The distribution of these substitutions, however, is different from that observed for HLA-A,B,C in that the HLA-G nucleotide variability is largely restricted to the α2 domain and only one of the substitutions in this domain (position 167) is at a functional residue of the peptide binding groove (Parham 1995). These new data indicate that HLA-G is not as monomorphic as it initially appeared to be. However, the observed polymorphism does not seem to be associated with peptide binding diversity although some of the substitutions which replaced conserved cysteine residues could affect the conformation of the molecule. It remains to be seen whether similar variations of HLA-G occur in other racial groups, and what may be the selection pressure that determines the pattern of HLA-G polymorphism.

HLA-G gene product

The full-length HLA-G transcript encodes a protein with an overall homology of 86% to the HLA-A,B,C protein consensus sequence, with the α3 region showing the highest degree of homology (91%) and the α1 and α2 regions showing 81% and 85% homologies respectively (Geraghty *et al.* 1987). The α3 region is highly conserved between class I loci and contains important residues for the non-covalent binding of the invariant light chain, β_2m, which is essential for cell surface expression. This region is also involved in binding to CD8[+] T cells. That this can occur with HLA-G is supported by the observation of Sanders *et al.* (1991) who transfected HLA-G into the HLA-null lymphoblastoid cell line LCL 721.221. They noted that these HLA-G transfectants were adherent to homodimeric CD8 transfected into COS7 cells with a level of binding similar to that occurring between similarly constructed HLA-A2 transfectants and CD8 transfectants. Immunoprecipitation studies have confirmed that HLA-G is indeed associated with β_2m and, therefore, can appear on the cell surface (Kovats *et al.* 1990). The α1 and α2 domains take part in the formation of the parallel α-helices between which foreign or self peptides are bound. In addition, classical class I HLA sequences show conservation of ten amino acids in the α1 and α2 domains which have side chains pointing into the antigen-binding groove and which are thought to serve as scaffolding for peptide binding and presentation to the T-cell receptor (Schmidt and Orr 1993). Nine of these ten amino acids are present in HLA-G which suggests that HLA-G would be able to bind peptides and present these peptides to T-cells. However, there is presently no documented evidence that HLA-G can actually take part in class I antigen-restricted cytotoxicity by CD8[+] T cells.

The work of Kovats *et al.* (1990) indicates that the HLA-G protein can occur in at least five isoforms with diverse molecular masses and isoelectric points. The 37 kDa acidic isoform appears to be secreted and not expressed on the cell membrane of trophoblast cells because it can be immunoprecipitated from culture supernatant, but cannot be identified by [^{125}I]lactoperoxidase surface labelling. Interestingly, the isoforms from a total of 13 individuals of unknown ethnic background show no variation, indicating that the HLA-G protein is not unduly polymorphic. Thus, in spite of variations detected at the genetic level, these do not affect the expressed HLA-G protein. This is in contrast to the highly polymorphic molecules encoded by the classical HLA-A,B,C loci. It will be of interest to look at protein isoforms from larger numbers of people of different ethnic backgrounds in view of the recent findings of van der Ven and Ober (1994).

Ishitani and Geraghty (1992) have also detected at least three different forms of HLA-G transcripts resulting from differential splicing. The largest mRNA (HLA-G1) is essentially similar to that which has been previously characterised, encoding a leader sequence, three external domains, a transmembrane region and a cytoplasmic tail. Of the two smaller transcripts, one (HLA-G2) excludes exon 3, thereby resulting in a predicted protein sequence with the α1 and α3 domains joined and the introduction of an asparagine residue at the point of joining which is not present in the HLA-G1. The third transcript (HLA-G3) does not contain exons 3 and 4, so the α1 domain is spliced directly to the transmembrane sequence. All three mRNA are expressed in placental tissue and trophoblast cell lines, and are translated into proteins in HLA-G transfectants. Because of the absence of the α3 domain, HLA-G3 protein does not react with Mab W6/32 but, surprisingly, the protein from HLA-G2 is also unreactive. Thus this Mab, which is the most frequently used antibody for studies on HLA expression by trophoblast, would not be able to detect the HLA-G2 and -G3 variants of this protein. Interestingly, the two external domains of the HLA-G2 protein bear a striking resemblance to the two external domains of an HLA class II protein, and the authors speculated that a non-polymorphic HLA-G2 homodimer could act as a surrogate class II molecule on trophoblast.

In addition to these three HLA-G isoforms, Geraghty's laboratory recently described two soluble variants of this molecule (Fujii *et al.* 1994). The unusual feature of these variants is that they contain a unique 21 amino acid carboxyl terminus and are generated by the retention of intron 4 with the presence of a stop codon which prevents readthrough into the transmembrane-encoding exon 5 instead of the more usual mechanism of splicing out exon 5. It was postulated that these soluble HLA-G molecules may serve to anergise alloreactive maternal T cells or inactivate NK cells at the implantation site. Further support that HLA-G may be shed from the cell surface is provided by the recent observation that the transporter protein, TAP1, which is required for the assembly of the HLA class I molecule, is expressed with high intensity by EVT while the class I antigen itself is not correspondingly elevated in these cells (Clover *et al.* 1995).

Kirszenbaum *et al.* (1994) have described another alternatively spliced form of HLA-G in trophoblast which is lacking in exon 4 and thus excludes the α3 domain in the deduced protein sequence. The resultant splicing of the α2 domain directly with the transmembrane region would again be expected to induce conformational changes in the cell surface protein. Thus, several different isoforms of HLA-G with potentially different functional attributes appear to be expressed by trophoblast. Their functions remain to be elucidated.

Pattern of tissue expression of HLA-G

Because of the lack of a specific HLA-G antibody, studies on the tissue distribution of this antigen are based on detection of mRNA. Results are rather confusing. Using sensitive PCR techniques, low levels of HLA-G mRNA have been reported in fetal eye, fetal thymus (Shukla *et al.* 1990), fetal liver (Houlihan *et al.* 1992), circulating T and B cells (Kirszenbaum *et al.* 1994) and adult skin biopsies (Ulbrecht *et al.* 1994). In contrast, Wei and Orr (1990), using an RNase protection assay, could not demonstrate HLA-G mRNA in resting T cells, PHA-transformed T cell blasts, fetal thymus, adult skin or liver, while abundant mRNA was present in placental tissues. The picture that emerges from these studies is that HLA-G transcripts are very difficult to demonstrate in non-trophoblast tissues except by highly sensitive detection systems.

We have recently succeeded in generating an HLA-G-specific antibody by immunising HLA-A2/β_2m double transgenic mice with HLA-G transfected into mouse Ltk⁻ cells (Chumbley *et al.* 1994a). The reactivity of this antibody on isolated first trimester extravillous trophoblast cells and on HLA-G transfectants is shown in Fig. 6.3. This antibody has permitted us to test a variety of fetal organs including those where HLA-G mRNA is reported to be present. HLA-G protein is not detectable in any of these tissues by immunohistology, including the fetal thymus. Only extravillous trophoblast (cytotrophoblast cell columns, interstitial trophoblast, placental bed giant cells) and not villous trophoblast (cytotrophoblast, syncytiotrophoblast) is stained by this antibody. In an earlier study, we have noted that mesenchymal cells of the chorionic villous core hybridised with an HLA-G-specific oligonucleotide (Chumbley *et al.* 1993), and others using an antisense probe have reported a similar finding (Yelavarthi *et al.* 1991). Using our antibody, however, HLA-G protein is again not detected in chorionic villous mesenchyme in spite of the presence of HLA-G mRNA.

Thus, it is clear that the presence of HLA-G transcripts does not guarantee that the corresponding protein is made. This is often found with non-classical class I molecules, possibly because of inefficient mRNA splicing mechanisms (Stroynowski and Lindahl 1994). However, it may be that the level of HLA-G expression in these other organs is below the level of detection by immunohistology, or that our antibody fails to recognise all the isoforms expressed (though being a polyclonal antiserum it is hoped that it would). Nevertheless, even if low levels of HLA-G protein were to be expressed by some other tissues, the overall conclusion still remains that this antigen is expressed significantly only by extravillous trophoblast. This suggests a tissue-specific function for the molecule. We have observed that trophoblast cells from an invasive complete hydatidiform mole also express HLA-G, which indicates that the paternal genome makes a contribution to the expression of this antigen because complete moles are androgenetic (Chapter 4).

Functions of HLA-G

The functions of HLA-G are not known and any discussion of this aspect of the antigen must be regarded as purely speculative (Le Bouteiller 1994; Parham 1995). Indeed, there are immunologists who believe that non-classical class I genes have no functions and are merely vestigial molecules left behind during

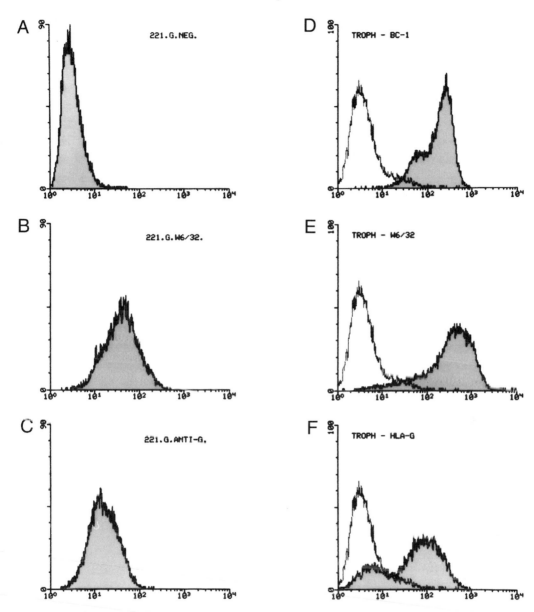

Fig. 6.3. Flow cytometric analysis of HLA-G transfectants stained with control mouse serum (**A**), Mab W6/32 (**B**) and HLA-G antibody (**C**), and of normal trophoblast stained with Mab BC-1 (reactive against extravillous trophoblast) (**D**), Mab W6/32 (**E**) and HLA-G antibody (**F**). In **C** and **F** it is apparent that the HLA-G antibody is staining HLA-G transfectants and the great majority of BC-1[+] and W6/32[+] trophoblast cells.

evolution. Even their restricted tissue distribution can be perceived as reflecting their declining functional importance. According to Klein and O'hUigin (1994), non-classical MHC genes are those kept in limbo while only a few genes of the set (the classical MHC genes) which best satisfy the environmental demands of that period are chosen to be functional. The selection of a small number of functional loci and their subsequent diversification by polymorphic variation is probably the optimal method to ensure variability. This system will guard against too much variation at the level of the individual, which would reduce the size of the T cell repertoire to dangerously low levels. Some of these non-classical genes in limbo may assume auxiliary functions. The evocative description of non-classical genes as 'rotting hulks in an evolutionary junkyard' is an allusion to the similarity of these genes to the retired warships from Lord Nelson's fleet which became prisons or hospitals once they had outlived their original purpose (Parham 1994a).

HLA-G may be an example of such a gene. Like other non-classical class I genes, HLA-G could either have evolved from a gene which was previously functional but has since been replaced by other newer genes, or is generated *de novo*. Either of these mechanisms implies that HLA-G may be a more recent invention than classical class I genes. Mutations acquired at appropriate promoter regions could then lead to a restricted tissue distribution in trophoblast. Such exile 'to obscurer corners of the body' (Parham 1994a) is frequently a reflection of the declining functional importance of a gene but, in the case of HLA-G, it could have assumed a new-found function in trophoblast which is related to reproduction. What this function is remains to be determined. Like other non-classical class I molecules, HLA-G is relatively non-polymorphic so the diversity of antigens it can present is likely to be limited. It is possible that HLA-G may have a specialised function analogous to the murine non-classical class I molecule, H-2M3, which preferentially binds to and presents peptides that have a formylated methionine (fMet) amino acid at the N terminus, adapting it to present N-terminal peptides from bacterial proteins such as *Listeria monocytogenes* (Hedrick 1992). In an analysis of the soluble form of the murine non-classical MHC Qa-2 antigen, Joyce *et al.* (1994) deduced that this molecule can bind at least 200 different naturally processed nonamer self-peptides. This implies that there is no restriction in peptide presentation by this non-classical MHC molecule, and that it can function just as effectively as classical class I molecules (Stroynowski and Lindahl 1994).

In the case of HLA-G, the peptides bound could be derived from intracellular stress-induced proteins which reflect the state of health of the cell, thereby providing a mechanism for surveillance by lymphocytes. There is evidence that the highly conserved family of heat-shock proteins (hsp) can function in a similar way as peptide-presenting molecules to primitive γδ T cells (O'Brien and Born 1991; Haas 1993). An evolutionary link between hsp and MHC is suggested by observations of structural similarities between the peptide-binding domains of hsp 70 and human MHC molecules (Rippmann *et al.* 1991).

Odum *et al.* (1991) reported that homotypic adhesion of HLA-G transfectants was inhibited by an antibody specific to HLA-G, indicating that this class I antigen may function as an intercellular adhesion molecule. As mentioned earlier, Sanders *et al.* (1991) observed that HLA-G transfectants were adherent to CD8+ transfectants. Since CD8 is a co-receptor with the T cell receptor for interaction with MHC and peptide, it was postulated that HLA-G could serve as a recognition molecule for CD8+ suppressor T cells and, thus, downregulate the immune response to trophoblast. We have found that T cells in decidua, like similar cells in other mucosal surfaces, are curiously unresponsive to allogeneic signals (Chapter 8). Wei and Orr (1990) have proposed a contrasting hypothesis that HLA-G may function as the MHC restricting element for the recognition of virally infected trophoblast by CD8+ cytotoxic T cells. Our recent observation that HLA-G protein is not demonstrable in fetal thymus would seem to preclude this molecule from influencing the selection of the αβ T cell repertoire and hence any active role in T cell recognition.

Our own hypothesis is that HLA-G interacts not with T cells but with the unusual population of decidual NK cells and that this interaction will result in either positive or negative signals which regulate trophoblast behaviour during implantation (King and Loke 1991; Loke and King 1991; Loke *et al.* 1993). This will be discussed in more detail in Chapter 8. Interestingly, we have found that a proportion of decidual NK cells (≈20%) express low levels of CD8 (unpublished). Some peripheral blood NK cells are known to express CD8α at a low level (Norment and Littman 1988).

Only human trophoblast appears to express HLA-G. This species restriction argues against this molecule having a fundamental role in mammalian reproduction. In some other species, such as the rat (Billington and Burrows 1986) and the horse (Donaldson *et al.* 1994), paternally derived class I antigens are present, indicating a completely different system of immune regulation during reproduction in these species. However, from the way non-classical class I genes are thought to have evolved, it is not surprising to find a distinct lack of correspondence between different species (Parham 1994a, b). Therefore, the absence of an HLA-G orthologue in other species does not invalidate the proposal that this antigen has a role to play in human reproduction. This is another instance where the human reproductive process is not directly comparable to that of other animals. It is possible that, in other species, amino acid substitutions in relevant conserved positions in another class I antigen could lead to the formation of a molecule with similar functional attributes to that offered by HLA-G, so that it may not be necessary for all species to have a close homologue of HLA-G. Geraghty has observed that HLA-G occurs in several isoforms due to differential splicing (Ishitani and Geraghty 1992; Fujii *et al.* 1994). It would be reasonable to suggest that alternative splicing of the primary transcript could also be a mechanism used to provide new forms of this molecule, and that these new forms will then be selected by evolutionary forces unique to individual species.

A principle that seems to be emerging from studies of non-polymorphic class I genes is that they are not always represented in all mammalian species even when they appear to be highly useful (Parham 1994c). For example, the ability of CD1b molecules to present mycolic acids to T cells in defence against mycobacteria is seen in humans and not in mice (Beckman *et al.* 1994). Conversely, H-2M3 which binds and presents peptides that have a formylated methionine at the amino terminus derived from bacterial proteins is a murine attribute not found in humans. In contrast to the above two examples, the monomorphic class I molecule (FcRn) which works as an Fc receptor for the transmission of IgG from mother to young is found in both mouse intestine and human placenta (Burmeister *et al.* 1994; Story *et al.* 1994). These examples also illustrate the functional diversity of the remarkably versatile class I molecule, and it is possible that additional roles will be discovered in the future (Ravetch and Margulies 1994).

Now that appropriate HLA-G probes are available, a valid approach to evaluate the function of this antigen is to look for any variations in its expression in pathological pregnancies. Colbern *et al.* (1994) have attempted to do this by correlating the mRNA level of HLA-G expression with pre-eclampsia. Although they did observe a lower level of HLA-G in chorionic tissue from pre-eclamptic term placentae compared with that from normal pregnancies, normalisation to mRNA for cytokeratin revealed that this was due to a smaller number of trophoblast cells present in pre-eclamptic placentae. Thus, there seemed to be no difference in HLA-G expression per trophoblast cell between normal and pre-eclamptic pregnancies. Examining the placenta at term is too late to detect events which occur early in gestation, such as aberrant trophoblast migration which is thought to be the basic pathology in pre-eclampsia (Chapter 11). Also, any alterations that might occur in HLA-G expression are unlikely to be detected by gross quantitative estimations of levels. The variations will be more subtle, such as the HLA-G gene mutations described by van der Ven *et al.* (1994) in African-American neonates with idiopathic intrauterine growth retardation.

The New World primate, the cotton-top tamarin (*Saguinus oedipus*), may give some insight into the possible nature of our ancestral HLA-G gene. The expressed MHC class I genes of this species show only limited polymorphism and their sequences are more similar to human HLA-G than to HLA-A,B,C (Watkins *et al.* 1990, 1991). Phylogenetic analyses suggest that the last common ancestor of humans and tamarins probably had both HLA-G and HLA-A,B,C so the two genes had already diverged by this stage of evolution, and it is from this ancestral G-homologue that the tamarin class I genes have evolved. Since tamarins can mount a CD8 T cell cytotoxic response, it must be assumed that their class I antigens can function in a similar way to human classical class I molecules. Two scenarios are possible during the evolution of these genes. The ancestral G-homologue was non-functional with respect to T cell presentation and only acquired functionality in the tamarin. Alternatively, the ancestral G was once functional and polymorphic, but these attributes were lost in humans when the molecule became adapted for use in trophoblast. The benefit of having a relatively neutral HLA class I molecule which does not readily trigger allorecognition at the feto-maternal interface could provide the required evolutionary pressures to select for the formation of such an antigen.

HLA-C

Immunoprecipitation with Mab W6/32 and SDS-PAGE analysis of trophoblast metabolically labelled proteins reveal two class I heavy chains of 39 kDa and 45 kDa in association with β_2m (Fig. 6.4) (Grabowska *et al.* 1990a). Others have observed a similar finding in the JEG-3 choriocarcinoma cell line (DeWit *et al.* 1990), so this appears not to be the result of the presence of contaminating non-trophoblast cells. The smaller molecule is HLA-G, but the nature of the larger one is still uncertain. A nucleotide sequence now known to be a subtype of Cw4 has been identified in the BeWo choriocarcinoma cell line (Ellis *et al.* 1989; Zemmour and Parham 1992), and we ourselves have obtained supporting evidence by staining trophoblast cells with HLA-C-specific antibodies (unpublished). Trophoblast cells, therefore, appear to express at least two HLA class I antigens: the non-classical HLA-G and the classical HLA-C. Interestingly, only the smaller molecule is expressed on the cell surface as shown by ^{125}I surface labelling (unpublished). Recent studies in our laboratory using HLA-C-specific antibodies revealed that the HLA-C antigen on the surface of trophoblast cells is mainly in the form of free heavy chains which would be unreactive with Mab W6/32 (unpublished). Thus, human first trimester trophoblast appears to express β_2m-associated HLA-G and non-β_2m-associated HLA-C heavy chains on its surface. Any discussion on the immunology of trophoblast must take these observations into account (Chapter 8).

For a classical class I gene the HLA-C locus is rather unusual. Zemmour and Parham (1992) have analysed the polymorphism and expression of this class I

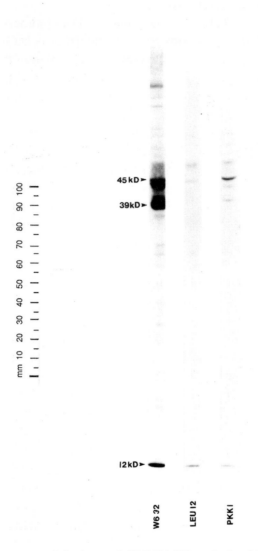

Fig. 6.4. Immunoprecipitation and SDS-PAGE analysis of [^{35}S]methionine metabolically labelled first trimester trophoblast cells with Mab W6/32. Heavy chains of 45 kDa and 39 kDa are identified together with a 12 kDa band which represents β_2m. Leu-12 and PKK1 are negative control Mabs.

molecule. They found that the total polymorphic positions of the HLA-C locus are comparable to that of HLA-B, but if just the α1 and α2 domains are analysed, then there is significantly less polymorphism in HLA-C than in either HLA-A or HLA-B. This difference is even more obvious if only the functional positions of the antigen recognition sites are considered. It seems, therefore, that HLA-C has less variation at the antigen binding site and more variation elsewhere. In addition, the amino acid residues at the antigen recognition site of HLA-C are mainly non-synonymous substitutions whereas synonymous substitutions predominate elsewhere, but the frequency of both types of substitutions at functional positions in HLA-C is about half that of HLA-B. The surface expression of HLA-C is about 10% of HLA-A or HLA-B, although the levels of mRNA and heavy chain proteins are the same. This suggests there could be inefficient assembly of this molecule, possibly due to failure to bind peptides, lack of availability of peptides or weak interaction with β_2m. Falk *et al.* (1993) have reported that HLA-C molecules are associated with peptides and, furthermore, the origin and processing of these peptides appear to be the same as for HLA-A or -B. Perhaps HLA-C can bind only to a restricted set of peptides and this could be a limiting factor for its surface expression. Thus, the properties of HLA-C would seem to put it half-way between a classical and a non-classical class I molecule.

Because of its low surface expression and relative lack of diversity, the question arises as to whether HLA-C is declining in functional efficiency or is a more recently formed locus that is still undergoing improvement (Zemmour and Parham 1992). Güssow *et al.* (1987) are of the opinion that HLA-C 'may be dispensable for proper functioning of the immune system'. However, recent observations that HLA-C may be an important ligand that determines resistance to lysis by NK cells indicate that this class I molecule may have a function (Chapter 8). Its low surface expression and presentation of a small selection of peptides are well suited for this role because any disturbance in the antigen processing machinery occurring inside the cell will be signalled to the outside by HLA-C. This would provide a sensitive monitoring system for NK cells to kill target cells infected with pathogens trying to evade the classical MHC-restricted host immune response by disrupting antigenic presentation by HLA-A or -B. Thus, it is too narrow to view HLA class I antigens solely in terms of their interaction with T cells. That some of these antigens can be recognised by NK cells has added a whole new dimension to our understanding of these molecules.

Regulation of MHC class I gene expression by trophoblast

In an earlier section of this chapter, three populations of trophoblast are described according to HLA class I expression: (1) villous syncytiotrophoblast (mRNA⁻, protein⁻), (2) villous cytotrophoblast (mRNA⁺, protein⁻), (3) extravillous trophoblast (mRNA⁺, protein⁺). This indicates that there is transcriptional and post-transcriptional regulation of this antigen in trophoblast (Le Bouteiller 1994). How this is achieved is not clear. When HLA-A or HLA-B α-chain genes were transfected into the MHC-negative JAR choriocarcinoma cell line, Boucrat *et al.* (1991) observed the expression of the exogenous product in association with endogenous β_2m after transfection, but the endogenous class I gene was not activated. These results indicate that those factors responsible for the extinction of endogenous class I genes in JAR do not affect similar transfected genes and are, therefore, consistent with the concept of *cis*-acting suppressive mechanisms, perhaps mediated through DNA methylation of appropriate areas of class I genes, such as CpG islands. Experiments using methylation-sensitive rare cutter enzymes have shown that endogenous class I genes are indeed methylated in the JAR cell line and *in vitro* treatment of these cells with the 5-azacytidine demethylating agent will induce re-expression of these genes (Le Bouteiller *et al.* 1991), so this could be an important mechanism involved in the control of class I gene expression in trophoblast.

Another mechanism for transcriptional regulation of class I genes operates through a complex array of nuclear DNA-binding proteins that specifically recognise several *cis*-acting regulatory elements in their promoter region. Some of the most studied are the enhancer A DNA-binding proteins of the KBF1/NF-κB/Rel family. Members of this family of proteins are present in first trimester human cytotrophoblast which transcribes class I antigens but not in syncytiotrophoblast which does not (Boucrat *et al.* 1993). The enhancer region of HLA-G shows conservation of 23 bp of the 29 bp HLA-A enhancer A region (Schmidt and Orr 1993), so the above KBF1/Rel family of DNA-binding proteins which bind to enhancer A may well have a role to play in the regulation of HLA-G expression. Furthermore, the DNA sequences associated with the TATA and CCAAT boxes of the promoter elements located 5′ to the coding sequences of the classical class I MHC genes are also conserved in HLA-G. These elements are the binding sites for RNA polymerase and are associated with the initiation of transcription. In contrast, the majority of the 30 bp long interferon response element (IRE) which has been demonstrated in all classical class I genes (Singer and Maguire 1990) is deleted from the HLA-G 5′ flanking sequence (Schmidt and Orr 1993). This implies that HLA-G will be insusceptible to the regulatory influence of these cytokines. However, we (Grabowska *et al.* 1990b) and others (Feinman *et al.* 1987) have observed that IFN-γ increases the surface expression of class I antigens on human trophoblast *in vitro*, albeit only to a small degree of approximately two-fold (Fig. 6.5) and Northern blotting has shown an increase in mRNA (Fig. 6.6).

IFN-α, on the other hand, had no effect on trophoblast class I expression (Chumbley *et al.* 1991). Furthermore, IFN-γ but not IFN-α was shown to protect first trimester trophoblast and JEG-3 choriocarcinoma cells from lysis by decidual effector cells, which is thought to be due to upregulation of surface class I

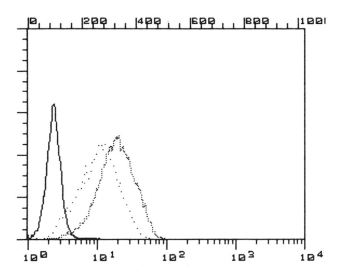

Fig. 6.5. Histogram showing the relative immunofluorescence of trophoblast cells labelled with Mab W6/32 following culture with (.........) and without (. . . . .) IFN-γ. Control (——).

antigens (King and Loke 1993). In the above studies the Mab used to identify class I expression was W6/32, which is directed at the monomorphic part of all class I molecules, and the probe was a full-length class I cDNA so it cannot be certain which trophoblast HLA class I molecule is specifically upregulated, as first trimester trophoblast is thought to express HLA-G and HLA-C. If HLA-G is indeed increased, then perhaps the small residual portion of IRE adjacent to the HLA-G enhancer A region is sufficient for binding of IFN-γ or HLA-G may have its own separate and as yet unidentified IREs. Alternatively, IFN-γ may not affect HLA-G transcription at all but merely acts to stabilise the HLA-G mRNA. Trophoblast cells do express IFN-γ receptors so they are potentially able to respond to this cytokine (Peyman and Hammond 1992).

Transgenic mice have provided useful tools for the study of the regulation of class I expression in trophoblast, particularly that of HLA-G. The first report was that of transgenic mice with HLA-B27 inserts where no expression of HLA-B transcripts was detected in any of the transgenic trophoblast populations (i.e. spongiotrophoblast, labyrinthine trophoblast and giant cells), while transcripts were present in the placental stromal cells and in the embryo (Oudejans *et al.* 1989). This suggests that the regulatory mechanisms controlling MHC expression in trophoblast are likely to be different from those operating in developing embryonic cells and these trophoblast control mechanisms appear to be conserved across species barriers. Interestingly, the cells of the yolk sac portion of the murine placenta, which is derived from primitive endoderm, do

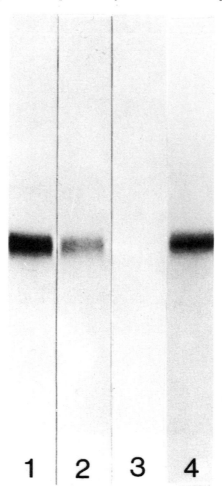

Fig. 6.6. Autoradiogram of a Northern blot probed with the class I HLA-specific cDNA, pWTCAII. The lanes show hybridisation of total RNA from: 1) trophoblast cells cultured for 3 days with 1000 units/ml IFN-γ; 2) trophoblast cells cultured for 3 days without IFN-γ; 3) mouse 3T3 fibroblasts; 4) EBV-transformed human B lymphocytes (WT49).

contain HLA-B27 mRNA so the absence of HLA-B transcripts is confined only to placental cells of the trophectoderm lineage. In humans, the yolk sac placenta is rudimentary.

   The presence of factors within murine extraembryonic tissues which can regulate human genes in a tissue-specific manner raises the hope that HLA-G transgenic mice could provide important insights into how the expression of this gene could be regulated in humans. Such experiments were conducted by Schmidt *et al.* (1993) using two HLA-G genomic fragments of 5.7 and 6.0 kb in length which included the entire HLA-G coding region, 1 kb of the 3′ flanking sequence and either 1.1 or 1.4 kb of the 5′ flanking sequence. Their results show that the 5′ upstream regions of HLA-G are largely responsible for the expression of this gene *in vivo*. However, while all the 5.7 kb HLA-G transgenic lines showed transgene expression in tissues such as thymus, testicle and brain, only extremely low levels of expression were seen in extraembryonic tissues. Since this 5.7 kb HLA-G fragment includes the enhancer A element known to be critical for tissue-specific expression of other human and murine class I genes, it seems that this fragment is insufficient to direct extraembryonic expression of HLA-G. In contrast, the 6.0 kb transgenic lines showed high levels of extraembryonic HLA-G expression which indicates that the extra 250 bp region present in the 6.0 kb HLA-G fragment provides the critical functional element for HLA-G expression in this tissue. This 250 bp region is located 1.1 kb upstream of the transcription start site, which is further upstream than any of the previously documented HLA class I regulatory elements. An additional finding of interest was that some of the HLA-G transgenic embryos were gestated successfully in non-transgenic mothers, which raises the question of why the recipient did not respond to this xenogeneic molecule (Yelavarthi *et al.* 1993). As yet, there is no clear evidence the HLA-G protein is made in these transgenic animals.

The most recent publication by Horuzsko *et al.* (1994) reported that transcription of HLA-G transgene begins at about day 7.5 post coitus. This is about 48 hours after implantation of the embryo, which takes place at 5.5 days post coitus in mice. Taken in conjunction with the data of Schmidt *et al.* (1993) that HLA-G transgene transcripts are detected at day 16.5 post coitus, it would appear that HLA-G transcription occurs almost continuously during development in HLA-G transgenic mice from early implantation up to term (day 19 post coitus). This is at variance with what is known in humans where HLA-G expression is very much reduced in third trimester trophoblast compared with first trimester (Kovats *et al.* 1990; Wei and Orr 1990). Therefore, until more information is available as to the exact developmental stages when HLA-G is expressed in both human and transgenic trophoblast, it is slightly premature to conclude that transgenic animals are appropriate experimental models for the study of HLA-G regulation in humans.

7

Uterine mucosal leucocytes

Leucocyte populations

Like other mucosal surfaces the uterus must be able to respond to antigenic challenge. Three different types of foreign antigen are encountered by the uterine mucosa: pathogenic organisms, seminal plasma including spermatozoa and trophoblast. Although the immune response to pathogens is likely to be similar to that encountered at other mucosal sites such as the respiratory tract or the gut, the uterine mucosa is different in undergoing cyclical proliferation and shedding under the control of sex hormones. Despite the loss of the stratum functionalis and mucosal integrity at menstruation, there is no diminution in the capacity of the endometrium to respond to pathogens at this stage of the cycle. This is presumably because the stratum basalis always remains as a stable component. Spermatozoa and seminal plasma do not appear to initiate any immune or inflammatory response in the human endometrium. This is perhaps surprising as, although spermatozoa do not express HLA antigens, seminal fluid does contain potentially immunogenic leucocytes. Usually it would seem that the surface epithelium provides an adequate barrier which may actually enhance the motility and capacitance of spermatozoa as they move past. Trophoblast provides a different sort of antigenic challenge since, in humans, breaching of the surface epithelium and infiltration into the decidual stroma and spiral arteries is essential for successful implantation. It might be expected that this invasion of semi-allogeneic cells into a host tissue will be reflected in the types of leucocytes present.

The advent of immunohistology meant that leucocyte populations present in tissues *in vivo* could be analysed using antibodies directed at appropriate markers. Localisation of the various leucocyte populations to the different compartments of the endometrium is now possible. Numerous immunohistological studies of both pregnant and non-pregnant endometrium have been performed (Kamat and

102

Table 7.1. *Leucocytes in uterine mucosa*

	Non-pregnant endometrium		Early decidua	
	Proliferative	Secretory	Basalis (trophoblast+)	Parietalis (trophoblast−)
Granulocytes				
Neutrophils	−	−/+	−/+	−
Eosinophils	−	−	−	−
Basophils	−	−	−	−
Lymphocytes				
B cells	−(+)	−(+)	−(+)	−(+)
T cells	+	+	+	+
NK cells (LGL)	+	+++	+++++	+++
Macrophages	+	+	+++	+

Isaacson 1987; Bulmer *et al.* 1988b, 1991; Marshall and Jones 1988; King *et al.* 1989b; Starkey *et al.* 1991) and a summary of the main findings is shown in Table 7.1 and Fig. 7.1 (between pp. 34 and 35). It should be noted that there are no quantitative studies comparing leucocytes in the decidua basalis (where trophoblast is present) with those in decidua parietalis (where trophoblast is absent). This is an important omission as immunohistology is the best method available to compare leucocyte populations in these two different parts of the decidua.

Although immunohistology using serial sections can give much information on phenotype of cells *in vivo*, a detailed phenotypic profile of uterine leucocytes requires the isolation of these cells from the tissues and analysis by dual immunofluorescence and flow cytometry (Chapter 5). This is necessary as double staining for two surface markers on leucocytes by immunohistology is unreliable. However, there are problems using isolated cells. Firstly, the method of extraction may damage surface antigens, particularly if enzymes are used (Ritson and Bulmer 1987a; Garcia *et al.* 1987). Secondly, it is difficult to rule out completely the presence of contaminating cells from maternal blood in the decidual leucocyte preparations. Careful washing of samples to remove all blood is essential. Routine quantification of the number of B cells present can give an indication of the degree of maternal blood contamination as these cells are scarce in the uterine mucosa. The percentage of B cells should be under 5%. Thirdly, the presence of cell debris, dead cells and macrophages may make analysis difficult, particularly as tissue cells generally exhibit much autofluorescence. Correct 'gating' out of dead cells and debris and use of Fab$'_2$ fragments as secondary reagents are critical for good analysis by flow cytometry.

T and B cells

Only a few B cells are present and these are confined to the lymphoid aggregates found in the basal layer of the endometrium throughout the menstrual cycle and during pregnancy. In humans, the uterus is normally sterile and true germinal centres and plasma cells are only found in uterine infections (More 1987). The uterus can therefore respond to pathogenic organisms in a similar manner to other mucosal sites. It is worth stressing that B cells are virtually absent from the implantation site in normal pregnancy making it unlikely that there is local anti-trophoblast antibody production.

T cells (defined by expression of CD3) are present in the uterine mucosa in both non-pregnant endometrium and decidua. They are found in three sites: basal lymphoid aggregates, scattered throughout the stroma, and in an intraepithelial location (Fig. 7.1). This distribution is reminiscent of other mucosal sites such as the bronchus and intestine. The numbers of CD3$^+$ T cells remain constant throughout the menstrual cycle and during early pregnancy. Both immunohistology and flow cytometric analysis have revealed that in early decidua CD3$^+$ cells account for about 10% of leucocytes although the proportion obtained varies between samples from 5% to 25% (Starkey *et al.* 1988; King *et al.* 1989b, 1991; K. Nishikawa *et al.* 1991) (Fig. 7.2C).

Although there have been some contradictory reports (Mincheva-Nilsson *et al.* 1992, 1994), it is now agreed that the majority of decidual CD3$^+$ cells express the αβ T cell receptor (TCR) with only very few γδ T cells present (Yeh *et al.* 1990; Chernyshov *et al.* 1993; Morii *et al.* 1993). A very small proportion (<5%) of decidual lymphocytes co-express CD56 and CD3 (Fig. 7.2C). These T cells have low CD56 expression and may represent the small γδ decidual T cell population. The relative proportions of αβ and γδ T cells are similar to those in blood, but analysis of decidual γδ T cell clones has

Fig. 7.2. Two-colour flow cytometric analysis of decidual lymphocytes. Freshly isolated decidual mononuclear cells were double-labelled with various antibodies to leucocyte differentiation antigens, conjugated to fluorescein isothiocyanate (FITC, horizontal axis) or phycoerythrin (PE, vertical axis), and analysed by flow cytometry. **A**. Simultest IgG$_{2a}$ (PE)/IgG$_1$ (FITC) negative control. **B**. CD14 (PE) versus CD45 (FITC). Ninety-four per cent of cells observed are leucocytes as shown by CD45 (leucocyte common antigen) staining. Seven per cent of cells are macrophages (CD14$^+$ and CD45$^+$). **C**. CD56 (PE) versus CD3 (FITC). Twenty four per cent of cells are CD3$^+$ T cells, although there is a small population (~4% of total cells) which are both CD3$^+$ and CD56^{dim+}. **D**. CD8 (PE) versus CD4 (FITC). Twenty-four per cent of total cells are CD8$^+$ and 16% are CD4$^+$. **E**. CD56 (PE) versus CD8 (FITC). Although a total of 23% of cells are CD8$^+$, 14% of total cells are double labelled for CD56$^+$ and CD8^{dim} (approximately 25% of total NK cells) and therefore only 9% of cells (CD8^{bright} CD56$^-$) are cytotoxic T cells. **F**. CD56 (PE) versus CD4 (FITC). Fifteen per cent of cells are CD4$^+$ and none of these are CD56$^+$.

revealed that fewer clones from decidua parietalis are V$\gamma9^+$/V$\delta2^+$ (42%) as compared with blood (72%), and a higher proportion are V$\delta1^+$ (Christmas *et al.* 1993). TCR expression by $\gamma\delta$ clones from decidua parietalis was found to be heterogeneous with seven receptor types. However, clones from decidua basalis were all V$\gamma9^+$/V$\delta1^+$. The reason for different $\gamma\delta$ TCR receptor usage in different areas of the decidua is unclear. In mice, percentages of $\gamma\delta$ T cells

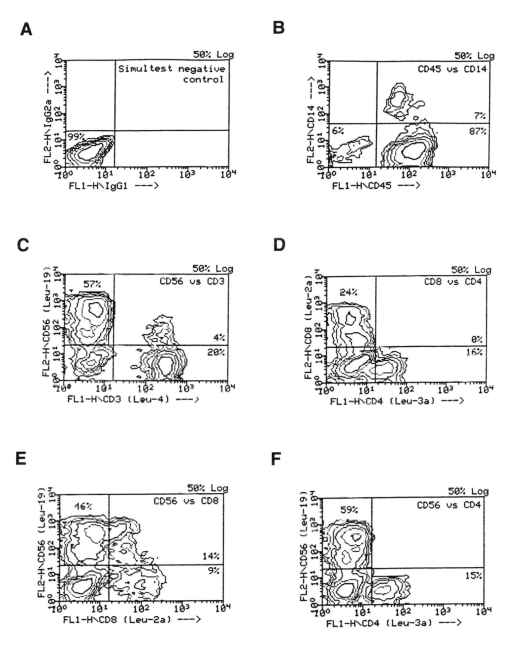

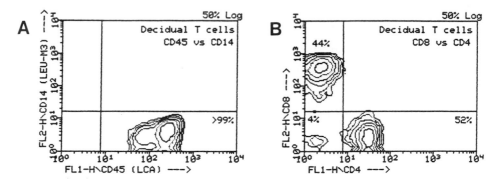

Fig. 7.3. Two-colour flow cytometric analysis of decidual T cells. T cells were isolated from a preparation of decidual mononuclear cells by panning over an anti-CD3 coated flask. **A.** CD14 (PE) versus CD45 (FITC). More than 99% of the cells obtained are CD45[+] CD14[-], indicating there is no macrophage contamination. **B.** CD8 (PE) versus CD4 (FITC). Forty-four per cent of cells are CD8[+] and 52% are CD4[+], indicating a CD4 : CD8 ratio of 1.2 : 1.

are higher at the feto-maternal interface compared with the spleen (Heyborne *et al.* 1992). These γδ T cells increase in numbers up to 100-fold during pregnancy when IL-2R becomes expressed. At least six distinct γδ receptor types were expressed, with Vγ1/Vγ6 being the predominant TCR (Heyborne *et al.* 1994). The exact localisation of these murine γδ T cells in the decidua in relation to the trophoblast is not clear.

Interesting, but unexplained, differences have been noted between CD3[+] cells circulating in blood and CD3[+] cells in decidua. There is apparently downregulation of the CD3-TCR in decidua as assessed by comparison of mean fluorescence intensity of blood and decidual cells (Chernyshov *et al.* 1993; Morii *et al.* 1993). The CD8 : CD4 ratio of isolated CD3[+] cells is almost equal (Fig. 7.3), but intraepithelial T cells are all CD8[+], as in the gut (Pace *et al.* 1991). The apparent CD8 : CD4 ratio of ~3 : 1 found by immunohistology (Bulmer *et al.* 1988b; Klentzeris *et al.* 1994) is due to weak expression of CD8 by a few CD56 cells (Chernyshov *et al.* 1993) (Fig. 7.2E).

There is negligible expression of IL-2Rα or IL-2Rβ on decidual T cells (Saito *et al.* 1992). Activation markers are also expressed by decidual T cells, notably CD69, and about 50% appear to be HLA-DR[+] (Saito *et al.* 1992). CD69 is a type II membrane glycoprotein with a lectin domain which is the earliest inducible cell surface glycoprotein acquired during T lymphocyte activation by a wide variety of stimuli (Borrego *et al.* 1993; Santis *et al.* 1994). Thymocytes also begin to express CD69 during T cell maturation (Jung *et al.* 1990). T lymphocytes in the inflammatory infiltrates *in vivo* of several diseases such as rheumatoid arthritis are also CD69[+] (Laffón *et al.* 1991). Whether the appearance of CD69 on decidual T cells is associated with interaction with putative carbohydrate ligands on target cells or whether CD69 is involved in migration and localisation to this specialised tissue compartment is unknown. The majority of decidual T cells also express the CD45RO antigen, indicating they are memory or activated T cells (Saito *et al.* 1994*b*).

All these surface phenotypic characteristics of decidual T cells suggest that they are activated and resemble pulmonary lymphocytes, lymphocytes from the synovial fluid in rheumatoid arthritis and gut lymphocytes in coeliac disease (Laffón *et al.* 1991; Halstensen and Brandtzaeg 1994; Marathias *et al.* 1994). Alternative explanations are that this phenotypic profile is a reflection of the maturity of these cells or is induced by tissue-specific factors. The expression of activation markers such as CD69 and CD45RO on T cells from non-pregnant endometrium needs to be examined to test whether the activated phenotype of uterine mucosal T cells is a pregnancy-related phenomenon or is found at all times in the endometrium. Furthermore, it would be of interest to determine whether similar T cells are to be found in virgin females.

To summarise, only small numbers of T cells and virtual absence of B cells at the site of trophoblast invasion in the first trimester indicate there is no influx of cells of the specific adaptive immune system. On these grounds alone it seems unlikely that a maternal classical immune response is generated to trophoblast in the decidua basalis. In contrast, in humans there is an accumulation of innate effectors, such as NK cells and macrophages, at the implantation site.

NK cells

The realisation that the maternal uterine leucotyes which preominate during early pregnancy are granulated CD56+ NK-like cells with large granular lymphocyte morphology has made a major impact on how we view the immunology of implantation (Chapter 8) (King and Loke 1991). This is not only true for humans as the granulated metrial gland (GMG) cells present in rodents during pregnancy are also NK-like cells (Croy and Kiso 1993; Liu *et al.* 1994; Stewart 1994). The presence of NK cells in the pregnant uterus may become a more universal finding as additional species are examined.

Distribution

In humans, granulated cells were noticed in both non-pregnant endometrium and decidua by histologists many years ago. These were labelled variously as endometrial granulocytes, Kornchenzellen or 'K' cells, globular leucocytes, specific endometrial granular cells or endometrial granulocytes (Weill 1921; von Numers 1953; Hamperl 1955; Hamperl & Hellweg 1958; Kazzaz 1972). Although the lineage of these cells was uncertain, the appearance and distribution of these granulated cells led Weill to conclude: 'Quoi qu'il en soit, ce qui est indiscutable c'est que ce sont des cellules à type lymphoïde propres à la décidua humaine'.

Histological studies have shown that the number of endometrial granulocytes is low in proliferative phase endometrium, but increases in the mid-luteal phase reaching a peak in the late secretory phase of the cycle. The recruitment of these cells therefore appears to be under hormonal control. In particular, progesterone seems essential for the appearance of endometrial granulocytes as they were found in ovariectomised women only after they had been treated with both estrogen and progesterone; estrogen alone was insufficient (Hamperl and Hellweg 1958). Endometrial granulocytes are also not a feature of conditions associated with unopposed estrogen such as endometrial hyperplasia and carcinoma (unpublished). Although these findings indicate progesterone is required for differentiation into granulated cells, it does not exclude the possibility that agranular cells, which are similar in other respects, appear under the influence of estrogen. Endometrial granulocytes are not found before menarche or post-menopausally, nor are they present in any other organs or tissues. The only exception is their appearance in foci of endometriotic endometrium, adenomyosis or areas of decidualisation occurring in the Fallopian tube, surface of the ovary or peritoneum. These observations indicate that the presence of endometrial stromal cells at whatever location supports the recruitment/development of endometrial granulocytes.

A few days before the onset of menstruation, the nuclei of endometrial granulocytes change from a round or reniform appearance to become fragmented. These nuclear changes of karyorrhexis and pyknosis indicate cell death by apoptosis is occurring, but this happens before there is breakdown of other endometrial cellular elements and the influx of neutrophils which are characteristic of menstruation (King *et al.* 1989b). The misnomer 'endometrial granulocytes' arose because these nuclear degenerative changes superficially resemble neutrophil nuclei. Possibly the only obvious difference between late secretory endometrium in a pregnant or non-pregnant cycle is that apoptosis of endometrial granulocytes does not occur in pregnancy and these cells persist in decidua until some time during the second trimester. Although they are very sparse in decidua at term, it is not known what their ultimate fate is in mid-gestation and this question should be explored further.

The bone marrow origin of endometrial granulocytes was established following the advent of monoclonal antibodies for leucocyte differentiation antigens. Bulmer observed that these cells stained for leucocyte common antigen (LCA)

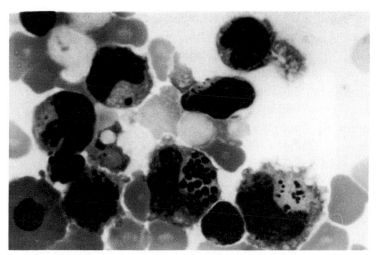

Fig. 7.4. A cytospin smear of decidual lymphocytes stained with Giemsa. Several cells with reniform nuclei and varying-sized cytoplasmic granules are visible. (Obj × 100)

(CD45) and expressed early T-lineage antigens (CD2, CD7, CD38) but not mature T cell markers (CD3, CD5, CD4, CD8) (Bulmer and Sunderland 1983, 1984; Bulmer and Johnson 1985, 1986). Using a Mab to the pan NK cell marker, CD56, it was finally established that these cells were NK-like cells with typical large granular lymphocyte (LGL) morphology (Ritson and Bulmer 1987b; King *et al.* 1989b): (1) The pattern and distribution of endometrial granulocytes and CD56$^+$ cells was similar. (2) Cytospin preparations of purified decidual lymphocytes showed similar numbers of granulated cells when stained with Giemsa (Fig. 7.4) and CD56$^+$ cells with immunohistological staining. (3) Immuno-electron microscopy confirmed granulated lymphocytes were CD56$^+$ and defined their ultrastructure (King *et al.* 1991).

CD56$^+$ cells have been quantitated in endometrium throughout the menstrual cycle (King *et al.* 1989b; Bulmer *et al.* 1991; Starkey *et al.* 1991) and a dramatic increase is noted from the proliferative to the secretory phase. The cells continue to be very abundant in pregnancy, accounting for at least 30% of all stromal cells in the decidua parietalis (Bulmer *et al.* 1991). Endometrial granulocytes (identified by the presence of cytoplasmic granules) were noted to be increased in areas of extensive interstitial trophoblast at the implantation site (Bulmer *et al.* 1987). We have found that CD56$^+$ cells (identified by immunohistology) are more abundant in the decidua basalis compared with the decidua parietalis, and in places seem to efface stromal cells (Fig. 7.5A–C between pp. 34 and 35). These CD56$^+$ cells are intimately associated with invading trophoblast (Fig. 7.5D). CD56$^+$ cells are found in all layers of the uterine mucosa, but predominate in the upper layers. They are found scattered throughout the stroma, but are preferentially located around spiral arteries and particularly around glands, where they often occur in small clusters (Fig. 7.1). The periglandular distribution of CD56[+] cells is more marked in decidua than luteal phase endometrium. In addition, they can be found in an intraepithelial location and ultrastructurally can be visualised moving through the epithelium (King *et al.* 1991; Pace *et al.* 1991). In proliferative phase endometrium, however, only a few CD56[+] cells are found scattered uniformly throughout the stroma.

The increase in CD56[+] cells in the luteal phase could be due to an influx of differentiated cells from blood or to proliferation of CD56[+] cells *in utero* from precursor cells. Proliferation has been shown to occur *in vivo* both by assessing mitoses of granulated cells (Pace *et al.* 1989) and more specifically by double immunohistology for CD45 or CD56 and the proliferation marker, Ki-67 (Tabibzadeh 1990; King *et al.* 1991). The CD56[+] cells were found to be actively proliferating both in the luteal phase and in decidua. These are phases when the other mucosal elements (epithelial glands and stromal cells) have ceased to proliferate and begin to differentiate, except for endothelial cells which continue to proliferate during this time. The stimulus for the *in vivo* proliferation of NK cells is still unknown.

Morphology and phenotype

Ultrastructurally, CD56[+] cells identified by immuno-electron microscopy, show features typical of large granular lymphocytes (King *et al.* 1991; Mincheva-Nilsson *et al.* 1994). The cells have a reniform nucleus, short stubby cytoplasmic projections, and membrane-bound granules of varying size with or without a peripheral rim (Fig. 7.6). CD56[+] cells are also seen in mitosis and in an intraepithelial location. The granules in uterine NK cells have now been shown to contain perforin, granzymes and TIA-1 (Lin *et al.* 1991; King *et al.* 1993). These potent cytolytic molecules are normally only found in NK cells and CTL in tissues in pathological conditions, so it is surprising to find such abundant, apparently lethal cells in a physiological situation. Perforin is also found in NK-like GMG cells in the uteri of pregnant mice (Parr *et al.* 1990). Recently, perforin-deficient mice have been generated which exhibit no NK activity against YAC-1 target cells (Clark 1994; Kägi *et al.* 1994). Homozygous mice had normal numbers of offspring, demonstrating that perforin is not essential for reproduction in this species. However, although the ability of these mice to clear a viral infection *in vitro* was severely impaired, lytic activity was still seen with both lymphohaematopoietic and fibroblast target cells indicating that, whilst perforin-mediated cytolysis is a mechanism of cell killing, alternative lytic pathways exist. The other cytolytic

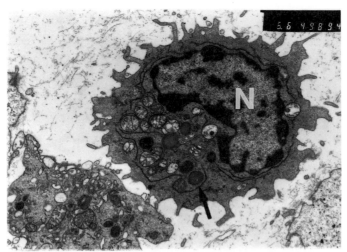

Fig. 7.6. Electron micrograph of a large granular lymphocyte in first trimester decidua. There is a reniform nucleus (N), short stubby cytoplasmic projections, long cisternae of rough endoplasmic reticulum, mitochondria and membrane-bound granules (arrow).

system, the Fas pathway, requires cell–cell contact between CTL/NK cells and Fas-antigen bearing cells (Lowin *et al.* 1994; Walsh *et al.* 1994). This Fas pathway may operate to regulate immune responses (Henkart and Sitkovsky 1994). Perhaps perforin may only be required in the uterus in abnormal pregnancies.

It can be concluded that the main population of decidual leucocytes is CD56$^+$ NK cells. However, subsequent flow cytometric phenotypic analyses have made it necessary to modify this conclusion somewhat because uterine NK cells are substantially different morphologically, phenotypically and functionally from circulating classical NK cells (Starkey *et al.* 1988; King *et al.* 1991; K. Nishikawa *et al.* 1991; Chernyshov *et al.* 1993). A histogram of PBL and isolated decidual lymphocytes stained for CD56$^+$ confirms that the majority of decidual CD45$^+$ cells are CD56$^+$ (Fig. 7.7). In addition, it is apparent that sub-populations can be identified in both blood and decidua on the basis of relative surface levels of the CD56 antigen (i.e. bright and dim). In blood, only 10% of CD56$^+$ cells are CD56^{bright} and these are more prominent in women (Nagler *et al.* 1989; King *et al.* 1991) (Fig. 7.8). In contrast, in decidua the majority of CD56$^+$ cells stain very intensely, ~5 times more than even the CD56^{bright} cells in blood. In decidua, about 10% of CD56 cells are CD56^{dim}. As shown by the scatter plot in Fig. 7.9, the CD56^{bright} cells in decidua are larger and more granular than similar cells in peripheral blood.

The CD56 antigen is NCAM, the neural cell adhesion molecule, which has been implicated in a variety of cell interactions during development (Goridis and Brunet 1992). NCAM is a cell surface glycoprotein consisting of a single

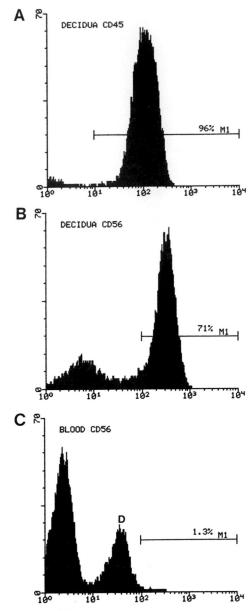

Fig. 7.7. Fluorescence histograms of single-colour FACS analysis of decidual and peripheral blood mononuclear cells. Cell number is represented on the vertical axis and fluorescence intensity on the horizontal axis. **A.** CD45. Ninety-six per cent of the decidual cells in this preparation are CD45[+] (leucocyte common antigen[+]). **B.** CD56. Seventy-one per cent of the decidual cells are CD56[+] indicating that 74% of decidual lymphocytes are CD56[+] NK cells. In addition, the fluorescence intensity of CD56 is high, indicating these are mainly CD56[bright] cells. **C.** CD56. In contrast, in peripheral blood, only 1.3% of mononuclear cells are CD56[bright]. There is also a population of CD56[dim] cells present (D) (~10%).

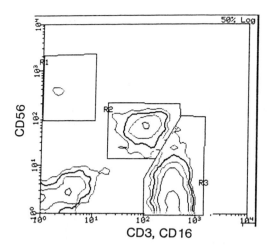

Fig. 7.8. Dual-colour flow cytometric analysis of peripheral blood lymphocytes stained for CD56 (PE, vertical axis) and both CD3 and CD16 (FITC, horizontal axis). A small CD56^{bright} CD16$^-$ CD3$^-$ population is seen in R1 (0.8%). In R2 the main NK population is seen (CD56^{dim} CD16$^+$) (10%). The T cell population is in R3 (CD56$^-$ CD3$^+$) (67%).

polypeptide chain. Considerable heterogeneity with respect to protein and carbohydrate structure is produced by differential splicing and post-translational modifications. Three major isoforms have been identified: a GPI-anchored form (120 kDa) and two larger isoforms with cytoplasmic domains (140 kDa and 180 kDa). Further complexity can be provided by the addition of α-2,8-polysialic acid (PSA). PSA influences not only NCAM homophilic binding, but also interactions of other adhesion molecules (Acheson *et al.* 1991). CD56/NCAM on circulating and decidual NK cells is characterised by the presence of the PSA moiety (Husmann *et al.* 1989). It is not known which isoforms of NCAM are present on decidual NK cells. All three isoforms were demonstrated in peripheral blood NK cells in one study (Husmann *et al.* 1989), but another report found only the 140 kDa form (Lanier *et al.* 1989). There is also an intriguing suggestion that multiple isoforms of NCAM are differentially expressed on NK lines and play a role in NK allorecognition, a finding which has obvious relevance to NK–trophoblast recognition (Suzuki *et al.* 1991). Initially, it was thought that NCAM interactions all involved homophilic binding, but this is now controversial, perhaps due to differences in behaviour between soluble and immobilised NCAM (Krog and Bock 1992).

The only other cell type to express NCAM at the implantation site is endovascular trophoblast (Burrows *et al.* 1994). These trophoblast cells are in close proximity to NK cells in the arterial wall at the site of medial destruction by trophoblast. Cellular expression of GPI-linked isoforms of NCAM may

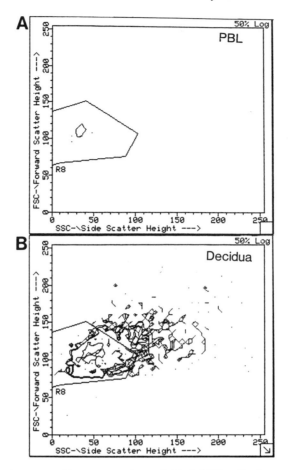

Fig. 7.9. Forward versus side scatter plots of CD56^{bright} cells from peripheral blood and decidua. The gate (R8) indicates the size and granularity of normal peripheral blood lymphocytes. **A**. The CD56^{bright} cells in blood are small and agranular. **B**. In contrast, in decidua, CD56^{bright} cells are variable in size with large granulated cells present.

regulate the secretion of metalloproteinases which might contribute to arterial medial destruction (Edvardsen *et al.* 1993). In addition, heterophilic adhesion of NCAM to heparin/heparan sulphate and collagen is possible, although integrins appear not to be involved as ligands (Kallapur *et al.* 1992; Murray and Jensen 1992). The expression of NCAM at such high density on decidual NK cells implies it is of functional significance. Besides function, there are many additional questions regarding this molecule. For example, what NCAM isoforms are present on decidual NK cells; what are the possible ligands for CD56/NCAM in decidua basalis; is CD56 capable of inducing signal transduction in NK cells; and what factors are responsible for the great increase in NCAM expression on these tissue NK cells?

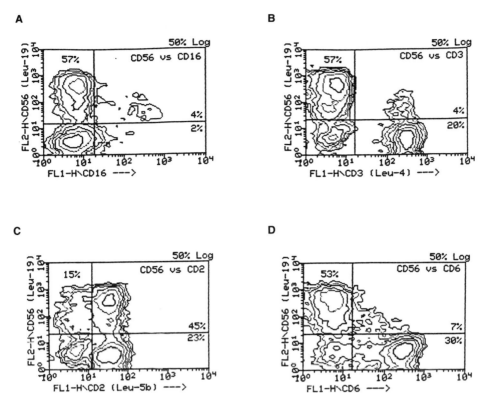

Fig. 7.10. Dual-colour flow cytometric analysis of decidual lymphocytes prepared as in Fig. 7.2. **A**. CD56 (PE) versus CD16 (FITC). Only a small number (4% of total cells) of decidual CD56⁺ NK cells are also CD16⁺ (7% of CD56⁺ cells). These CD16⁺ cells are all CD56^{dim}. **B**. CD56 (PE) versus CD3 (FITC). In this sample 24% of cells are CD3⁺ T cells although there is a small population (~4% of total cells) which are CD3⁺ and CD56⁺. **C**. CD56 (PE) versus CD2 (FITC). Sixty per cent of cells are CD56⁺. Of these 75% are CD2⁺. **D**. CD56 (PE) versus CD6 (FITC). The great majority of CD56⁺ cells are CD6⁻.

In extensive studies of peripheral blood NK cells, Lanier's group have identified sub-populations of NK cells not just by the antigenic density of the NK cell marker, CD56, but also by levels of the other classical NK marker, CD16 (Lanier *et al.* 1986; Nagler *et al.* 1989). CD16 is the FcγRIII, a low-affinity receptor for aggregated IgG. In blood, 90% of CD56⁺ NK cells are CD56^{dim} CD16^{bright} and 10% are CD56^{bright} CD16⁻. This is in complete contrast to decidua where 90% of decidual NK cells are CD16⁻ with only ~10% CD16⁺ cells identified by flow cytometric analysis of decidual isolates (Starkey *et al.* 1988; Manaseki and Searle 1989; K. Nishikawa *et al.* 1991; Chernyshov *et al.* 1993) (Fig 7.10) and ~2% by immunohistology (King *et al.* 1989b; Bulmer *et al.* 1991; Klentzeris *et al.* 1992). This means that only 1% of circulating lymphocytes are phenotypically similar (CD56^{bright} CD16⁻) to the majority of lymphocytes in the

Table 7.2. *Phenotype of main population of CD56^{bright} decidual cells*

NK cell markers	Activation markers
CD16$^-$	CD69$^+$
CD57$^-$	Kp43$^+$
CD56^{bright}	HLA-DR$^-$
	CD45RA$^+$
Early T cell markers	
CD2$^\pm$	*Cytokine receptors*
CD7$^\pm$	IL-2Rβ^+
CD38$^+$	IL-2Rα(CD25)$^{-/+}$
	c-kit$^-$
Mature T cell markers	IL-7R$^-$
mCD3$^-$	IL-6R$^-$
CD4$^-$	IFN-R$^-$
CD6$^-$	IL-1R$^-$
	TFNR$^-$
	GM-CSFR$^-$

uterus. CD57, another NK marker present on some adult NK cells, is always absent from decidual NK cells.

It has been suggested that the larger numbers of CD16$^+$ cells found in decidual isolates compared to those detected by immunohistology are due to the presence of contaminating cells from maternal blood (Christmas *et al.* 1990; Chernyshov *et al.* 1993). This is a valid point, but there is a possible alternative explanation for this discrepancy. In sections of endometrium and decidua we have found that CD16$^+$ cells are preferentially localised in the lumina of arteries. The CD16$^+$ cells are particularly prominent in the spiral arteries of the decidua basalis, and they are also found in the cytotrophoblast shell overlying these vessels. Furthermore, by flow cytometry the CD16$^+$ cells in decidua can be divided into two populations on the basis of fluorescence intensity: CD16^{bright} and CD16^{dim}. The mucosal lymphocyte marker, HML-1 (CD103) (Cerf-Bensussan *et al.* 1987), is only co-expressed on the decidual CD16^{dim} population. These findings indicate that CD16^{dim} CD103$^+$ CD56$^+$ cells are a sub-population of decidual NK cells. The other CD16^{bright} population, however, may be contaminants from blood (unpublished).

A detailed phenotypic profile of other leucocyte antigens present on decidual CD56$^+$ NK cells can be drawn from several studies (Table 7.2). Of T lineage markers, early T antigens such as CD2 (Fig. 7.10C) and CD7 are found on the majority of CD56^{bright} decidual cells although small CD2$^-$ and CD7$^-$ populations are also present (King *et al.* 1991; K. Nishikawa *et al.* 1991). A similar proportion of fetal liver and thymic CD56$^+$ cells are also CD2$^-$ and CD7$^-$ (Sánchez *et al.* 1994).

Mature T cell markers CD3 (Fig. 7.10B), CD4 (Fig. 7.2F), CD5 and CD6 (Fig. 7.10D) are not expressed on the surface of decidual CD56^{bright} cells apart from the finding that CD8 is present at low density on ~20% (Fig. 7.2E). A minor fraction of circulating NK cells do express CD8α and not CD8β chains (Norment and Littman 1988; Nagler *et al.* 1989). The differential expression of CD8α/α and CD8α/β by NK and T cells suggests they are functionally distinct and may differ in their relative affinity for MHC class I molecules (Giblin *et al.* 1994). *In vivo*, CD56$^+$ CD8$^+$ and CD3$^+$ CD8$^+$ cells are found in an intraepithelial location in the endometrium and decidua. Although CD3 proteins are not found on the surface of CD56^{bright} decidual NK cells, immunohistology using an antiserum to CD3ϵ and Western blotting of highly purified CD56$^+$ CD3$^-$ decidual lymphocytes shows there is cytoplasmic expression of CD3ϵ (unpublished). CD3ϵ mRNA has also been identified in highly purified decidual CD56$^+$ cells (Hayakawa *et al.* 1994). This is a further difference from adult classical NK cells which are cytoplasmic (cy) CD3ϵ^- unless activated by IL-2 (Lanier *et al.* 1992a). Fetal CD56$^+$ NK cells, isolated from fetal liver, also express cyCD3ϵ but, in addition, cyCD3δ and γ protein subunits are present which can form CD3$\epsilon\delta$ and CD3$\epsilon\gamma$ complexes in the cytoplasm (Lanier *et al.* 1992a; Phillips *et al.* 1992). These observations indicate either that decidual NK cells are activated *in vivo* or that they resemble fetal NK cells appearing before other lymphocytes in ontogeny (see below).

Recombination activating genes (RAG-1 and RAG-2) are expressed together in pre-B and pre-T cells, cell types expressing V(D)J recombinase activity. Both RAG-1 and RAG-2 are found in gut intraepithelial lymphocytes (IEL) (Guy-Grand *et al.* 1992) and decidual CD56$^+$ CD16$^-$ cells, which has given rise to the suggestion that extrathymic differentiation may occur in the decidua (Hayakawa *et al.* 1994). Decidual CD3$^-$ clones had both TCR γ and δ genes in the germ line configuration (Christmas *et al.* 1990). Fetal liver NK cell clones also show no evidence of TCR rearrangement, but it is not known if they express RAG genes (Phillips *et al.* 1992). The significance of RAG-1 and RAG-2 expression in decidual lymphocytes is not yet clear.

Besides cyCD3ϵ there are other markers which indicate that decidual NK cells are in an 'activated' state (Table 7.2). The intermediate affinity IL-2R (p75) is expressed on all decidual NK cells while the high affinity IL-2R (p55) (CD25) is expressed on a proportion (~15%) of these cells (K. Nishikawa *et al.* 1991; Saito *et al.* 1993a). HLA-DR is also present on a few (~20%) CD56$^+$ decidual cells. CD69 is particularly interesting as this molecule is induced on T lymphocytes and NK cells rapidly after *in vitro* activation, and is found on both decidual CD56$^+$ NK cells and CD3$^+$ T cells. CD69 is not present on circulating adult NK cells, but is found on fetal liver NK cells (Phillips *et al.* 1992). CD69 is a member of the Ca^{2+}-dependent (C-type) animal lectins. These are type II integral membrane proteins with a carbohydrate-recognition domain. Other members of this family include members of the NK-gene complex in rodents and humans although CD69 expression is unlike these other NK-associated genes as it can be inducibly expressed on many haematopoietic lineages (López-Cabrera *et al.* 1993; Santis *et al.* 1994). Expression of CD69 involves activation of the Ras protein and cross-linking of CD69 triggers intracellular signals resulting in NK cell cytolytic activity. It is of interest that although CD69 is only transiently expressed after activation, both gut lymphocytes and decidual T cells and NK cells express CD69. As mentioned, this might reflect persistent antigen restimulation as T cells from the gut are refractory to stimulation via CD3/TCR *in vitro* and have an elevated cytoplasmic [Ca^{2+}] (De Maria *et al.* 1993). CD69 may interact with carbohydrate ligands via the lectin-like domain, but putative carbohydrate molecules have so far not been identified (Hamann *et al.* 1993). However, some members of this supergene family (CD23 and CD72) are not necessarily involved in carbohydrate recognition as protein ligands have been identified (Van de Velde *et al.* 1991; Aubry *et al.* 1992). Alternatively, the expression of CD69 by both fetal and decidual NK cells may not mean that these specific NK populations are 'activated', but is rather a reflection of developmental or tissue-specific function.

Ontogeny

In contrast to the extensive studies on T cell development, particularly in the thymus, much less is known about NK ontogeny and differentiation. NK cells do show many similarities to T cells with respect to surface phenotype and effector functions, suggesting they might have a common origin. However, unlike NK cells, T cells rearrange TCR genes and always require the presence of MHC class I or class II antigens to recognise their targets (Lanier *et al.* 1992b). It now seems likely that a common NK/T cell progenitor does exist, but how and when the developmental pathways diverge in fetal life remains a mystery. Haematopoietic cells migrate into the fetal liver from the blood islands of the yolk sac as early as 5 weeks gestation (Fig. 7.11). By 6 weeks gestation, membrane (m) CD3$^-$CD56$^+$ lymphocytes are identifiable in the fetal liver (Phillips *et al.* 1992). T cells (mCD3$^+$) are not observed until 16 weeks gestation, and by 24 weeks equal proportions of CD56$^+$ NK and mCD3$^+$ T cells are found.

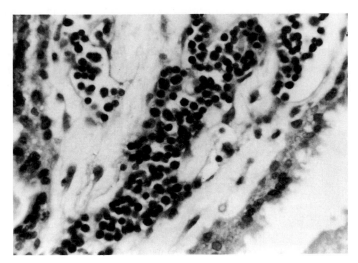

Fig. 7.11. Blood islands present in the yolk sac at 6 weeks gestation. (Obj × 40)

Thus, NK cells (which are capable of spontaneous cytotoxicity) are the earliest lymphocytes to appear in fetal life and are certainly present before the development of the thymus.

Interestingly, fetal liver CD56' NK cells closely resemble the uterine NK population in adults. Many features are shared which distinguish fetal and decidual NK cells from the main population of CD56^{dim} circulating adult NK cells (Table 7.3): lack of expression of CD16 and CD57; high surface density of CD56; lower constitutive cytolytic activity against the K562 cell line; expression of the activation marker CD69; and response to low concentrations

Table 7.3. *Characteristics of NK cells from blood, decidua and fetal liver*

	Blood	Decidua	Fetal liver
NK markers	CD56^{dim} CD16^{bright} CD57$^{\pm}$	CD56$^{bright+++}$ CD16^{-} CD57	CD56^{bright} CD16$^{-/dim}$ CD57^{-}
Cytoplasmic CD3	cyCD3^{-}	cyCD3^{+}	cyCD3^{+}
Activation markers	CD69^{-}	CD69'	CD69^{+}

NK activity	High
	Respond to high-
	    dose IL-2
		Low
		Respond to low-
		    dose IL-2
			Low
			Respond to low-
			    dose IL-2

Cytokine production	GM-CSF^{-} CSF-1^{-}	GM-CSF^{+} CSF-1^{+}	GM-CSF^{+} CSF-1?

of IL-2 due to the expression of the high affinity IL-2R (CD25) (Phillips *et al.* 1992). Furthermore, cyCD3 proteins (ϵ, δ & γ) are detectable in fetal CD56 cells, and we have also found cyCD3ϵ in decidual CD56$^+$ cells (unpublished). The presence of intracytoplasmic CD3 proteins in fetal NK cells is intriguing, and the functional significance is unknown. The development of both T and NK cells is disrupted by the introduction of the gene encoding human CD3ϵ into transgenic mice (Wang *et al.* 1994). An aberrant signal appears to be generated by expression of transgenic CD3ϵ protein in pre-NK cells. These findings support the idea that T and NK cells share a common precursor. Furthermore, correct CD3ϵ expression appears critical for normal NK development. Avian NK cells also express cyCD3ϵ and the preservation of this complex over such a long period of vertebrate evolution suggests it is more than just an ancient relic (Göbel *et al.* 1994).

On the basis of all these findings, a hypothesis for the relationship between T and NK cell development has been proposed (Lanier *et al.* 1992b). A putative common NK/T cell progenitor present in embryonic liver receives signals which induce either thymic homing, TCR gene rearrangement and expression of CD1, or induce CD56 and/or CD16 expression and downregulation of cyCD3. Later in fetal life, these common NK/T cell progenitors from the liver migrate to the thymus, bone marrow and possibly other sites, since NK or T cells can be generated from CD34^{bright} CD3$^-$ CD4$^-$ CD8$^-$ CD1$^-$ thymocytes depending on the *in vitro* microenvironment (Sánchez *et al.* 1994). However, the thymus is not essential for NK cell differentiation. Perhaps before the thymus is present, the fetal liver bipotential NK/T cell progenitors mainly differentiate along the NK pathway.

Two possible NK differentiation pathways can be proposed (Fig. 7.12). In the first hypothetical scheme (A) the CD56^{bright} cyCD3$^+$ fetal cells are immature NK cells which will mature into adult CD56^{dim} CD16^{bright} cells losing cyCD3$^+$ as they move along a common differentiation pathway (Phillips *et al.* 1992). Decidual NK cells could then undergo tissue-specific homing and inductive differentiation from uterine signals resulting in a different phenotype. Decidual NK cells exhibit upregulation of CD56 compared with fetal NK cells and may have lost cyCD3δ and γ. Nonetheless, their close resemblance to fetal NK cells does give rise to a second possible pathway of NK differentiation (B) which is perhaps more attractive. There could be intrinsic differences in NK cell progenitors at different time points during development. The CD56^{bright} cells in the uterus may represent a distinct NK cell population which arises from fetal NK stem cells and is completely separate from the differentiation pathway used by adult circulating CD56^{dim} NK cells. Additional support for this is provided from studies in the beige mouse (*bg/bg*) which has a genetic defect in NK cells resulting in giant

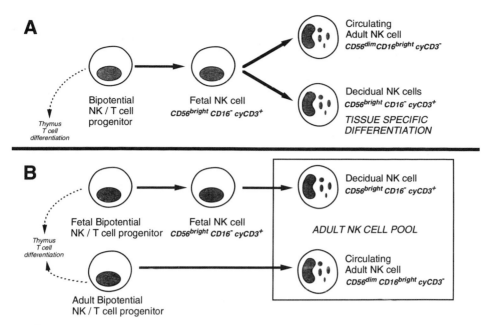

A

Bipotential NK / T cell progenitor

Thymus T cell differentiation

Fetal NK cell
$CD56^{bright}$ $CD16^-$ $cyCD3^+$

Circulating Adult NK cell
$CD56^{dim}$$CD16^{bright}$ $cyCD3^-$

Decidual NK cells
$CD56^{bright}$ $CD16^-$ $cyCD3^+$
TISSUE SPECIFIC DIFFERENTIATION

B

Fetal Bipotential NK / T cell progenitor

Thymus T cell differentiation

Fetal NK cell $CD56^{bright}$ $CD16^-$ $cyCD3^+$

Decidual NK cell
$CD56^{bright}$ $CD16^-$ $cyCD3^+$

ADULT NK CELL POOL

Adult Bipotential NK / T cell progenitor

Circulating Adult NK cell
$CD56^{dim}$ $CD16^{bright}$ $cyCD3^-$

Fig. 7.12. Hypothetical pathways of natural killer (NK) cell differentiation.

NK granules. Despite this, the NK-lineage GMG cells in the uterus are morphologically normal (Croy 1994). The mutation in the beige mice results in a failure of lysosomal membrane fusion. This defect might arise only after a developmental switch from fetal to adult NK stem cell progenitor and this could explain why the uterine NK cells appear normal.

There are precedents in mice supporting this second NK developmental hypothesis which involve other lymphocyte lineages. B cells generated in fetal ($CD5^+$) and adult ($CD5^-$) life are different. $CD5^+$ B cells (B-1) generated during early ontogeny can persist and maintain their progeny only in the peritoneal cavity during the life time of the animal. Stem cell enriched adult bone marrow will not generate $CD5^+$ B cells, but only adult $CD5^-$ B cells (B-2), supporting the concept that a developmental switch has occurred in the B progenitor cells (Lam and Stall 1994). A counterpart in the T cell lineage is seen in the waves of T cells produced in fetal life which are biased for particular T cell receptors and which may also result from developmental switches (Ikuta *et al.* 1990). Some of these fetal T cells with uniform expression of a particular TCR persist in adult life at specific sites such as the skin. These dendritic epidermal Vγ3 T cells which are the first to develop in the thymus can develop from fetal but not adult stem cells (Havran and Allison 1990). The presence of T and B cells at surface locations in the adult which have arisen from fetal progenitors raises the question of the specificity of their Ig or TCR receptors. Interestingly, both murine $CD5^+$

peritoneal B cells (B-1) and skin γδ T cells seem to respond preferentially to self antigens, and for the T cells, these are particularly antigens which are present in the tissues in which they reside (Kroemer *et al.* 1993). The biological significance of this is hard to understand, but the view that the immune system is present during embryonic and fetal life to monitor changes in self rather than to combat foreign antigens, as in the adult, is appealing (Kroemer *et al.* 1993; Hardy and Hayakawa 1994) (Chapter 2).

If this second view of NK development is correct, inevitably several questions arise. Firstly, do fetal and decidual NK cells recognise the same target ligands as adult blood NK cells? Elucidation of the several newly described NK receptors (Chapter 8) will eventually answer this question. Linked to this is the ancillary question as to why fetal NK cells are present so early in embryonic development, as this may shed light on the potential function of decidual NK cells. In the fetus, NK cells have been proposed to regulate early haematopoiesis thereby having a homeostatic role in monitoring self (Phillips *et al.* 1992). An analogous function of decidual NK cells in regulating cyclic endometrial renewal and/or trophoblast proliferation/differentiation seems highly plausible.

Secondly, at what stage of development is the uterine mucosa seeded with stem cells, or does the stem cell population reside elsewhere with maturing cells moving into the uterine mucosa during each menstrual cycle? Since granules are presumably a marker of terminal differentiation and only appear under the influence of progesterone, the fact that endometrial granulocytes have not been identified in premenarche human endometrium does not necessarily mean the stem cells are absent. In mice, the uterine NK-lineage cells, GMG cells, also differentiate under the influence of progesterone, perhaps acting via decidual stromal cells (Stewart 1987). GMG precursors (identifiable by LGL-1$^+$ staining) were detectable postnatally at 2 weeks of age with a further increase at the time of puberty (5–7 weeks) (Kiso *et al.* 1992). It may be that an earlier NK cell precursor population lacking LGL-1 seeds the fetal or neonatal uterus. Dendritic epidermal γδ T cells are seeded to the skin only in fetal life (Havran and Allison 1990). No similar immunohistological studies have been performed in humans.

A third question is, how does the small CD56^{bright} CD16$^-$ cyCD3$^-$ population circulating in adult blood fit with either of the proposed NK differentiation pathways? Although phenotypically sharing many features with decidual NK cells, these cells show two differences. They are agranular small lymphocytes not showing the typical LGL morphology. Secondly, they do not express cyCD3 proteins. It seems most likely that they represent an immature stage of adult NK cells, but at present their relationship with other tissue and circulating NK cells is unclear.

The construction of the immune system during ontogeny reflects phylogenetic progression and the very early appearance of NK cells in the embryo indicates they can be regarded as primitive in origin. It is misleading, therefore, to view all recognition systems solely within the framework of the much more advanced adult immune system (Chapter 2).

Proliferation and survival

Little is known about the recruitment and life-span of NK cells *in vivo*. NK cells are mainly found in the circulation and so the proliferation of uterine NK cells and their survival in the decidua right into the second trimester is an unusual feature. So far the only cytokine which will induce proliferation of decidual NK cells *in vitro* is IL-2 (K. Nishikawa *et al.* 1991; King *et al.* 1992). The stimulus for the vigorous proliferation of CD56$^+$ cells in the luteal phase and in early decidua is unknown, but *in vivo* it cannot be IL-2 as this cytokine has not been found in the decidua (Saito *et al.* 1993c; Jokhi 1994). Furthermore, IL-2 induces activation of NK cells into potent lymphokine-activated killer (LAK) cells which could damage trophoblast (King and Loke 1990). *In vivo* in mice NK cells can be expanded by both an IL-2 dependent and IL-2 independent pathway; the latter is associated with high levels of IFN (Welsh and Vargas-Cortez 1992; Su *et al.* 1994). Prolactin, secreted by decidual stromal cells, is a possible candidate for stimulation of decidual NK proliferation, particularly as prolactin levels rise and are maintained over the same time period that CD56$^+$ cells are present in the uterus (Handwerger and Brar 1992). The prolactin receptor belongs to a family which includes receptors for a number of cytokines such as IL-2Rβ (Kelly *et al.* 1991) (Chapter 10). Prolactin is mitogenic for lymphocytes in some species (Viselli *et al.* 1991), and has been regarded as an evolutionary precursor of IL-2. *In vitro*, however, proliferation of decidual NK cells is not observed when the cells are plated onto a monolayer of stromal cells, and we have not found evidence for expression of the prolactin receptor on the majority of CD56$^+$ cells (unpublished).

The number of cells in a tissue is a reflection of both cell proliferation and death. Uterine NK cells morphologically are seen to undergo apoptosis on day 26–27 of the menstrual cycle and in the decidua of failing pregnancies. These are both times of falling progesterone levels, indicating that uterine NK cell survival in the tissues may be progesterone dependent. However, progesterone itself does not induce proliferation of decidual NK cells (unpublished), and it is not known if the progesterone receptor is expressed by CD56$^+$ cells. The expression of *bcl*-2, a proto-oncogene product which is able to suppress apoptosis, in decidual CD56$^+$ cells shows survival factors for NK cells are present in the decidual environment (unpublished). In the late secretory phase when NK cell death occurs, *bcl*-2 expression is downregulated. These survival factors could be growth factors/hormones secreted by stromal cells or macrophages, or they may be extracellular matrix proteins such as fibronectin and laminin. Integrin–matrix–stromal interactions are likely to be of importance in development and survival of tissue NK cells. The contact between NK precursors and bone marrow stromal cells is essential for normal NK development in this tissue (Delfino *et al*. 1994). Development of uterine NK cells may utilise similar mechanisms within the uterine microenvironment.

Expression of integrins

Many lymphocyte functions, such as cytokine secretion, effector-target interactions and binding to endothelial cells or extracellular matrix, are dependent on adhesion molecules, particularly the integrins (Allavena *et al*. 1991; Dustin and Springer 1991; Hemler 1991; Shimizu and Shaw 1991). Immunohistology and flow cytometric analysis have shown that CD56$^+$ cells from first trimester decidua all express the α_1, α_4, α_5 and β_1 integrin subunits but not the α_2, α_3, α_4, α_v or β_4 (Burrows *et al*. 1993b; Burrows 1994). Similar findings were reported by Dietl *et al*. (1992). Decidual CD56$^+$ cells also express strongly the HML-1 antigen (CD103) (King *et al*. 1991) which is now recognised to be the $\alpha_E\beta_7$ integrin (Cerf-Bensussan *et al*. 1992; Parker *et al*. 1992). We have observed that HML-1$^+$ cells staining with the strongest intensity are near the mucosal surface or in the epithelium. This integrin, therefore, may be responsible for lymphocyte–epithelial interactions rather than homing to the mucosa as HML-1 inhibits binding of gut IEL to a colon cell line (Cepek *et al*. 1993). The adhesion molecules expressed by decidual CD56$^+$ cells compared with similar cells in peripheral blood are summarised in Table 7.4.

Abundant fibronectin (FN), of either trophoblast or decidual origin, is present in decidua (Chapter 9). Binding to this matrix protein via appropriate receptors could influence the migration of CD56$^+$ cells within decidua. FN has been reported to facilitate the migration of freshly isolated blood NK cells through Nucleopore filters *in vitro* (Somersalo and Saksela 1991) and integrin-mediated matrix interactions have been implicated in the specific positioning of lymphocytes in tissues (De Sousa *et al*. 1990; Ratner 1992). Indeed, decidua is the only adult tissue which is so heavily populated by NK cells. This interaction may also induce NK cell proliferation because FN has been observed to augment

Table 7.4. *Adhesion molecules expressed by the major population of CD56$^+$ cells*

	Decidua	Blood
Fibronectin receptors		
$\alpha_4\beta_1$	++	+
$\alpha_5\beta_1$	++	++
$\alpha_4\beta_7$	++	+
Laminin receptors		
$\alpha_6\beta_1$	–	++
$\alpha_1\beta_1$	++	–
HML-1		
$\alpha_E\beta_7$	+++	–
Ig superfamily		
ICAM-1	++	+
NCAM (CD56)	++++	+
β_2 integrins		
CD11a	+	++
CD11b	+	++
CD11c	++	I

T cell proliferation via binding to $\alpha_4\beta_1$ and $\alpha_5\beta_1$ receptors (Shimizu *et al.* 1990; Klingemann and Fred 1991). Decidual CD56$^+$ cells do express the nuclear proliferation marker Ki-67 (King *et al.* 1991). The production of cytokines by decidual NK cells may also be regulated by interactions with FN as binding to extracellular matrix (ECM) protein via integrins is demonstrated to be involved in cytokine gene expression by lymphocytes (Yamada *et al.* 1991; Miyake *et al.* 1993). Since FN is secreted by trophoblast, the additional possibility arises that these integrins could mediate trophoblast–NK cell interaction.

Recent *in vitro* studies in our laboratory have shown that decidual NK cells readily bind to purified FN *in vitro* and that this adhesion can be disrupted by specific antibodies to α_4, α_5 and β_1 integrin subunits and also by synthetic peptides containing the tri-amino acid RGD sequence (Burrows 1994). Interestingly, decidual NK cells do not bind to laminin (LM) *in vitro*, which may be due to the absence of expression of the $\alpha_6\beta_1$ LM receptor by these cells. However, decidual NK cells do bind to type IV collagen; this binding is probably mediated by the $\alpha_1\beta_1$ integrin because the adhesion can be blocked by Mabs to the α_1 and β_1 subunits. We have observed that decidual NK cells also bind strongly to monolayer cultures

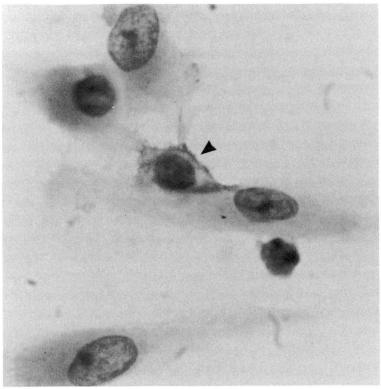

Fig. 7.13. Binding of decidual NK cells to stromal cells. Decidual lymphocytes were incubated with a monolayer of decidual stromal cells for 60 minutes. After washing, the slide was stained with anti-CD56. A CD56 NK cell is seen (arrowhead) with elongated pseudopodia firmly adherent to a stromal cell.

of decidual stromal cells, where they elongate and extend pseudopodia over the stromal cells (Fig. 7.13). Thus, if all the above *in vitro* findings reflect the *in vivo* situation, it may be concluded that decidual NK cell interaction with FN and collagen via appropriate integrin receptors is likely to play an important regulatory role in the biology of these uterine leucocytes.

As observed for trophoblast (Chapter 9), decidual NK cells also secrete matrix metalloproteinases (MMP) which will presumably facilitate their migration through the decidual ECM. Martelli *et al.* (1993) have reported the production of a 92 kDa gelatinase by CD45[+] lymphoid cells from first trimester decidua. We have recently demonstrated by gel zymography that first trimester decidual CD56[+] cells secreted two MMP of 96 and 94 kDa which are likely to represent different isoforms of 92 kDa collagenase (gelatinase B) and an MMP of 67 kDa which is likely to be the 72 kDa collagenase (gelatinase A) (Burrows 1994). Of these, the 96 kDa band was the more intense. In addition to the soluble forms, two membrane-bound MMP of 96 and 94 kDa were also detected. The secreted 67 kDa MMP was significantly increased after IL-2 stimulation. Others have reported that cytokines enhance the expression of collagenase synthesis by human monocytes (Wahl *et al.* 1993).

In addition to β_1 integrin receptors for ECM, decidual NK cells also express many members of the β_2 family of integrins which mediate cell–cell interactions, such as CD11a/CD18 (LFA-1), CD11b/CD18 (Mac-1) and CD11c/CD18 (gp150/95) heterodimers (Burrows *et al.* 1993b; Slukvin *et al.* 1994). LFA-1 is now accepted as one of the important receptors mediating NK adhesion and target cell lysis (Storkus and Dawson 1991; Zarcone *et al.* 1992) so could play an important role in NK–trophoblast interaction. We have observed that this integrin is upregulated in decidual NK cells by IL-2, which could explain our previous finding that this cytokine transforms decidual NK cells into potent LAK cells which lyse isolated trophoblast cells while unstimulated NK cells do not (King and Loke 1990) (Chapter 8).

Macrophages

Immunohistological studies have indicated that ~20% of leucocytes in both the endometrium and decidua are macrophages, identifiable by Mabs to CD14 (Fig. 7.1; Table 7.1). They express the class II MHC molecules HLA-DR, -DP and -DQ and contain acid phosphatase, non-specific esterase and lysozyme, and have been shown to contain haemosiderin granules. When disaggregated from the endometrium, they show adherence to glass, emission of cell processes, and the ability to phagocytose opsonised red blood cells. Endometrial macrophages, therefore, have the typical features of tissue macrophages, and are probably involved in scavenging and degradative functions associated with menstruation.

Macrophages in the endometrium do not appear to be under hormonal control as their numbers are relatively constant throughout the menstrual cycle with only a small rise in numbers premenstrually. In the pregnant uterus, however, macrophages are greatly increased in number at the implantation site in the decidua basalis. The difference in morphology between macrophages and CD56+ decidual cells is clearly evident in Fig. 7.14. They are in intimate contact with the cytotrophoblast shell and invading trophoblast populations, whilst much smaller numbers are found in the decidua parietalis where there is no trophoblast. Numerous macrophages are also found at sites of ectopic implantation in the Fallopian tube, but in this situation there does not seem to be preferential localisation at areas of trophoblast invasion.

Whether decidual macrophages have any specific functions related to successful pregnancy is unknown. Indeed, it is remarkable how little they have

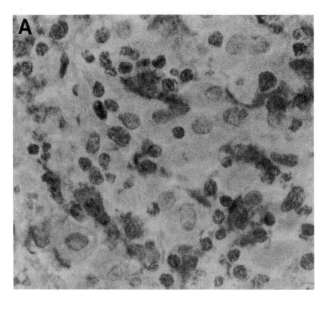

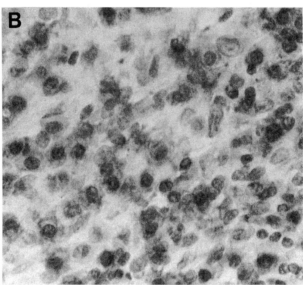

Fig. 7.14. Serial frozen sections of the implantation site stained for macrophages (**A**) and natural killer (NK) cells (**B**). A serial section from the same block identifying the presence of trophoblast is shown in Fig 7.5A. Macrophages, identified by an antibody to CD14 (**A**), are abundant. The macrophages are large with long cell processes. They have a different morphology from the CD56⁺ NK cells, which are large rounded cells (**B**). (Obj × 40)

been studied. In general terms, macrophages can act either by phagocytosis, which may result in MHC class II antigen presentation, or by production of a wide range of soluble products. Phagocytosis of dying trophoblast, which may have undergone apoptosis after interactions with NK cells, could be one important function. Macrophages are abundant around the zone of necrosis present at the feto-maternal interface (Nitabuch's layer). The significance of Nitabuch's layer is obscure, but it is likely that resolution of the necrotic tissue occurs by decidual macrophages. It is also possible that these HLA-DR⁺ macrophages are capable of antigen presentation and, in addition, a few CD1⁺ professional antigen presenting cells (APC) are present close to epithelial glands. Theoretically, therefore, decidual macrophages could process molecules secreted by trophoblast or derived from phagocytic ingestion of trophoblast. Antigen presentation of allogeneic proteins (particularly HLA proteins) processed by recipient APC is an indirect mechanism of graft rejection in transplantation. Therefore, the absence of class II molecules on trophoblast does not necessarily infer that antigen processing of trophoblast HLA class I and other proteins cannot take place. Decidual macrophages can present alloantigens in a standard mixed lymphocyte reaction (MLR) (Oksenberg *et al.* 1986; Dorman and Searle 1988). Despite this, we have not found any evidence of a lymphocyte proliferative response in the presence of decidual macrophages when irradiated HLA class I⁺ trophoblast cells are used as stimulators (unpublished). So far there is no evidence that indirect presentation of trophoblast antigens by decidual macrophages can take place.

Macrophages are also capable of producing, and respond to, a wide range of soluble products (Chapter 10). Decidual macrophages express several cytokine receptors, GM-CSF-R (Jokhi *et al.* 1994b), CSF-1R, (Jokhi *et al.* 1993), IFN-γR (Jokhi 1994). In addition, apparently uniquely among tissue macrophages all decidual macrophages express c-*kit*. The kit ligand (KL), also known as stem cell factor (SCF), is secreted by the media of spiral arteries and by extravillous trophoblast (Sharkey *et al.* 1992, 1994). Therefore, the large numbers of macrophages at the implantation site may be recruited and activated by locally produced cytokines secreted by trophoblast. There is little information to date on what decidual macrophages produce. A recent report has indicated the newly described cytokine, vascular endothelial growth factor (VEGF), is transcribed by macrophages in the decidua basalis (Sharkey *et al.* 1993). The receptor for VEGF, known as *flt*, is present on extravillous trophoblast, illustrating how alternative interactions between macrophages and trophoblast might occur.

8

Maternal systemic and local immune response to trophoblast

Background

Ever since Medawar recognised the paradox that the fetus is (in genetic terms) a semi-allograft which escapes rejection, a search has been made to understand how the maternal immune system functions during pregnancy (Medawar 1953). The first question which needs to be addressed is: Is there any evidence of maternal immune recognition of the feto-placental unit? If evidence of such a response is found, it can then be asked: Is this maternal immune response beneficial or potentially harmful to both mother and fetus unless modulated in some way? Regrettably, the first question has been largely ignored and what evidence exists is shaky. Attempts to answer the second question before the first has led to the controversy and confusion which exists at present. In this chapter, the evidence for maternal recognition of the feto-placental unit will be reviewed. Because placental trophoblast is the cell population which forms the ultimate interface with the mother, these are the cells which are most relevant to the present discussion. Trophoblast cells which gain access to maternal blood are likely to encounter a systemic response, whereas those invading into the uterine wall will meet with a local immune response.

Maternal systemic immune response to trophoblast

Major Histocompatibility Complex (MHC) antigens

Circulating maternal B cells and T cells are able to respond to paternally encoded HLA antigens, but these responses are sporadic and clearly unrelated to trophoblast antigen expression (Antczak 1989; Sargent 1993; Billington 1993). Sera from multiparous women are a major source of anti-HLA sera used for cross-matching in tissue-typing laboratories, and T cells from occasional women show sensitised responses to paternal lymphocytes in mixed lymphocyte reactions (Sargent *et al.* 1987, 1988). However, the immunogenic source of maternal sensitisation is unlikely to be trophoblast because villous syncytiotrophoblast, which is in contact with maternal blood, does not express MHC class I or class II antigens even after treatment with IFN-γ. In contrast, extravillous trophoblast does express the class I antigens, HLA-G and probably HLA-C (Chapter 6). We have recently investigated their possible immunogenicity to circulating T cells by assaying [^{3}H]thymidine uptake by maternal peripheral blood lymphocytes (PBL) co-cultured with irradiated HLA class I-positive extravillous trophoblast. No proliferative response was seen, confirming that both extravillous and villous trophoblast are non-immunogenic to maternal PBL (unpublished). Maternal anti-HLA antibodies occur late in first pregnancies (Regan 1992; Regan *et al.* 1991) and are more easily detectable in multiparous women (Ahrons 1971). These findings suggest that the source of immunisation is either by fetal cells from feto-maternal bleeds, which tend to occur particularly at delivery, or due to breaks in the syncytium exposing HLA-positive villous mesenchymal cells. It should be emphasised that the presence or absence of maternal anti-HLA antibodies and sensitised T cells directed at fetal HLA class I specificities has no discernible influence on the outcome of pregnancy. This is not surprising since no trophoblast cells express the relevant target antigens.

The situation in rodent pregnancy is somewhat different in that paternally derived MHC antigens are reported to be expressed by certain rat placental trophoblast populations (Billington and Burrows 1986), and there is a class switch in antibody response towards a mainly non-complement-fixing isotype in pregnant mice (Bell and Billington 1980). In a recent study with pregnant transgenic mice expressing a T cell receptor specific for the murine histocompatibility antigen H-2K^b carrying a K^b positive conceptus, K^b-specific T cells were characterised by reduced expression of the TCR and CD4/8 co-receptors. K^b-specific T cells remained normal during H-2^k syngeneic or H-2^s allogeneic pregnancies. The changes in T cell phenotype suggest a functional shift towards tolerance specifically for paternal alloantigens (B. Arnold, personal communication). Thus, there appears to be a degree of systemic immune modulation in murine pregnancy that is not seen in human pregnancy.

Trophoblast antigens

Since a maternal systemic response to classical MHC class I antigens does not appear to be relevant to reproduction in humans, attempts have been made to identify other trophoblast-specific molecules which might be immunogenic.

There are reports that such anti-trophoblast antibodies do exist (Davis and Brown 1985; Kajino *et al.* 1988; McCrae *et al.* 1993). However, none of these studies tested the sera from women before they became pregnant. When we did this and looked for the presence of antibodies to both syncytiotrophoblast plasma membranes and to extravillous cytotrophoblast cells using ELISA and Western blotting, we could not detect any anti-trophoblast antibodies which were specifically pregnancy related (Grabowska 1989). The suggestion that all the anti-trophoblast antibodies have already been bound to the placenta and are therefore undetectable in the systemic circulation (Jalall *et al.* 1989) seems unlikely as anti-trophoblast antibodies were also not observed immediately post partum.

In spite of these negative findings, there are reproductive immunologists who continue to harbour the belief that the pregnant mother does generate a classical immune response to trophoblast. Opinions differ as to how this response would affect pregnancy. Some investigators consider this response to be beneficial, perhaps even necessary, for successful pregnancy. This concept has been the basis for present regimes of treating women with recurrent spontaneous miscarriages by 'immunotherapy' whereby the patients are immunised by husbands' or third party lymphocytes in order to boost this putative response. A discussion of the evidence for or against the efficacy of such regimes is beyond the scope of this chapter. Interested readers can make up their own minds by analysing the data from double-blind trials that have been published (Coulam *et al.* 1994). Others believe that this maternal immune response, like any allogeneic response, is detrimental to trophoblast survival and, therefore, needs to be altered or suppressed. Clinical regimes based on these conflicting views seem premature. There is a paucity of convincing evidence demonstrating that a systemic classical immune response to trophoblast occurs in all pregnancies. It would seem logical to establish this before moving to therapeutic intervention.

Complement regulatory proteins

A group of molecules expressed by trophoblast which may be relevant to trophoblast survival are members of the family of complement regulatory proteins. The first of these to be detected in trophoblast was CD46, or membrane co-factor protein (MCP), by Purcell *et al.* (1990) when they observed that this protein shared physical, immunological and biochemical properties with a trophoblast antigen previously described as TLX. Since then, two additional members of this family – CD55 which is decay accelerating factor (DAF) and CD59 which is the inhibitor of the membrane attack complex (MAC) – have also been localised to trophoblast (Hsi *et al.* 1991; C. Holmes *et al.* 1992). With some slight quantitative variations, these proteins are present in all trophoblast sub-populations from early gestation to term, so they appear to be ubiquitous.

These regulatory proteins control complement activation on the surface of the cell which expresses them and not on bystander cells (Oglesby *et al.* 1992), although Vanderpuye *et al.* (1994) have recently shown that CD46 can also occur in a soluble form. This soluble CD46 could contribute to the regulation of complement in the fluid phase in the intervillous space. CD46 and CD55 act at the level of C3 convertase with the former serving as cofactor for inactivation of C3b by factor I, while the latter acts to inhibit the assembly and accelerate the decay of C3 convertase. In contrast, CD59 directly regulates the formation and function of the terminal cytolytic MAC by interacting with the terminal complement components C8 and C9 (Walsh *et al.* 1992). These regulatory proteins have a glycosyl-phosphatidylinositol (GPI) anchor rather than a transmembrane domain. This may allow greater lateral mobility of the proteins on the cell membrane and, thus, could be important for rapid movement towards sites of complement attack before lytic plugs can form.

CD46 expression is heterogeneous due both to a genetic polymorphism and to an extensive tissue polymorphism, with 14 different mRNA transcripts, coding for different protein isoforms, identified in 16 tissues (Russell *et al.* 1992). This heterogeneous nature of CD46 tissue expression is due to exquisite control of mRNA splicing. In placenta, a unique isoform (termed e) has been identified in addition to other forms. The effects of this extensive polymorphism on the biological role of CD46 acting as a cofactor in the complement cascade are unknown, particularly as the variations described are distal to the functional site. CD46 variants may have additional functions which affect interactions with other molecules.

Because of their complement inhibitory activity, it has been proposed that the expression of these regulatory proteins by trophoblast is to gain protection from lysis by maternal complement. Indeed, CD59 appears to be expressed by cells which are most in need of protection from homologous lysis, such as blood cells and endothelial cells, whereas those tissues with less access to complement, such as liver parenchyma, pancreatic islet cells and CNS oligodendrocytes, do not express CD59 (Walsh *et al.* 1992). Tedesco and colleagues (1993) have provided supporting evidence that CD46 and CD59 expressed by isolated human trophoblast cells do protect these cells against antibody- and complement-mediated lysis by demonstrating that masking of these regulatory proteins by specific Mabs will abrogate this protection. The antibody used in this experiment is from a male patient with Addison's disease which fortuitously happened to cross-react with trophoblast, so it is unclear whether this model really depicts the *in vivo* situation because, as previously mentioned, potentially cytolytic anti-trophoblast antibodies have never been convincingly demonstrated in all normal pregnant women nor in women with miscarriages, and trophoblast does not have the appropriate antigens to bind to anti-HLA antibodies. As discussed earlier, it is still doubtful whether a classical humoral immune response against trophoblast is generated. However, Tedesco *et al.* (1993) have shown that CD46 and CD59 also protected trophoblast against reactive lysis mediated by C5b6 complexes triggering C7, C8, C9. This would be a more attractive hypothesis as trophoblast is then protected against lysis by complement generated by unconnected antigen–antibody reactions which may occur in the vicinity of the implantation site, such as infections. Another possibility is that the function of the complement regulatory proteins is to protect trophoblast from complement generated via the alternative pathway through the clotting and fibrinolytic systems, thereby preventing inappropriate thrombotic episodes occurring in the intervillous space.

The demonstration by Finberg *et al.* (1992) that CD55 (DAF) can also protect target cells from NK lysis defines a new role for this complement regulatory protein, and is also the most relevant because NK cells are the main lymphoid cell type present in human decidua. These investigators reported that the following manipulative procedures would influence NK cell lysis of the prototype target cell line K562: (1) DAF$^-$ clones of K562 were more susceptible to NK lysis than the DAF$^+$ parental cell line. (2) Exogenous DAF restored DAF$^-$ clones' resistance to lysis to the same level as for DAF$^+$ parent. (3) Masking of the regulatory molecule by F(ab')$_2$ anti-DAF increased the susceptibility of DAF$^+$ cells to lysis. At present, it is not clear how DAF provides resistance to NK cytolysis. There are obvious parallels between complement-mediated lysis and NK-cell-mediated lysis. For example, C9, the terminal membrane attack protein of the complement cascade, shares sequence homology with perforin, the channel-forming protein present in the granules of NK cells. However, there is as yet no evidence that the complement proteins involved in the C3 stage of complement activation can influence perforin-mediated killing.

Maternal local immune response to trophoblast

The outcome of contact between maternal leucocytes and trophoblast in the uterine wall is likely to be very different from the systemic situation. Not only is the composition of leucocytes present in the uterus completely different from that in blood, but in addition all the infiltrating extravillous trophoblast (EVT) populations express HLA class I antigens (Chapters 6 and 7). At present the functions of decidual bone marrow-derived cells in relation to pregnancy are unknown, but unravelling of these EVT–maternal leucocyte interactions must lie at the heart of the control of trophoblast invasion and thus ultimately the vital feto-placental blood supply.

T and B cell responses

There have been surprisingly few attempts at establishing whether a classical immune response is generated to extravillous trophoblast in the placental bed, yet there is an avalanche of reports supposedly demonstrating ways of suppressing such a response. Despite the absence of obvious polymorphic HLA-A,B class I antigens and the complete lack of class II antigens, in theory an immune response could still be generated by the presentation of trophoblast organ-specific or paternally encoded polymorphic molecules by maternal decidual HLA-DR$^+$ macrophages to decidual CD3$^+$ T cells (indirect antigen presentation) (Benichou *et al.* 1992). Such a response would not be likely to result in T cells producing B cell stimulatory cytokines (Th2 response), as B cells are virtually absent from the implantation site and plasma cells are never found. Generation of anti-trophoblast antibodies locally thus seems improbable.

Another mechanism for T cell stimulation has recently been described. Tumour antigens expressed on non-haematopoietic cells can be transferred to host antigen presenting cells and be presented in association with class I molecules to CD8$^+$ T cells (Huang *et al.* 1994). It is difficult to isolate enough T cells from the decidua to answer the question as to whether these cells can recognise trophoblast *in vitro*, because CD3$^+$ T cells only account for 10% of decidual leucocytes (Chapter 7). However, we have performed assays analogous to a mixed lymphocyte reaction using a mixture of all leucocytes isolated from decidua (which include NK cells, HLA-DR$^+$ macrophages and T cells) as responders and with either irradiated first trimester extravillous trophoblast or allogeneic peripheral blood lymphocytes as stimulators. No proliferation of decidual lymphocytes was seen to trophoblast (unpublished). As mentioned earlier, these trophoblast cells also did not stimulate proliferation of peripheral blood lymphocytes so, using this *in vitro* assay, they would appear to be non-immunogenic to both maternal systemic and local immune cells. Interestingly, we and others have found that decidual lymphocytes also do not respond to allogeneic blood lymphocytes (Mincheva-Nilsson *et al.* 1992; Deniz *et al.* 1994).

It seems that T cells from the uterus behave like T cells from other mucosal sites, notably the gut, where proliferative responses to allogeneic signals are deficient (De Maria *et al.* 1993). It is a well-known phenomenon that antigens introduced into the gut tend to be tolerogenic. The gut-associated lymphoid tissue (GALT) appears to have unique properties that favour tolerance induction rather than sensitisation. This is highly likely to be an evolutionary adaptation to prevent host reaction to ingested proteins. The possible mechanisms could involve active suppression or clonal anergy/deletion (Weiner 1994). Perhaps the uterine mucosal system, which is related to GALT, also responds to antigen in a similar way. This would explain the lack of decidual T cell reactivity to trophoblast HLA-G even though this class I molecule is not expressed in the fetal thymus to influence T cell selection (Chapter 6).

It should be emphasised that, although there is no evidence that any local classical immune response is generated to human trophoblast, the only end-point that has been measured so far is lymphocyte proliferation. To be absolutely certain, additional parameters, such as production of IL-2 and other cytokines, need to be studied. Ideally, pure T cell populations, free of CD56$^+$ cells, should also be used although new techniques will need to be developed to obtain such preparations. In mice, Vγ1$^+$ hybridomas derived from $\gamma\delta$ T cells are observed to respond to placental cells by cytokine release (Heyborne *et al.* 1994). Nevertheless, the relative unimportance of T and B cell responses in pregnancy is supported by the demonstration that several types of immunodeficient mice (nude, thymectomised and SCID) continue to reproduce normally (Croy and Chapeau 1990; Croy *et al.* 1991a).

Uterine NK cells

Instead of T and B cells, the leucocyte populations which predominate in the early decidua are NK cells and macrophages. These cells represent the innate rather than the specific arm of the immune response. NK cells lyse a variety of target cells in the absence of prior stimulation including tumour cells, virus infected cells and, in some cases, normal cells (Trinchieri 1989; Storkus and Dawson 1991; Lanier and Phillips 1992). They represent the first line of defence against infections, tumour spread and pathogenic alterations in the normal homeostasis of the organism. In addition, NK cells play a role in the regulation of haematopoiesis (Kärre 1993).

NK cells are generally found circulating in the blood, and whilst some NK cells are found in the spleen they are very sparse in lymph nodes. The only other tissues where very small numbers of NK cells are found are all mucosal in nature, namely the liver and lung, and a few have also been described in the gut. However, the mucosal lining of the progesterone-primed uterus is the only tissue where they are present in great abundance and here they form an integral part of the tissue stroma. In the uterine mucosa, the increase in numbers during the luteal phase of the menstrual cycle and the further increase at the implantation site in the first trimester strongly suggests these uterine NK cells are involved in the maintenance of normal pregnancy. It is highly likely that at least a part of the defensive capabilities of decidua against trophoblast over-penetration reside in these cells. This might not be their only role. It has been difficult to ascribe a function to lymphocytes at other mucosal sites. In the gut, where mucosal lymphocytes are very numerous (although mainly CD3$^+$), they may serve to regulate epithelial cell growth and integrity. Murine Thy-1$^+$ dendritic epidermal T cells which express an invariant $\gamma\delta$ T cell receptor and which recognise a self antigen on keratinocytes in a non-MHC restricted fashion uniquely secrete the epithelial growth factor, keratinocyte growth factor (KGF). They may act to maintain the integrity of epidermis (Boismenu and Havran 1994). Perhaps the uterine NK cells serve a similar function during the normal cyclic renewal and differentiation of the endometrium. In the event of pregnancy, they could also help to avoid disintegration of the mucosa at menstruation, and prolong mucosal survival into decidua. Certainly, the dramatic variation in numbers reflects the cyclic change in epithelial growth seen in the uterus. The possibility that uterine NK cells may regulate endometrial growth and differentiation has not been addressed experimentally.

On recognition of a target cell, NK cells may respond by proliferation, killing of the target cell or cytokine production. Cytolysis is the effector mechanism which is easiest to measure *in vitro* and which has been studied most, but *in vivo* it may be a much less important phenomenon than NK cytokine production. The remainder of this chapter will discuss the possible functions of the distinctive uterine NK cells.

Decidual NK cell cytotoxicity

NK activity is generally measured by the ability of the effector cells to kill the K562 erythroleukaemic cell line which lacks surface expression of MHC molecules. Decidual CD56$^+$ cells do kill K562 cells but at lower levels than adult NK cells freshly isolated from blood (King *et al.* 1989a; Manaseki and Searle 1989; Ferry *et al.* 1990) (Fig. 8.1). A single-cell conjugate between decidual CD56$^+$ effector and K562 is shown in Fig. 8.2. It has been suggested that this low level of NK activity is due to the presence of the minor CD16$^+$ population, and that CD56^{bright} CD16$^-$ decidual cells cannot lyse K562 (Chernyshov *et al.* 1993). This was because when CD3$^-$ clones were generated from decidua, only the CD16$^+$ clones obtained showed NK activity, whilst CD16$^-$ clones had negligible activity (Christmas *et al.* 1990). In contrast, we (unpublished) and Saito *et al.* (1993a) have observed that decidual CD56$^+$ CD16$^-$ cells sorted to

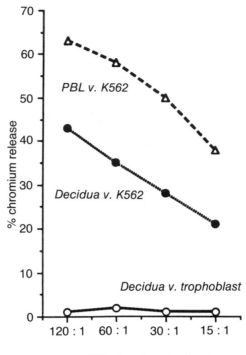

Fig. 8.1. A 4 hour chromium release assay using the K562 cell line and normal first trimester trophoblast as targets. The effector cells were either peripheral blood lymphocytes (PBL) or decidual lymphocytes. Levels of cytotoxicity against K562 cells are lower with decidual effectors compared with blood at all effector:target ratios. Trophoblast cells are resistant to lysis by freshly isolated decidual effectors.

>99% purity had demonstrable NK activity at equivalent levels to unsorted cells. Furthermore, $CD56^{bright}$ $CD16^-$ blood NK cells also show equivalent levels of cytolytic activity to decidual NK cells (Nagler *et al.* 1989), so it may be concluded that the $CD16^-$ decidual NK cells are capable of lysing K562 cells. We have also noted that levels of decidual NK killing of other HLA class I negative cell lines such as LCL.221 were as high as those obtained from PBL (Chumbley *et al.* 1994b).

The finding of NK cells capable of killing K562 inevitably led to the question of whether these cells could kill extravillous trophoblast. This is particularly pertinent as there is a striking temporal and spatial association between decidual NK cells and trophoblast invasion. Lysis of unduly invasive trophoblast cells could be one mechanism of control. It had been difficult to answer this question for a variety of reasons. Firstly, it is necessary to obtain normal trophoblast targets which are sufficiently free of mesenchymal contaminants. Secondly, cells which phenotypically resemble extravillous trophoblast *in vivo*, particularly in HLA class I expression, are required. Thirdly, there are problems associated with

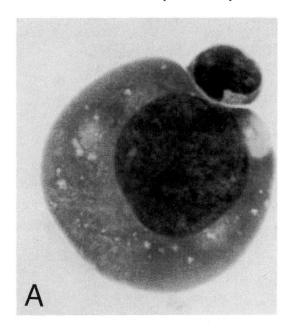

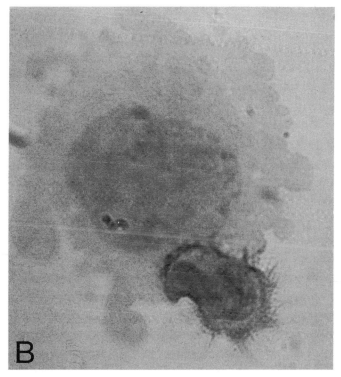

Fig. 8.2. Conjugates formed between decidual effector cells and K562 cells stained with Giemsa (**A**) or immunostained for CD56 (**B**). The target cells are indented by the smaller CD56+ cells.

labelling adherent cells with ^{51}sodium chromate (^{51}Cr) for use in the cytotoxicity assays. If the cells are kept in suspension, there are high levels of spontaneous ^{51}Cr release and, in addition, the nature of the surface putative NK target molecules may be altered. We have attempted to overcome these problems by using first trimester trophoblast isolated to a high degree of purity which stains positively for W6/32, and hence expresses HLA class I antigens. These cells were ^{51}Cr-labelled *in situ* in 96-well plates, which resulted in low levels of spontaneous lysis. These trophoblast targets were not lysed by freshly isolated decidual NK cells (King *et al.* 1989a) (Fig. 8.1). Similar results have been found with other trophoblast targets such as JEG, JAR and BeWo choriocarcinoma cells, and term chorionic plate trophoblast (Ferry *et al.* 1991).

Decidual CD56$^+$ cells will proliferate in response to low-dose IL-2. All the cells express IL-2Rβ with ~15% of the cells expressing IL-2Rα, the high-affinity IL-2 receptor. After culture in IL-2, the cytotoxicity of decidual NK cells against K562 is greatly enhanced and these IL-2 stimulated cells then become capable of killing first trimester EVT (Fig. 8.3) and JEG-3 choriocarcinoma cells (King and Loke 1990). In a similar study by Ferry *et al.* (1991), some slight killing of BeWo choriocarcinoma cells by IL-2 stimulated decidual effectors was observed, but chorionic plate term trophoblast was not killed. The different gestational age and source of the trophoblast used may explain these conflicting findings. First trimester extravillous trophoblast is obviously the most relevant target for activated decidual NK cells *in vivo*. It is not surprising that normally most trophoblast cells escape killing by maternal NK cells, but whether occasional overexuberant cells are lysed is unknown. This has been suggested to occur in mice (Stewart and Mukhtar 1988). It can be concluded that decidual NK cells do have the *potential* to kill trophoblast when appropriately activated by IL-2 or other cytokines. A powerful defensive system is thus in place for protecting the mother, but the circumstances when it is used are unclear.

NK recognition of target cells

Despite intensive research, it has been difficult to define both the receptors used by NK cells and the ligands on target cells, in contrast to what is known about T cells (Fig. 8.4). Nonetheless, several general principles are emerging (Moretta *et al.* 1994b; Trinchieri 1994; Yokoyama 1995):

(1) The appearance of NK cells in SCID mice and in recombination activating gene (RAG) deficient mice suggests that NK receptors do not require gene rearrangement for expression and function (Hackett *et al.* 1986; Shinkai *et al.* 1992). Instead, NK cells are likely to use several receptor systems in one cell, rather than the T cell

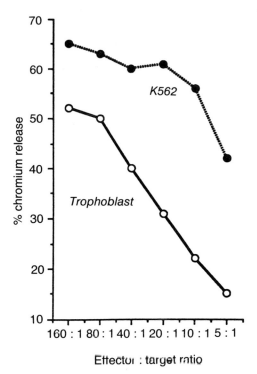

Fig. 8.3. A 4 hour chromium release assay using normal first trimester trophoblast and K562 cells as targets. The effectors were decidual lymphocytes which were cultured with 100 U/ml IL-2 for 5 days. High levels of killing of K562 are seen even at low effector:target ratios (compare with Fig. 8.1). Trophoblast cells are killed by these activated decidual lymphocytes.

system where each different T cell expresses one variant of only one receptor system. Thus NK cell heterogeneity probably arises from the combination of several NK receptors expressed, in complete contrast to the exquisite specificity conferred by the T cell receptor alone.

(2) Although specific receptors used in a certain situation are undefined, both stimulation and inhibition dictate the lytic activity of the NK cell. A balance between positive and negative signals received by different receptors influences the behaviour of the NK cell.

(3) Carbohydrates were proposed to have a role in NK cell recognition several years ago (McCoy and Chambers 1991), and this has always been an attractive proposition because of the observed changes in cell surface glycoconjugates in tumour cells (Feizi 1985). Proteins of the C-type lectin family, characterised by the presence of a carbohydrate-recognition domain (CRD), have been found expressed on NK cells in mice, rats and man (Chambers *et al.* 1993; Yabe *et al.* 1993; Yokoyama and Seaman 1993). NKR-P1, found on rodent NK cells, binds to several oligosaccharide ligands and this interaction leads to activation of the lytic machinery of the NK cells

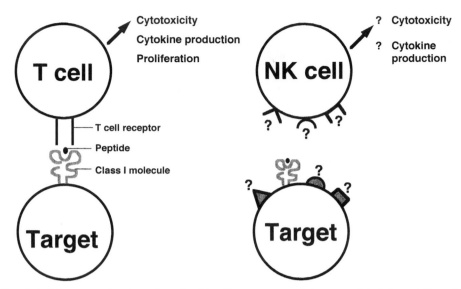

Fig. 8.4. Diagram showing that the T cell receptor and its associated target ligand are known, but the equivalent structures for NK cells have not been established.

(Bezouška *et al.* 1994). The multispecificity for oligosaccharides is a feature of other endogenous lectins (e.g. selectins). The highest affinities of NKR-P1 are towards the acidic oligosaccharides derived from heparin and chondroitin sulphate. Of interest is that lower-affinity binding to α2-3-linked sialic acid on Lewis^a and Lewis^x was observed. Sialyl-Le^x has been shown to be expressed by extravillous trophoblast, particularly endovascular trophoblast (King and Loke 1988) (Fig. 8.5). Clearly the identification of possible NK carbohydrate ligands on trophoblast will be an important line to pursue.

(4) There is now general acceptance that MHC class I molecules on target cells profoundly influence NK function and generally provide an inhibitory signal to the NK cell (Kärre 1993). Thus the possibility that decidual NK cells could recognise and be influenced by trophoblast class I molecules becomes very attractive, and this must be one of the most important and interesting hypotheses to test at the present time.

NK cells preferentially kill target cells which have low or absent class I MHC expression. This is predominantly a feature of haematopoietic target cells, but can be seen with solid tumour cells and even normal cells both *in vivo* and *in vitro* (Trinchieri 1994). This finding led to the 'missing self' hypothesis which postulated that NK cells eliminated cells not expressing class I molecules (Ljunggren and Kärre 1990). NK cells are thus operating in exactly the opposite manner to T cells, which kill cells expressing self-MHC molecules associated with non-self peptides. The missing self hypothesis required some modification when it became clear that distinct NK clones could discriminate between different

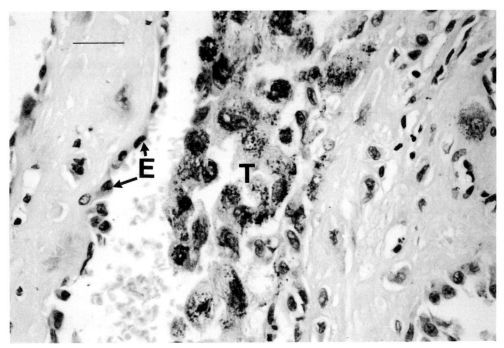

Fig. 8.5. An artery from the decidual basalis in the first trimester lined by both endovascular trophoblast (T) and by endothelial cells (E). The section is immunostained for sialyl-Le^x which is expressed strongly in the endovascular trophoblast. (Obj × 25)

class I alleles. There is thus a higher degree of functional complexity than originally expected. The mechanism of class I recognition by NK cells has been explained by two hypotheses (Fig. 8.6): (a) the effector inhibition theory which postulates that the presence of class I will deliver a negative signal to NK cells, or (b) the target interference hypothesis which postulates that class I molecules mask target ligands that stimulate NK lysis (Raulet 1992; Kärre 1993; Moretta *et al.* 1994b). Currently, the effector inhibition theory is more favoured. If MHC class I molecules were to block NK cell recognition of target cells, then early cell signalling events should be inhibited. Kaufman *et al.* (1993) could find no decrease in phosphoinositide turnover or calcium signalling after NK cells interacted with class I molecules, indicating that these molecules can initiate inhibitory signals in NK cells without blocking access to target structures. NK cytolytic function in any particular situation represents a balance between complex stimulatory and inhibitory signals and, although class I MHC molecules are only one target ligand, in general it appears that class I mediated inhibition will overrule other stimulatory signals (Correa *et al.* 1994). The molecular mechanisms of MHC-mediated protection could be unravelled by identifying the receptors on NK cells that can monitor variation in MHC.

Models for Class I protection against NK lysis

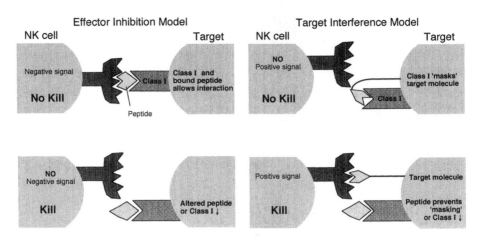

Fig. 8.6. Possible mechanisms of class I recognition by NK cells.

To date, several putative NK receptors have been found in both humans and rodents. Some receptors recognise class I target ligands, but other target ligands have not yet been defined. The first receptor identified was Ly-49 which is present on a subset of murine NK cells (Karlhofer *et al.* 1992). Ly-49+ cells do not kill target cells expressing H-2D^d or H-2D^k and Ly-49 binds directly to the α_1/α_2 domains of the class I molecule with a negative signal then being delivered to the NK cell (Daniels *et al.* 1994a). The protein is a homodimer of two 44 kDa subunits, and is a type II integral membrane protein expressing an extracellular domain with similarities to the carbohydrate recognition domain (CRD) of C-type (Ca^{2+}-dependent) animal lectins (Yokoyama *et al.* 1989, 1990). Ly-49 is part of a multigene family of genetically linked loci, termed the NK gene complex, on mouse chromosome 6. The original Ly-49 isolate is now designated Ly-49A as several novel Ly-49 cDNAs have recently been cloned which appear to be derived from distinct genes. These NK cell antigens bind to different repertoires of MHC class I molecules (Brennan *et al.* 1994; Smith *et al.* 1994). Interestingly, another member of this C-type lectin family, NKR-P1, structurally related to Ly-49, activates NK activity in contrast to the inhibitory signal delivered by Ly-49. Ligands for NKR-P1 have now been identified to be oligosaccharides (Bezouška *et al.* 1994). NK-associated antigens with similar type II membrane protein structure have been demonstrated in humans suggesting an NK gene complex is also present (Table 8.1). These include CD69 (López-Cabrera *et al.* 1993), the NKG2 gene cluster (Yabe *et al.* 1993; Chambers *et al.* 1993) and NKR-PIA (Lanier *et al.* 1994). Ligands for CD69, and the NKG2 and NKR-PIA

Table 8.1. *Recently described human NK cell receptors*

Name	Structure	Ligand	Comment	Reference
NKB1	70 kDa glycoprotein	HLA-B alleles Bw4	–	Litwin *et al* (1994)
Kp43 (CD94)	Disulphide-linked homodimer	HLA-B alleles Bw6	Structurally related to murine Ly-49 family	Moretta *et al.* (1994a)
p58	p58 kDa homo/ heterodimer associated with CD3ζ chain	HLA-C alleles	Defined by Mabs GL183 and EB6	Moretta *et al.* (1993)
NKG2	C-type lectin	?	Defined by cDNA cloning only	Yabe *et al.* (1993)
NKR-PIA	C-type lectin	?	Homologue of rodent NKRP-1 which recognises carbohydrates	Lanier *et al.* (1994)
CD69	C-type lectin	?	Expression is not restricted to NK cells	López-Cabrera *et al.* (1993)

gene products are unknown, but there is no evidence to date that they recognise HLA class I molecules.

Recently, several human NK receptors with different molecular structures which do recognise HLA Class I molecules have been identified (Trinchieri 1994; Yokoyama 1995) (Table 8.1). Kp43 (CD94) has been shown to be the receptor on human NK clones for certain HLA-B alleles (Moretta *et al.* 1994a). The HLA-B alleles (HLA-B7, -B8 and -B14) recognised by Kp43 belong to the supertypic specificity Bw6, but another recently recognised NK receptor recognises a different set of HLA-B alleles (HLA-B*5101 and -B*5801) of supertypic specificity Bw4 (Litwin *et al.* 1994). This receptor NKB1 is a 70 kDa glycoprotein which is still poorly characterised. The finding that human NK receptors for class I MHC molecules have broad specificity may partially explain the difficulty in recognising simple patterns of HLA recognition when multiple HLA alleles are used (Litwin *et al.* 1993). A third set of clonally heterogenous NK receptors to HLA-C alleles leads to a similar conclusion. This 58 kDa family of molecules, termed p58, present on NK clones is recognised by Mabs EB6 and GL183, and is non-covalently linked to the CD3ζ chain (Moretta *et al.* 1993).

Using HLA-C transfectants it appears that HLA-C alleles specifically inhibit lysis depending on dimorphism at positions 77–80. Thus, two groups of NK clones (NK1 and NK2) specifically recognising either Cw4 and related alleles, or Cw3 and related alleles were defined (Colonna *et al*. 1993). A third group of NK clones, NK3, was generated which recognises HLA-Bw4 but not HLA-Bw6 allotypes (Cella *et al*. 1994). Similar to the HLA-C alleles, these HLA-B alleles show a polymorphism at residues 77–83 although the differences are more complex than those found in HLA-C. Only HLA-Bw4 alleles with isoleucine at position 80 were inhibitory to NK3 clones. It remains to be seen if the receptor on these NK3 clones is the same as NKB1 identified by Litwin *et al*. (1994) which also recognises HLA-Bw4 alleles (see above).

A more public and probably primordial polymorphism of the class I alleles seems to be used by NK cells, compared with the fine specificity of T cells. This is further supported by the observation that ancestral MHC haplotypes maintained *en bloc* from remote ancestors define NK allospecificities (Christiansen *et al*. 1993). Additional NK receptors for other class I molecules are likely to be found. To summarise, at present it appears that NK cells have generated receptor diversity by using several receptors of different molecular structure rather than somatic recombination as used by T and B cells. Different combinations of these receptors on NK cells will give a NK repertoire capable of recognising both major changes in conformation or level of surface expression of class I molecules and other still undefined target ligands.

MHC molecules are generally present on the cell surface in association with β_2-microglobulin (β_2m) with a peptide lodged in the groove. Which part of this tri-partite molecule does the NK cell recognise? There are several possibilities:

(1) Several lines of evidence point to the α_1/α_2 domains and the peptide binding groove in the modulation of NK sensitivity, but it is still unclear whether the peptide and the binding region are recognised directly or whether indirect effects such as conformational changes are important. Experimental manipulations affecting the peptide and the antigen binding groove by either single amino acid substitutions of the class I molecules, or alteration of endogenous peptide by feeding exogenous peptides, are found to modulate target cell sensitivity to natural killing, giving rise to suggestions that the nature of the peptide may affect NK recognition (Kärre 1993). However, no difference was observed at the C-terminal position 9 of peptides isolated from the two dimorphic variants of HLA-C that determine resistance to NK1 and NK2 clones (Falk *et al*. 1993). Perhaps neither the groove nor the peptide is directly involved and the effects seen with exogenous peptides are a reflection of how the contents of the groove affect the structure of the whole molecule. Similarly, cell lines with a defect in the mechanisms for transport and loading endogenous peptide into class I MHC molecules are NK sensitive *in vivo* and *in vitro*, but this effect may be secondary to the reduced levels of surface expression of class I molecules

(Kärre 1993; Salcedo *et al.* 1994). More recently, a direct role for peptides complexed with class I molecules in providing protection from NK-mediated lysis has been suggested (Kärre 1995). In a study with a human NK cell clone, only one of several self peptides bound to HLA-B27 conferred protection against lysis (Malnati *et al.* 1995). In contrast, in a murine system, virtually all H-2D^d binding peptides protected target cells against a Ly-49$^+$ NK cell subset (Correa and Raulet 1995). Perhaps some NK cell receptors can recognise the class I molecule itself while others require the presence of a specific self peptide.

(2) MHC molecules can occur on the surface of cells either associated with β_2m or in the form of free heavy chains which can occur as a dimer (Bix and Raulet 1992; Carreno and Hansen 1994). The equilibrium between free heavy chains and the β_2m-associated form can be modified by incubating cells with exogenous β_2m. Experiments where the β_2m-associated complex on target cells was increased after exposure to exogenous β_2m resulted in loss of NK protection, suggesting that free heavy chains were the important elements conferring protection (Carbone *et al.* 1993). However, in another study, acid treatment of target cells which results in loss of β_2m with retention of the free heavy chains (Polakova *et al.* 1993), the opposite result was found indicating that NK resistance required the presence of the β_2m-associated molecule (Ciccone *et al.* 1994a). This question therefore needs clarification.

(3) Soluble forms of the class I molecule may block NK cytotoxicity by binding to appropriate NK receptors and inhibit lysis without a requirement for cell contact (Roth *et al.* 1994). Soluble forms of HLA-G have been identified in trophoblast (Kovats *et al.* 1990; Fujii *et al.* 1994).

(4) As discussed previously, many NK-associated molecules have a CRD so there is a possibility that the recognition site on class I MHC molecules is a carbohydrate. Studies using tunicamycin, which inhibits the formation of N-linked carbohydrates, showed inhibition of binding of Ly-49 to H-2D^d (Daniels *et al.* 1994b). The carbohydrate motif is highly conserved at position 87 which is close to the region of the class I molecule which affects NK sensitivity (Parham 1994b). In addition, the peptide itself may be glycosylated and since glycopeptide can elicit a specific CTL response this might also alter NK recognition (Haurum *et al.* 1994).

In summary, the exact nature of NK–MHC recognition remains elusive despite growing evidence that NK cell function is modulated (in many systems but by no means all) by the presence of class I proteins. NK cells do not lyse autologous normal cells expressing a full complement of self MHC alleles. How the NK repertoire is 'educated' is a mystery, but seems at least to be partly determined by self-MHC alleles. Self-reactive NK cells expressing low levels of Ly-49 are present *in vivo*. Experiments using MHC-congenic mice have shown that this is due to downregulation of the receptor after interaction with specific host MHC class I molecules (Karlhofer *et al.* 1994). The regulatory mechanism, therefore, is distinct from the negative selection of self-reactive T cells, which results in permanent deletion.

Apart from the lack of a clonally distributed receptor generated by gene rearrangement, NK cells do show resemblance to γδ T cells. As for NK cells it has been hard to define the general rules for γδ T cell recognition. There is a fundamental difference in the way αβ T cells and γδ T cells recognise antigen. Although class I molecules (including non-classical molecules) can be involved in γδ T cell recognition, the site of interaction is at the side of the MHC molecule away from the peptide binding groove (Schild *et al.* 1994). Furthermore, there is no evidence that peptides bound to class I molecules are involved in recognition (Weintraub *et al.* 1994). Other MHC-like molecules (such as heat-shock proteins) or structurally unrelated carbohydrate antigens may also act as ligands. These features are reminiscent of recent findings from NK cells but are obviously not characteristic of αβ T cells. γδ T cells are also found in surface locations similar to NK cells. Possibly γδ T cells and NK cells play a similar role in immunity that is different from classical αβ T cells.

Decidual NK cell recognition of trophoblast HLA class I antigen

Trophoblast class I molecules might be one recognition system used by decidual NK cells to prevent destruction of placental cells by NK cells. Perturbations in the surface levels of HLA-G/HLA-C due to factors such as the availability of peptide, or the activation state of decidual NK cells, could influence trophoblast sensitivity to lysis.

The data supporting this hypothesis are still rather limited. Pre-treatment of trophoblast target cells with IFN-γ does partially protect the cells from IL-2 stimulated decidual NK cells (King and Loke 1993). IFN-γ increases surface expression of trophoblast class I molecules approximately two-fold (Grabowska *et al.* 1990b), and this could be responsible for protection, particularly as similar resistance to lysis was not induced by IFN-α pre-treatment which has no effect on trophoblast class I expression (Chumbley *et al.* 1991). This is only indirect evidence that trophoblast class I molecules are important. More direct proof has been obtained using class I-deficient cell lines transfected with HLA class I genes. Using polyclonal freshly isolated decidual effectors, HLA-G did provide partial protection, but not as much as was seen with a classical class I gene, HLA-A2 (Chumbley *et al.* 1994b) (Fig. 8.7). Decidual NK clones were the effectors used against HLA-G and HLA-B8 transfectants in another study (Deniz *et al.* 1994). Decreased killing of HLA-G$^+$ cells was found compared with the parent HLA null cells.

Thus, there is some preliminary evidence that decidual NK cells have receptors for HLA-G. Surprisingly, in the report from Deniz *et al.*, HLA-B8 was not protective to either decidual or blood NK clones. As Kp43 is expressed at high

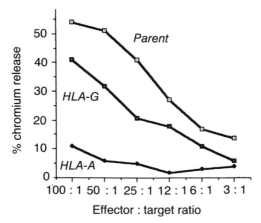

Fig. 8.7. A 4 hour chromium release assay using freshly isolated decidual effector cells at various effector:target ratios. The target cells are LCL.221 HLA-null cells (parent) or LCL.221 cells transfected with class I HLA-G or HLA-A genes. Partial protection from NK cytolysis is provided by HLA-G and significant protection by HLA-A.

levels on decidual NK cells, it would be expected to inhibit cytolysis against HLA-B8 (Litwin *et al.* 1994). The role of the putative trophoblast HLA-C molecule in NK recognition is completely unknown, but there is good evidence that classical NK cells can recognise sets of HLA-C alleles in a clonal manner (see above). It may be that the co-ordinated expression of both HLA-G and HLA-C are required to provide a set of trophoblast HLA class I molecules, which act together for optimal NK recognition in the same way that the full complement of autologous class I molecules provides the best protection against any host NK cell (Ciccone *et al.* 1994b). We have recently observed that HLA-G expressed on the surface of trophoblast is complexed with β_2m while HLA-C appears to be mainly in the form of free heavy chains (Chapter 6). How these molecules interact with decidual NK cells is not known. As yet we also have no idea how NK recognition could modify trophoblast behaviour. The possibility that the signal mediated by NK class I receptors affects not only cytotoxicity but also

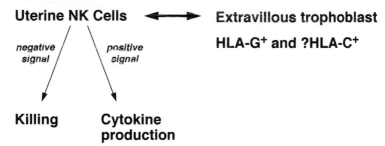

Fig. 8.8. A hypothetical model of the possible outcome of interaction between uterine NK cells and extravillous trophoblast at the implantation site.

cytokine production should be considered (Fig. 8.8). NK cells have been observed to alter their repertoire of cytokine production after contact with a target cell (Trinchieri 1994). This is likely to be a far more relevant effector mechanism by which NK cells can influence trophoblast migration and differentiation.

Cytokine production by NK cells

NK cells are known to produce a variety of cytokines, but most of the evidence reported to date has been obtained *in vitro*. The stimuli inducing NK cytokine production and the relative importance of these cytokines in physiological and pathological states have been difficult to ascertain. There is evidence that NK cells produce cytokines upon binding to recognisable cell types and may contribute to bone marrow haematopoiesis. NK cells may mediate a variety of homeostatic functions and regulate activity of many cell types by cytokines. In these situations, NK cell targets are generally rapidly proliferating and differentiating cells. The cycling endometrium and trophoblast cells at the implantation site are also both rapidly proliferating and differentiating. Furthermore, several cytokine receptors have been identified on extravillous trophoblast and on cells in the decidua such as macrophages and glandular epithelial cells (Chapter 10). Classical NK cells are known to produce a variety of cytokines such as TNF-α, IFN-γ, GM-CSF, CSF-1 and TGF-β so it is pertinent to ask under what situations they might be produced by decidual NK cells. As a first step to screen for which cytokines are expressed by maternal decidual lymphocytes, the reverse-transcriptase polymerase chain reaction (RT-PCR) has been used to look for cytokine mRNAs in highly purified CD56$^+$ and CD3$^+$ decidual lymphocytes (Chapter 10). In the studies using this technique, G-CSF, GM-CSF, CSF-1, TNF-α, LIF, IL-8 and IFN-γ mRNA were detected in CD56^{bright} CD16$^-$ cells (Saito *et al.* 1993c, 1994a; Jokhi *et al.* 1994d). IL-1β, IL-2, IL-3, IL-4, IL-5 and IL-6 mRNAs were looked for but were not found. This repertoire was different from those produced by circulating NK cells. Protein production has now been assayed by both ELISAs and/or bioassays for many of these cytokines (Saito *et al.* 1993c; Jokhi 1994). The main products produced *in vitro* are GM-CSF and CSF-1. IL-2, IL-7 and IL-12 have been shown to induce different patterns of cytokine expression in blood CD56$^+$ NK cells, indicating that specific stimuli activating NK cells may alter their biological role (Naume *et al.* 1993). Indeed, NK cells may both positively and negatively regulate haematopoiesis. It would be interesting to establish whether trophoblast can similarly alter the cytokine repertoire of uterine CD56^{bright} cells. It would also be pertinent to investigate the effect of NK cell cytokines on extravillous trophoblast, as well as on other cells in the placental bed, particularly macrophages which express many of the receptors for decidual NK cell cytokines.

9

Trophoblast interaction with extracellular matrix

Introduction

At the site of implantation, placental trophoblast cells undergo a series of transformations. Cytotrophoblast cells surrounding chorionic villi occur as a single, polarised epithelial layer resting on basement membrane (villous trophoblast). At the tips of anchoring villi clumps of trophoblast cells form into non-polarised cellular aggregates (trophoblast columns and shell) from which individual cells (interstitial trophoblast) eventually disperse to invade uterine decidua. On histological sections, many interstitial trophoblast cells are observed to have elongated morphology resembling mesenchymal cells, and we have previously reported the acquisition of mesenchymal characteristics by these cells, such as expression of vimentin microfilaments and production of the enzyme leucine amino-peptidase (Loke and Butterworth 1987). The concept of epithelial to mesenchymal transition is well established in embryogenesis (Hay 1991), and in malignant transformation (Birchmeier and Birchmeier 1994). In functional terms, the change from villous to extravillous trophoblast is a transformation from a sessile to a motile phenotype. In many biological systems, cell migration is dependent on adhesion to extracellular matrix (ECM) proteins for anchorage and traction (Fleming 1991; Hynes 1992). For example, the physiological migration of neural crest cells during embryonic development or that of epithelial cells in wound healing, as well as pathological invasion of cancer cells, all require cell–matrix interaction (Ruoslahti and Pierschbacher 1987; Hynes and Lander 1992; Albelda 1993; Grinnell 1992, 1994). In addition to mediating adhesion, matrix also imparts signals for growth and differentiation (Hay 1991).

Thus, it is now widely accepted that a cell's behaviour is controlled not only by its developmental lineage but also by the extracellular material surrounding it, so that a functional unit in higher organisms has been defined as the cell plus its ECM (Lin and Bissell 1993). It is likely that ECM binding to specific transmembrane receptors could also affect the pathways of other regulators of

151

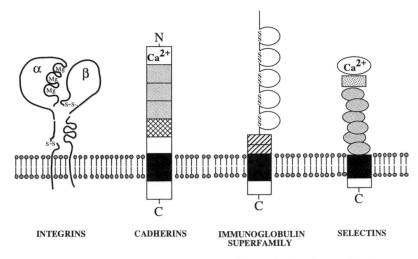

Fig. 9.1. Basic structures of the four major families of adhesion molecules.

cellular function, such as growth factors and hormones, resulting in significant influence on cell behaviour. Accumulating evidence indicates that trophoblast behaviour during implantation may similarly be influenced by the ECM proteins in decidua (Graham and Lala 1992).

Integrins as receptors for extracellular matrix

Cells bind to ECM proteins by appropriate cell surface receptors called adhesion molecules (Hynes 1994). Fig. 9.1 shows the basic structures of the four families of adhesion molecules. Of these, the main receptors which mediate adhesion to ECM are the integrins (Hynes 1992; Kühn and Eble 1994). Integrins are transmembrane glycoproteins consisting of non-covalently associated α and β sub-units. Several α and β subunits have now been identified. Presently, fifteen α subunits and eight β subunits are known and more are likely to be discovered in the future. Both subunits have a large extracellular domain, a transmembrane segment and a cytoplasmic tail. The extracellular domains of both subunits contain calmodulin-type divalent cation-binding sites which serve to explain the divalent cation dependency of integrin function. The cytoplasmic portions of the β subunit are relatively short sequences, ranging from ~40 to 60 amino acids in length, with the exception of β_4 which has 1000 amino acids. The primary sequences of β subunit cytoplasmic domains are highly conserved through evolution, showing 100% homology between human, avian, murine and amphibian sequences. Individual β subunit cytoplasmic domains also share sequence similarities. Like the β subunit, the α subunit cytoplasmic sequences are also highly conserved among different species but, interestingly, show little homology between the subunits themselves in contrast to the findings with the β subunit. These observations suggest that the α and β subunit cytoplasmic domains may have unique functions. The cytoplasmic portions interact with components of the cytoskeleton and this interaction is probably regulated by phosphorylation of the β subunit cytoplasmic tail. In this way, signals are transmitted from the ECM into the cell.

The ligand specificity of the heterodimer is determined by the combination of the various α and β subunits. For example, $\alpha_1\beta_1$ and $\alpha_6\beta_4$ are both receptors for the ECM protein laminin, whereas $\alpha_5\beta_1$, $\alpha_4\beta_1$ and $\alpha_4\beta_7$ bind fibronectin (Ruoslahti and Pierschbacher 1987; Yamada 1989; Dedhar 1990; Albelda and Buck 1990; Hynes 1992). However, it should be pointed out that many integrins are promiscuous and are capable of binding to several different ligands, and the reverse is also the case in that individual ligands can be recognised by more than one integrin (Hynes 1992). In addition, the same integrin on different cell types will bind to different ligands, demonstrating a degree of tissue regulation of integrin specificity. The $\alpha_6\beta_4$ heterodimer also binds to other components of the lamina lucida of the basement membrane, such as the proteoglycan 19-DEJ-1 and the trimeric protein BM600 (Legan *et al.* 1992).

The recognition site for many integrins is the tripeptide arginine-glycine-aspartic acid, or RGD sequence in molecular nomenclature, which is present in a large number of ECM proteins including fibronectin, type I collagen, vitronectin, tenascin, laminin and entactin. Evidence for the role of the RGD sequence is derived from making progressively smaller fragments of ECM proteins which can promote cell adhesion, and then constructing synthetic peptides which will simulate these properties. Synthetic peptides containing the RGD sequence will also compete with ECM proteins for their receptors. Changes in these peptides, such as replacing arginine with a lysine residue, alanine for glycine or glutamic acid for aspartic acid will all eliminate the binding properties of the peptides. Conformation of the RGD sequence within the protein may be important in determining its receptor specificity, which could explain why various ECM proteins bind to different integrins despite their shared RGD sequence. Besides the RGD sequence, other binding sites have also been identified, such as the GPEILDVPST sequence which is the target sequence for the $\alpha_4\beta_1$ integrin present in one of the alternatively spliced segments of fibronectin.

Integrins not only bind cells to matrix, but they also help to shape the matrix around the cell. Thus, the assembly of fibronectin requires the expression of $\alpha_5\beta_1$ integrins by the cell although the precise molecular mechanisms of this matrix assembly are not known. Possibly integrin–matrix interaction initiates subsequent steps of fibronectin–fibronectin binding followed by fibronectin–fibronectin cross-linking resulting in the deposition of a pericellular layer of insoluble fibronectin which is the functional form of this ECM protein.

The concept that cell adhesion molecules act as signalling receptors is now well accepted (Juliano and Haskill 1993). However, extracellular ligand-induced signalling through integrins does not follow the same pathway as for classical signalling receptors such as growth factor receptors (Sastry and Horwitz 1993). Integrin cytoplasmic domains do not possess intrinsic kinase or phosphatase activities so they have to interact either directly or indirectly with cellular initiators of signalling cascades such as the tyrosine kinases in order to transmit message into the cell. The recently discovered novel cytosolic tyrosine kinase, called focal adhesion kinase (pp125^{FAK}), present in abundance in adhesion plaques could be the tyrosine kinase involved (Schaller and Parsons 1994). The substrates for FAK include tensin and paxillin, two adhesion plaque proteins whose phosphorylation leads to cytoplasmic signalling to the nucleus. Integrin-mediated tyrosine phosphorylation of FAK occurs within 30 seconds of adhesion to fibronectin and remains high as long as the cells are adherent (Williams and Kieffer 1994). Integrin binding to ECM may expose a FAK-binding site within the integrin cytoplasmic domain leading to enzymic activation (Schaller and Parsons 1994). Phosphorylation of FAK can be triggered by β_1, β_2 and β_3 integrin subunits. Experiments with synthetic peptides mimicking the cytoplasmic domains of these subunits have shown that binding occurs primarily via the highly conserved, membrane proximal 13 amino acids, and this region appears to bind directly to the amino-terminal non-catalytic domain of FAK. In addition to binding to FAK, the cytoplasmic portion of integrins can provide a direct physical link between the ECM and the cytoskeleton. The β_1 subunit of integrins has been observed to interact directly with talin and α-actinin. A diagrammatic representation of possible intracellular pathways of integrin-mediated signalling is shown in Fig. 9.2. Thus, it can be seen that integrins are not merely receptors which a cell uses for anchorage or migration over its surrounding matrix, but are central to our understanding of how a cell detects and responds to signals from its external environment.

Expression of integrins by trophoblast

We and others have investigated the expression of integrins by different populations of trophoblast using immunohistological staining of tissue sections of the implantation site with Mabs directed against various integrin subunits (Korhonen *et al.* 1991; Damsky *et al.* 1992; Burrows *et al.* 1993a). The

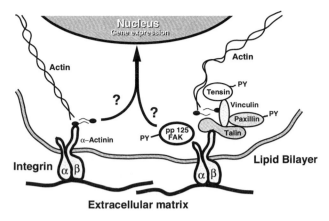

Fig. 9.2. Possible intracellular pathways of integrin-mediated signalling.

overall conclusion is that the layer of villous cytotrophoblast expresses the $\alpha_6\beta_4$ heterodimer (Fig. 9.3). This integrin remains on cytotrophoblast cells of the cell columns nearest the villous core, but is no longer present further out in the cell columns. These latter trophoblast cells together with interstitial trophoblast which has invaded decidua are observed to express the $\alpha_5\beta_1$ heterodimer. Thus, there appears to be a progressive downregulation of the $\alpha_6\beta_4$ laminin receptor with a concomitant upregulation of the $\alpha_5\beta_1$ fibronectin receptor as trophoblast is transformed from a sessile to a motile phenotype. In addition to the α_5 subunit, interstitial trophoblast has also been reported to express the α_1 and α_6 subunits although no other β subunits have been detected, so it is possible that these migrating trophoblast cells may express additional heterodimers coupled to β_1 besides $\alpha_5\beta_1$ such as $\alpha_1\beta_1$ and $\alpha_6\beta_1$ (Damsky *et al.* 1992; Burrows *et al.* 1993a) (Table 9.1).

The $\alpha_6\beta_4$ laminin receptor is widely distributed among epithelial cells, where it functions to anchor the cells to the underlying basement membrane (Sonnenberg *et al.* 1990). A similar role may be postulated for this integrin in villous trophoblast because laminin is the major component of the chorionic villous basement membrane. As referred to earlier, β_4 is unusual among β subunits in having a relatively long cytoplasmic domain. This could provide a stable anchor by interacting with trophoblast intracellular filaments. Interestingly, Aplin (1993) has observed $\alpha_6\beta_4$ also at the interface between villous trophoblast and syncytiotrophoblast, which seems to suggest that this integrin may function in cell–cell as well as cell–basement membrane interaction. Although $\alpha_6\beta_4$ is eventually lost as trophoblast migrates into decidua, this integrin is, nevertheless, still present in the proximal portion of the cytotrophoblast columns nearest the chorionic villi. This implies that the sequence of events is the loss of $\alpha_6\beta_4$

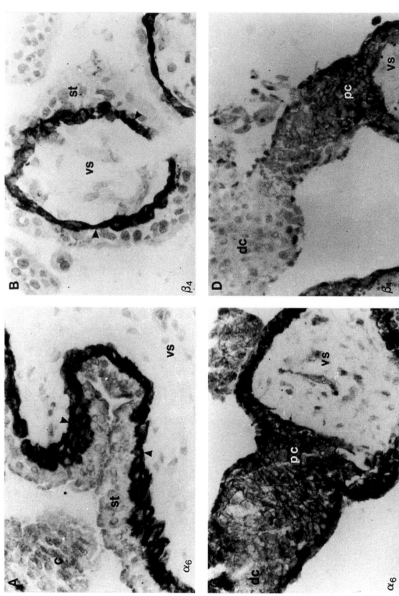

Fig. 9.3. Frozen sections of first trimester chorionic villi stained with Mabs to the α_6 and β_4 integrin subunits. A. The α_6 subunit is strongly expressed by villous cytotrophoblast (arrowheads), but not by the overlying syncytiotrophoblast (st), attached piece of cell column (c) and villous stroma (vs). B. The β_4 subunit is similarly expressed by the villous cytotrophoblast only (arrowheads). C. The α_6 subunit is expressed by cells of the proximal part of the cell column (pc) but there is a reduced expression by cells of the distal part of the cell column (dc). D. The β_4 subunit is also expressed by cells of the proximal part of the column (pc), but there is a complete loss of expression by cells of the distal column (dc). (Obj × 25)

Table 9.1. *Immunohistological analysis of integrins expressed by first trimester trophoblast*

Integrin subunit	Villous syncytio-trophoblast	Villous cytotro-phoblast	Proximal column	Distal column	Interstitial trophoblast	Endovascular trophoblast
α_1	−	−	−	+	+	+
α_2	−	−	+	−	−	−
α_3	−	−	−	−	−	−
α_4	−	−	−	−	−	−
α_5	−	−	−	+	+	+
α_6	−	++	+	+	+	−
α_v	−	−	−	+	?	?
β_1	−	−	−	+	+	+
β_4	−	++	+	−	−	−

following trophoblast migration, rather than the downregulation of this integrin initiating the onset of migration by detaching trophoblast from the basement membrane.

The acquisition of the $\alpha_5\beta_1$ fibronectin receptor by migrating interstitial trophoblast closely parallels that seen in the healing of a skin wound where $\alpha_6\beta_4$-positive sessile keratinocytes forming the normal epithelial surface are transformed into $\alpha_5\beta_1$-positive motile cells which migrate over the gap in the wound onto a substrate of fibronectin produced in the wound matrix. Fibronectin and its receptors are also implicated in various cell migrations during embryonic development. Thus, the expression of the $\alpha_5\beta_1$ fibronectin receptor appears to be associated with cell motility. The $\alpha_1\beta_1$ and $\alpha_6\beta_1$ heterodimers (which are also expressed by interstitial trophoblast) are generally considered to be laminin receptors so a variety of additional signals are likely to be transmitted to migrating trophoblast. There is evidence that integrin subunits may also occur in variant forms. The laminin receptor expressed by murine embryonic stem cells consists of a novel isoform of α_6 whose cytoplasmic domain differs significantly in amino acid sequence from that normally reported for other cells (Cooper *et al.* 1991). This increases the complexity of integrin–matrix interaction.

Zhou *et al.* (1993) recently reported that invading trophoblast within the placental bed of pre-eclamptic patients fails both to downregulate β_4 and to upregulate α_1 integrin subunits, as seen in normal pregnancy, indicating that there is disregulation of these adhesion molecules in this pathological condition (Fig. 9.4). A characteristic of pre-eclampsia is inadequate or shallow invasion of decidua and its spiral arteries by trophoblast, so one possible explanation is that the expression of appropriate adhesion molecules is required for the correct

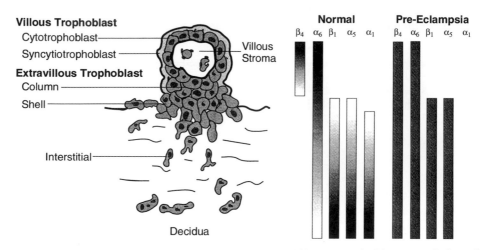

Fig. 9.4. The changes in integrin expression by different trophoblast populations in normal pregnancy and in pre-eclampsia. The main differences described to date are failure to downregulate the β_4 subunit expression and to upregulate α_1 subunit expression by invading trophoblast in pre-eclampsia.

degree of trophoblast invasiveness. What factors determine the switch from one integrin to another as trophoblast changes from villous to extravillous phenotype are not known. Other diseases besides pre-eclampsia, such as intrauterine growth retardation, are also characterised by shallow trophoblast invasion. Further delineation of trophoblast integrin expression in pathological pregnancies should be very rewarding.

We have observed that trophoblast adhesion to fibronectin *in vitro* can be inhibited by Mabs to the α_5 and β_1 integrin subunits as well as by synthetic RGD peptides in a dose-dependent manner (Burrows 1994). Similarly, trophoblast adhesion to laminin is inhibited by Mabs to α_1, α_6 and β_1 subunits. These observations provide supporting evidence that these particular integrin heterodimers could be the ones involved in trophoblast–matrix interaction *in vivo*. In addition, we have noted that trophoblast cells, in the absence of serum, will adhere only to laminin and not to fibronectin (Burrows *et al.* 1993a). Similar findings have been reported for isolated skin keratinocytes where adhesion to fibronectin is dependent on exposure of the cells to certain unknown serum factors (Kim and Grinnell 1990; Grinnell 1992). Expression of integrin receptors, therefore, does not necessarily imply that they are fully functional. Many need to be activated (Mercurio and Shaw 1991; Hynes and Lander 1992) and trophoblast fibronectin receptors could require such activation. Furthermore, the activation and deactivation of integrins are dynamic processes which allow a cell to alternate between adhesive and non-adhesive states. This regulation of adhesion will provide a mechanism whereby integrin molecules at the leading edge of a cell could be activated to bind ligand while those at the trailing edge are deactivated, allowing detachment and retraction. In this way, cell migration can proceed (Diamond and Springer 1994). The difference between an adhesive or a non-adhesive phenotype appears to be correlated with either a quantitative or a qualitative change in integrin molecules. There are Mabs now available that can recognise neoepitopes on activated integrin molecules, implying that structural or conformational changes do occur (Diamond and Springer 1994). Such alterations could modulate the affinity of the integrin to its ligand. Thus, the expression of fibronectin receptors by migrating trophobast is only one step towards their acquisition of the relevant function. It would be important now to determine the signal responsible for their activation.

Recently, Moss *et al.* (1994) demonstrated that the β_1 integrin from first trimester trophoblast, in contrast to that from term trophoblast, exhibited high levels of polylactosamine-containing oligosaccharides, indicating a temporal control of this glycosylation. The functional implication of this finding is unclear. The most interesting possibility would be that the polylactosamine residues would enable trophoblast to interact with lectin-like molecules on other cells. The discovery that one member of the NK lectin family in rats, NKR-P1, can bind oligosaccharides (Bezouška *et al.* 1994) (Chapter 8) could be a mechanism whereby NK cells interact with trophoblast, thus conferring an additional role for trophoblast integrin molecules.

Trophoblast expression of other integrin subunits may also be relevant to function. By immunohistology, we have observed that trophoblast of the cell columns weakly expresses the α_v subunit (Burrows 1994). The α_v subunit is promiscuous and can form heterodimers with numerous β subunits, such as β_1 and β_3, which bind to several ligands (e.g. vitronectin and fibronectin). Expression of α_v is associated with the acquisition of invasive properties of melanoma cells and ligands for the $\alpha_v\beta_3$ integrin enhance tumour cell migration, so this subunit could similarly facilitate trophoblast migration (Albelda 1993; Seftor *et al.* 1992).

The cytotrophoblast cells at the base of the columns express the α_2 integrin subunit. This is an area where many mitotic trophoblast cells are found. This is in accord with other cell systems where $\alpha_2\beta_1$ is observed to be expressed strongly by proliferating cells at the periphery of a wound site and also by aggressive melanoma cells (Albelda 1993).

Our laboratory has recently investigated tyrosine phosphorylation of proteins in trophoblast after binding to laminin or fibronectin using Western blotting with a Mab to phosphotyrosine residues (Burrows 1994). We found that the predominant tyrosine phosphorylated protein in trophoblast after adhesion to both laminin or fibronectin was a 115 kDa protein together with a weaker 125 kDa band. This is consistent with the observations of Guan *et al.* (1991) who documented tyrosine phosphorylated proteins between 115 and 130 kDa in NIH/ 3T3 fibroblasts after binding to fibronectin. We have also observed that ligation of integrin subunits by Mabs to α_5 or β_1 resulted in similar bands of 125 kDa and 115 kDa tyrosine phosphorylated proteins. Clustering of β_1 integrins with anti-β_1 Mab has been reported to increase tyrosine phosphorylation of proteins between 115 and 130 kDa in fibroblasts and ligation of α_4 integrin subunit with Mabs has also been shown to stimulate tyrosine phosphorylation in human B cells (Kornberg *et al.* 1991; Freedman *et al.* 1993). Thus, trophoblast interaction with ECM via integrins appears to lead to activation of similar signal transduction pathways that are utilised by other cells.

Earlier in this chapter the role of paxillin as a substrate for FAK protein was discussed. Recently, paxillin has been shown also to complex with the proto-oncogene product, pp60[c-src], and triggering of FAK can repress the enzymic activity of pp60[c-src] (Murphy *et al.* 1993; Eck *et al.* 1994; Schaller and Parsons 1994). In the context of trophoblast biology, it is interesting that pp60[c-src] might influence the formation of multinucleated giant cells *in vitro* because inhibition of pp60[c-src] with herbimycin-A prevented this process (Rebut-Bonneton *et al.* 1993). It may be proposed that when trophoblast migrates through decidua, the suppression of pp60[c-src] by integrin-mediated signal transduction from decidual matrix would prevent the premature differentiation into placental bed giant cells. At the decidual–myometrial junction, this signal transduction is interrupted, perhaps by the secretion of tenascin, which has the ability to interfere with cellular adhesion to ECM proteins, thus leading to giant cell formation. This is the site where these cells are particularly numerous *in vivo* in normal pregnancy.

Distribution of extracellular matrix (ECM) proteins in placental bed

Fibronectin (FN)

Changes in the pattern of integrin expression as trophoblast migrates into decidua are accompanied by a parallel alteration of ECM production by these cells. In the proximal portion of the cytotrophoblast columns FN cannot be detected, but it appears in the distal portion of the columns (Earl *et al.* 1990; Damsky *et al.* 1992). Since no other cell types are present in these areas, the FN is likely to be made by trophoblast. This conclusion is supported by *in vitro* observation of cultured extravillous trophoblast synthesising FN (Burrows *et al.* 1993a). Highly migratory cells such as transformed or tumour cells have been described to secrete FN into their immediate surroundings (Humphries *et al.* 1991), and this endogenously produced matrix protein could provide a platform from which invading cancer cells derive the necessary traction for movement. Perhaps a similar mechanism is utilised by migrating trophoblast. The decidual stroma is also rich in FN. Progesterone is reported to be a major stimulant of FN synthesis by non-pregnant endometrial stromal cells *in vitro* (Zhu *et al.* 1992). This increase in biosynthesis is accompanied by an increase in the cellular level of transcription. The stimulation is also dose dependent, which indicates that the induction of FN is mediated through a saturable mechanism, probably via progesterone receptors expressed on endometrial stromal cells. This conclusion is supported by the observation that RU486, which is known to compete with progesterone for binding to its receptor, inhibits progesterone's stimulatory effect on FN synthesis.

Although encoded by only one gene, FN exists in a number of variant forms generated by alternative splicing of its precursor mRNA (Potts and Campbell 1994). This can occur at three sites called ED-A, ED-B and IIICS. The antibodies used by Damsky *et al.* (1992) detected both the ED-A and ED-B isoforms. These FN isoforms are normally found in embryogenesis where they mediate embryonic cell migration (ffrench-Constant and Hynes 1988). Interestingly, there is a reappearance of this embryonic pattern of FN splicing during wound healing in the adult animal where it has been observed that the FN in the wound is ED-A$^+$, ED-B$^+$ while that in normal skin is ED-A$^-$, ED-B$^-$ (ffrench-Constant *et al.* 1989). Further support that trophoblast FN is an embryonic isoform is provided by Feinberg *et al.* (1991b) who used Mab FDC-6 directed at a unique *O*-linked glycosylated hexapeptide within the type III connecting segment of embryonic FN which is not present in adult plasma FN. Thus, it seems that trophoblast migration during implantation together with embryonic cell migration during development and epithelial cell migration during wound healing may all use the same or closely related class of FN as a substrate.

What role FN plays in trophoblast migration is not clear. We have observed that human extravillous trophoblast cells exhibit a totally different morphology when cultured on a substrate of FN compared with laminin, indicating that these two matrix proteins transmit different signals (Burrows *et al.* 1993a). Trophoblast cells on FN display numerous pseudopodia and projections and time lapse photography shows them to be highly motile. There are now many studies in a variety of cellular systems that show the FN receptor family of integrins and its FN ligand are involved in cell migration through a process of motility-driven adhesion. This is probably mediated by localisation of the integrin and cytoplasmic talin at sites of membrane–matrix positive contacts (Mueller and Chen 1991). However, Damsky *et al.* (1994), using an *in vitro* assay of trophoblast invasion into Matrigel, observed the opposite finding that perturbing interactions between FN and the $\alpha_5\beta_1$ receptor accelerated trophoblast migration, whereas interruption of $\alpha_1\beta_1$ binding to laminin/collagen inhibited migration. They, therefore, concluded that laminin/collagen provide the invasion-promoting signal via $\alpha_1\beta_1$ and FN the invasion-restraining signal via $\alpha_5\beta_1$.

Besides influencing cell migration, there is evidence that FN can affect cellular differentiation. *In vitro* experiments with human skin keratinocytes have shown that methylcellulose will stop DNA synthesis and induces expression of involucrin (a marker for terminal differentiation). The addition of FN will inhibit the latter but not the former in a concentration- and time-dependent manner and this is mediated by the $\alpha_5\beta_1$ integrin (Adams and Watt 1989). Thus, in this epithelial system, binding of FN via its receptor can inhibit terminal cell differentiation without affecting DNA synthesis. This is precisely the regulatory mechanism that could explain the findings at the implantation site where the migrating interstitial trophoblast cells no longer show any evidence of proliferative activity as measured by the absence of mitotic figures and of the nuclear proliferation marker Ki-67 (Bulmer *et al.* 1988a), and yet do not become terminally differentiated until they reach the decidual–myometrial zone when they become placental bed giant cells. Indeed, premature terminal differentiation might lead to inadequate trophoblast migration which is the major cause of unsuccessful implantation (Chapter 11). FN could play a crucial role in this process. Signal transduction from ECM mediated by tyrosine phosphorylation of cellular proteins is now a well-recognised phenomenon (Kornberg *et al.* 1991; Juliano and Haskill 1993). It is interesting that we have recently observed increased levels of tyrosine phosphorylation of intracellular proteins in trophoblast cultured on a substrate of FN (Burrows 1994).

It must be emphasised that all the experiments described above are performed with plasma FN, because this is currently the only source easily available. Since embryonic FN appears likely to be the major isoform secreted by trophoblast in the implantation site, some care is needed in the interpretation of available *in vitro* data. Furthermore, decidua also produces its own FN. Invading trophoblast, therefore, will come into contact with both adult maternal FN as well as its own endogenously produced fetal FN. High concentrations of adult FN have been observed to promote cell spreading but to retard migration while embryonic FN supports migration (Madri *et al.* 1988). Thus, trophoblast invasion would come within the sphere of influence of both types of FN.

Laminin (LM)

Laminin is found in great abundance in decidua and much of this is probably produced by the maternal stromal cells (Chapter 3). The distribution of this matrix protein is unusual in that it surrounds the decidual cells as a distinct pericellular layer (Fig. 9.5A) which is observed to be a continuous linear membrane under the electron microscope (Charpin *et al.* 1985; Wewer *et al.* 1985; Faber *et al.* 1986). Decidual stromal cells in culture also lay down LM in a similar pericellular fashion, but very little LM is secreted into the culture medium (Loke *et al.* 1989b) (Fig. 9.5B). In the non-pregnant endometrium, LM around stromal cells cannot be detected in the proliferative phase of the menstrual cycle (Fig. 9.5C) but this matrix protein begins to accumulate in the cytoplasm and as a pericellular layer in stromal cells at the early secretory phase. By late secretory phase, the amount of LM present is equivalent to that seen in decidua (Faber *et al.* 1986; Loke *et al.* 1989b). This cyclical variation suggests that some hormonal influence at or shortly following ovulation may be the stimulus for LM synthesis.

Interestingly, the reciprocal finding is observed for type VI collagen, which is present as a dense microfibrillar network in the stroma of pre-implantation endometrium but is no longer detectable in first trimester decidua (Mylona *et al.* 1995). It was postulated that this loss of collagen VI would lead to the formation of a more flexible decidual matrix that will allow for easier trophoblast invasion. Because the appearance of LM coincides with the time of implantation, this matrix protein could also influence trophoblast migration. While LM was strongly expressed by the basement membrane underlying villous cytotrophoblast, we did not detect LM in trophoblast cell columns. Trophoblast cells isolated from first trimester placentae also did not produce LM *in vitro* but did produce FN (Burrows *et al.* 1993a). In contrast, Damsky *et al.* (1992) observed LM in both proximal and distal parts of the trophoblast columns, with the A, B1 and B2 chains being all present. It is possible that the antibodies directed at individual LM chains used by Damsky's group are more sensitive than the one employed by us which is a pan-LM antibody generated by a combination of A, B1 and B2 chains as immunogen.

The LM molecule is made up of three genetically distinct chains: A (α1), B1 (β1) and B2 (γ1). These are linked together by disulphide bonds into a cross-shaped structure (Mercurio 1990; Kleinman and Weeks 1989). The cruciform molecule has one long arm and three short arms comprising one heavy chain and two light chains. Seven different heterotrimers are now recognised, designated as laminin 1 to 7 according to the new nomenclature (Burgeson *et al.* 1994). The relationship of these isoforms to the old nomenclature and chain composition is shown in Table 9.2 (Aplin and Church 1994). Most of the work done so far on the characterisation of LM is on extracts of this matrix protein synthesised by the Englebreth-Holm-Swarm (EHS) murine tumour (laminin 1). Recent data have suggested that the LM in other tissues may not be the same,

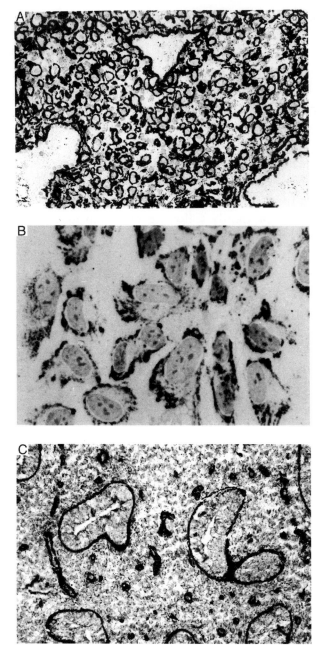

Fig. 9.5. **A**. Frozen section of first trimester decidua stained for laminin showing distinct pericellular distribution around individual stromal cells. (Obj × 16) **B**. Decidual stromal cells in culture also produce pericellular deposits of laminin. (Obj × 40) **C**. Frozen section of proliferative phase endometrium showing laminin in basement membranes of glands and blood vessels but very little around stromal cells, in contrast to decidua. (Obj × 16)

Table 9.2. *New nomenclature for laminin isoforms*

Name	Previous name	Chain composition
Laminin 1	EHS laminin	$\alpha1\beta1\gamma1$
Laminin 2	Merosin	$\alpha2\beta1\gamma1$
Laminin 3	S-laminin	$\alpha1\beta2\gamma1$
Laminin 4	S-merosin	$\alpha2\beta2\gamma1$
Laminin 5	Kalinin/nicein	$\alpha3\beta3\gamma2$
Laminin 6	K-laminin	$\alpha3\beta1\gamma1$
Laminin 7	K-S-laminin	$\alpha3\beta2\gamma1$

From Aplin and Church (1994).

so there seems to be a degree of tissue-specificity in the expression of LM (Mercurio 1990). At present, it is not clear what LM variants are present in the implantation site. Damsky *et al.* (1992) did not detect merosin (laminin 2) or S-laminin (laminin 3). J. Aplin *et al.* (personal communication), however, using Mabs specific for subunits, detected $\alpha2$, $\beta1$ and $\gamma1$ around decidual stromal cells indicating that merosin (laminin 2) is present.

As described earlier, migrating trophoblast expresses the $\alpha_1\beta_1$ and $\alpha_6\beta_1$ laminin receptors. The major cell-binding site of LM is located in the long arm of the cruciform structure, known as the E8 fragment, which is the domain recognised by the $\alpha_6\beta_1$ integrin (Hall *et al.* 1990; Mercurio 1990). The other cell-binding site is the E1/P1 fragment, which is located at the centre of the cross where the short arms of the three subunits meet. This forms the binding site for $\alpha_1\beta_1$. However, this domain is cryptic and only becomes exposed after proteolysis, so its physiological significance as an integrin-binding site is unclear.

Laminin has diverse biological activities. How it may influence trophoblast behaviour has not yet been elucidated. *In vitro*, the adhesion characteristics of trophoblast binding to LM differ markedly from binding to FN (Burrows *et al.* 1993a). Trophoblast cells become flattened and phase dark within 5 minutes of seeding on a substrate of FN, whereas cells seeded onto LM remain rounded and phase bright even after 120 minutes (Fig. 9.6A,B). This indicates that trophoblast adheres and spreads more readily on FN than on LM. After a few days in culture, trophoblast cells seeded on LM form a uniform layer of large polygonal cells which are closely packed in the manner of paving stones. In contrast, trophoblast cells plated onto FN adhere in a more irregular pattern with many cells possessing pseudopodia and long extensions, some of which communicate with other cells (Fig. 9.6C,D). The impression given is that trophoblast cells assume a sessile phenotype on LM and a motile phenotype on FN. Cultures of other cell types

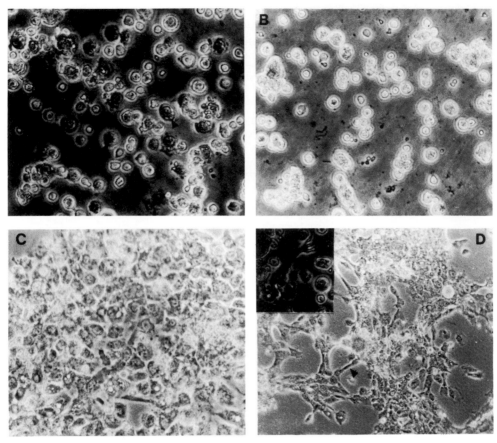

Fig. 9.6. Phase contrast photomicrographs of trophoblast cells cultured on a substrate of laminin (LM) or fibronectin (FN). **A.** Trophoblast cells 15 minutes after seeding on FN showing numerous flattened phase dark cells (arrowhead). (Obj × 20) **B.** In contrast, all trophoblast cells seeded onto LM remain rounded and phase bright after 15 minutes. (Obj × 20) **C.** After 5 days in culture, trophoblast cells seeded on LM form a uniform layer of polygonal-shaped cells resembling paving stones. (Obj × 20) **D.** After 5 days in culture, trophoblast cells seeded on FN consist of elongated cells many of which possess extending pseudopodia (inset). (Obj × 20)

have been reported to remain stationary on LM and become migratory on FN (Hynes and Lander 1992). However, not all cells behave in this fashion. Myoblasts, for example, are reported to move rapidly over LM and only poorly over FN (Goodman *et al.* 1989). The situation is further complicated by the observation that myoblast locomotion over LM decreases significantly at high concentrations of the matrix protein. In addition, when myoblasts move over a mixed substrate of LM and FN, the FN effect predominates. Since both these matrix proteins are present in the placental bed in unknown concentrations, it would be difficult to predict how trophoblast will behave *in vivo*.

There is increasing evidence that ECM proteins possess mitogenic properties (Levesque *et al.* 1991). Fragments from the inner segments of the short arms of LM consist of cysteine-rich epidermal growth factor (EGF)-like repeats which are capable of stimulating thymidine incorporation in cultured cells possessing EGF receptors, indicating that LM could have mitogenic effects on certain cell types (Panayotou *et al.* 1989). Since villous trophoblast expresses EGF receptors, these cells are potentially able to respond to LM (Bulmer *et al.* 1989; Jokhi *et al.* 1994a). In this case, the LM would be derived from the underlying villous basement membrane.

That LM is an important ECM inducer of cellular differentiation has been demonstrated for a variety of cell types such as mammary gland epithelium, hepatocytes and skin keratinocytes (Lin and Bissell 1993). Endothelial cells grown on a matrix of Matrigel have also been observed to undergo morphological differentiation and capillary tube formation. This effect is abrogated by preincubation of endothelial cells with an anti-laminin antibody or with synthetic peptides derived from the B1 (β1) LM chain (Kubota *et al.* 1988). Migrating trophoblast undergoes ultimate differentiation into placental bed giant cells at the implantation site and it would be tempting to suggest that LM could have a part to play in this process.

In Chapter 8, we have discussed the interaction between invading trophoblast and decidual NK cells. LM may influence this interaction. A LM-like molecule closely resembling the B2 (γ1) subunit is observed to be expressed by resting CD56+ CD3− peripheral blood NK cells and this expression is increased after IL-2 transformation into LAK cells. Anti-LM antibodies will inhibit the NK cell cytolysis of target cells so LM could function as a receptor utilised by NK cells in non-MHC restricted cytotoxicity (Schwarz and Hiserodt 1988). At the level of the target cell, NK-sensitive cell lines are found to express LM receptors and are able to bind ^{125}I-labelled LM while NK-resistant ones do not bind LM (Laybourn *et al.* 1989). Thus, the expression of LM receptors by target cells and of laminin by NK cells could form reciprocal structures for interaction. The presence of exogenous laminin may inhibit this interaction, either by competing for the NK cell recognition structure on the target cell or by steric hindrance. It has been shown that murine tumour cells which express high levels of surface LM tend to be highly metastatic and that the addition of LM to LM-receptor-positive murine tumour cells increases their metastatic activity. These observations could be the result of LM on the surface of tumour cells interfering with NK effector cell binding. It could be envisaged that the amount of LM present in the implantation site and the number of unbound LM receptors on trophoblast could have an important influence on trophoblast interaction with decidual NK cells.

Tenascin (TN)

Tenascins are a family of three related ECM proteins: tenascin-C (TN-C), tenascin-R (TN-R) and tenascin-X (TN-X). All share a distinctive pattern of four types of domain: an N-terminal containing oligomerisation sites where the subunits are connected to form tenascin trimers and hexamers; a region of EGF domains; a segment containing a series of FN type III domains; and finally a C-terminal domain (Erickson 1993). TN is mainly expressed during morphogenesis in embryonal life and reappears in adults during inflammation, tissue repair and in malignant tumours. Its function is unknown, but a variety of activities have been proposed which have a bearing on cell adhesion, migration, growth and differentiation (Chiquet-Ehrismann 1990; Sage and Bornstein 1991; Pesheva *et al.* 1994).

In the placenta, Damsky *et al.* (1992) detected TN in the chorionic mesenchyme directly underneath the developing trophoblast cell columns. Similar localisation of TN has been observed in the mesenchyme adjacent to growing epithelial structures during organogenesis and also at the dermal–epidermal junction in a wound site, suggesting that this ECM protein may facilitate epithelial–mesenchymal interactions (Chuong and Chen 1991; Sage and Bornstein 1991). We have observed strong expression of TN in first trimester uterine myometrium, particularly in areas associated with placental bed giant cells (Burrows 1994). Functional antagonism between TN and FN has been reported (Lotz *et al.* 1989) and TN has been observed to retard cell attachment to FN (Erickson and Bourdon 1989). Furthermore, loss of adhesion to FN results in terminal differentiation of keratinocytes (Watt *et al.* 1993). It could be proposed, therefore, that TN may have an important influence on interstitial trophoblast to stop invasion, and to differentiate into giant cells when the boundary of the myometrium is reached.

Endovascular trophoblast

Besides invading into decidua, trophoblast cells also migrate down the lumina of the spiral arteries (Chapter 4). These endovascular trophoblast cells consist of plugs of loosely cohesive cells which move down the wall of the vessel like 'wax dripping down the side of a candle' (Ramsey and Donner 1980). The plugs are thought to act as valves which only allow plasma to seep into the intervillous space at low pressures during early gestation protecting the fetus from the effects of maternal blood being delivered at high pressure (Hustin 1992). Endovascular trophoblast cells subsequently replace the vascular endothelial lining and may become embedded in the walls of the arteries. This phenomenon is also observed in non-human primates such as the macaque and baboon (Enders and King 1991), and in the golden hamster (Fuller *et al*. 1994). The mechanisms involved are not known, but the process bears a resemblance to events leading up to the transvascular migration of leucocytes into an inflammatory site (Butcher 1991). Preliminary evidence suggests that the two processes may indeed utilise similar adhesion molecule–ligand interactions.

Selectins are the most recently identified family of cell adhesion molecules (Vestweber 1992). Three members of this family have been identified – L-, E- and P-selectins – which are all involved in the initial binding of leucocytes to endothelial cells. The extracellular part of all selectins is composed of three different types of protein domain. At the N-terminal is a domain related to the calcium-dependent (C-type) animal lectin domain. This is followed by a domain related to a repeating structure found in EGF which, in turn, is succeeded by protein motifs found in the complementary regulatory proteins. All three selectins are anchored in the membrane by a single transmembrane region followed by a short cytoplasmic tail of only 17–35 amino acids depending on the selectin. The genes for all three selectins have been mapped to chromosome 1 in the human as well as in the mouse, suggesting that the selectins have arisen by multiple gene duplications which happened before the divergence of mouse and man. The ligands for E- and P-selectins are established to be carbohydrates containing the $\alpha(1$–$3)$ fucosylated lactosaminoglycan structure, known as Lewis X (Le^x), in particular the sialylated derivative, sialyl-Le^x (Dejana *et al*. 1992; Lasky 1992). These structures are found on cell surface glycolipids as well as in *O*- and *N*-linked carbohydrates of glycoproteins. We have observed that endovascular trophoblast expresses the blood-group-related carbohydrate antigen, sialyl-Le^x (King and Loke 1988).

Currently, both E- and P-selectins have been localised to vascular endothelial cells in decidua basalis but not parietalis, so that the relevant surface molecules are present for endovascular trophoblast to adhere to decidual endothelial cells (Tortosa *et al*. 1993; Burrows *et al*. 1994) (Table 9.3). This interaction is the initial event in neutrophil recruitment to an inflammatory site (Osborn 1990; Sugama *et al*. 1992). During acute inflammation, P-selectin, which is pre-packaged within Weibel–Palade bodies in endothelial cells, is rapidly translocated to the cell surface under the influence of inflammatory mediators such as histamine and leukotrienes, while E-selectin is actively synthesised by endothelial cells when stimulated by inflammatory cytokines, such as IL-1 and TNF-α (Vestweber 1992). Leucocytes, which express sialyl-Le^x, then adhere to these selectins via this ligand. The importance of P-selectin is confirmed by recent studies in 'knock-out' mice with deletion of the P-selectin gene. These animals exhibit deficient leucocyte adhesion to endothelium in inflammatory sites

Table 9.3. *Expression of cell adhesion molecules by endovascular trophoblast and decidual endothelial cells*

Monoclonal antibody	Reactivity	Endothelial cells (decidua parietalis)	Endothelial cells (decidua basalis)	Endovascular trophoblast
QBEND/40	Endothelial cells	+	+	−
MCA796	P-selectin	−	++	−
BBA-1	E-selectin	−	+	−
YTH 79.6	ICAM-1	++	++	+
BBA-5	VCAM-1	−	+	−
MAB 1954	α_4 integrin subunit	−	−	−
Leu-19	NCAM	−	−	++
ERIC-1	NCAM	−	−	++
735	PSA (polysialic acid)	−	−	++

(Mayadas *et al.* 1993). Vascular invasion by trophoblast during implantation, therefore, could be regulated by the expression of appropriate adhesion molecules which will permit interaction between endovascular trophoblast and decidual vascular endothelial cells as is seen in leucocyte migration at an inflammatory site, lymphocyte recirculation across high endothelial venules, and tumour metastases in distant organs (Osborn 1990; Springer 1990; Turner 1992). This hypothesis remains to be tested by functional assays *in vitro*.

In addition to sialyl-Le^x, we have observed endovascular trophoblast to express strongly the polysialylated (PSA) form of NCAM (CD56) (Burrows *et al.* 1994). The neural cell adhesion molecule (NCAM) consists of a large family of glycoprotein isoforms which are the product of a single gene. NCAM is a member of the immunoglobulin family of recognition molecules (Buck 1992). The protein products of the NCAM gene fall within three main size groups: 180, 140 and 120 kDa. In addition, the degree of glycosylation can considerably alter the molecular size (Walsh and Doherty 1991; Goridis and Brunet 1992). NCAM is one of only a few proteins that express long chains of α-2,8-polysialic acid (PSA) (Alcaraz and Goridis 1991). NCAM from embryonic brain is high in PSA and this moiety is also present on the endovascular trophoblast.

The presence of the PSA residue decreases the extent, duration or intimacy of cell–cell contact so this property of the molecule may modulate adhesion and disadhesion between trophoblast and endothelium and, thus, allow the correct degree of trophoblast movement within the vessel. In addition, NCAM–NCAM homotypic adhesion could be a mechanism for the formation of the loosely cohesive trophoblast plugs at the mouths of the spiral arteries which play such an important role in regulating blood flow to the fetus in early pregnancy. Besides cell–cell interaction, NCAM is also known to bind to components of the ECM such as collagen, heparin and heparan sulphate proteoglycans (Cole *et al.* 1986; Probstmeier *et al.* 1989). It can be envisaged that endovascular trophoblast may use this adhesion molecule to bind to these matrix proteins in the vessel wall once the overlying layer of endothelium is breached.

Matrix-degrading proteinases

In the preceding sections, the importance of cell–matrix interaction in basic cellular processes such as adhesion, migration, proliferation and differentiation has been discussed. It is clear, therefore, that any alteration of this interaction will greatly influence these cellular processes. Enzymes that can digest matrix proteins would be expected to play an important role (Kliman 1994). There are two main families of enzymes that have been implicated in the degradation of the protein components of the ECM (Alexander and Werb 1989; Matrisian 1992; Kleiner and Stetler-Stevenson 1993) (Fig. 9.7). The two families of enzymes are interactive, initiating a cascade of proteolytic events that result in matrix degradation. This process is similar to both the clotting cascade and complement activation and serves to mount a powerful but controlled mechanism coordinating the complete breakdown of various components of the ECM.

The first of these families include the plasminogen activators. In this system of serine proteases, inactive plasminogen is converted to active plasmin either by a tissue-type plasminogen activator (tPA) or urokinase plasminogen activator (uPA), and these activators are controlled by a series of specific plasminogen activator inhibitors (PAI-1, 2, 3).

The second important family of enzymes are the metalloproteinases. These are usually secreted as latent proenzymes which need to be activated and uPA has been implicated as an important physiological activator. Metalloproteinases are usually described under three subclasses – collagenases, gelatinases and stromelysins – with distinctive but overlapping substrate specificities (Table 9.4). As its name suggests, the collagenase subclass (MMP-1, MMP-5) acts on fibrillar collagens and has the ability to cleave alpha chains of types I, II and III collagens into smaller fragments. The substrates for the gelatinases (MMP-2, MMP-9) is gelatin (denatured collagen) as well as intact type IV basement membrane collagen and type V collagen. The stromelysins (MMP-3, MMP-10, MMP-7) are so named because of their relatively broad substrate specifities which include proteoglycans and glycoproteins such as fibronectin and laminin. Type IV

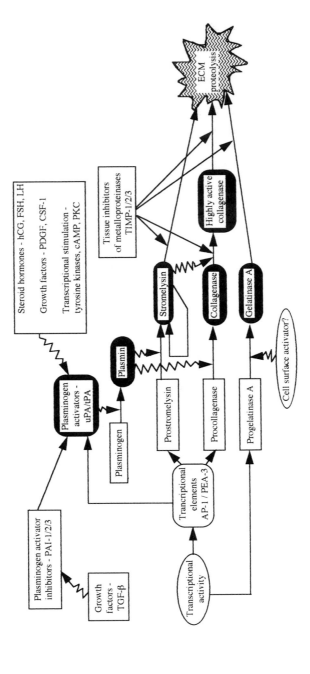

Interaction between serine protease and metalloproteinase cascades

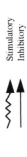

Stimulatory

Inhibitory

Fig 9.7. Interaction between serine protease and metalloproteinase cascades.

Table 9.4. *Members of the metalloproteinase family*

Names	Deduced mass (kDa)	ECM substrate
Collagenases		
MMP-1 (interstitial collagenase)	54.1	*Collagens I, II, III, VII, X
MMP-5 (neutrophil collagenase)	53.4	*Collagens I, II, III
Gelatinases		
MMP-2 (gelatinase A, 72 kDa IV collagenase)	73.9	*Gelatins, collagens IV, V, elastin
MMP-9 (gelatinase B, 92 kDa IV collagenase)	78.4	*Gelatins, collagens IV, V, elastin
Stromelysins		
MMP-3 (stromelysin 1, proteoglycanase)	54	Proteoglycans, fibronectin, laminin, gelatin, collagens III, IV, V, X
MMP-10 (stromelysin 2)	54.1	Proteoglycans, fibronectin, laminin, gelatin, collagens III, IV, V, X
MMP-7 (matrilysin, uterine metalloproteinase)	29.7	*Proteoglycans, collagen IV, fibronectin, gelatin, elastin
Other		
Stromelysin 3	54.6	?
Metalloelastase	53.9	Elastin, fibronectin

Members of the metalloproteinase family divided into three main categories depending on substrate specificity.
? substrate unknown.
* preferential substrates.

collagen is also cleaved by the stromelysins in the globular, but not the helical, domain. Like the plasminogen activators, the activities of metalloproteinases are subject to tight control by a special class of tissue inhibitors of metalloproteinases (TIMP) which complex with the enzymes and thus inhibit their proteolytic action. Interestingly, TIMP can be transcriptionally activated by many of the same agents that activate metalloproteinases so that both protease and its inhibitor appear to be co-ordinately induced. This could be a mechanism by which the extent of ECM degradation is limited and excessive proteolysis prevented.

The spatial and temporal control of proteinase activity can be mediated by a variety of mechanisms which are beginning to be unravelled. In the past few years, the identification of specific cell surface receptors for the proteases plasmin and plasminogen as well as for their activators has provided insights into mechanisms for regulation of cell-associated proteolytic activity (Testa and Quigley 1988; Saksela and Rifkin 1988). The uPA receptor is widely distributed in tissues whereas the tPA receptor is restricted to endothelial cells. The receptor for uPA also localises to the focal contacts beneath cells cultured *in vitro* which are the sites of cell–matrix interaction. When bound to its specific receptor, uPA is not internalised and thereby retains its enzymic activity. It has been shown that only receptor-bound and cell-surface associated urokinase influences cell motility while the secreted form does not (Ossowski 1988). This may be because the receptor-bound proteinase is protected from its inhibitor. These observations indicate that binding of the enzyme to a particular cell surface receptor could be an important means of spatial regulation of its activity. Temporal regulation is exemplified by the endothelial-type plasminogen activator inhibitor PAI-1, which is constantly produced in fully active form and shed from the cell membrane into the ECM where it is quickly denatured into an inactive form.

The ECM itself can influence proteinase activity by altering the transcription of the genes for these enzymes. It has been observed that ligation of the fibronectin receptor by specific antibody induces the expression of genes encoding the ECM-degrading metalloproteinases, collagenase and stromelysin in rabbit synovial fibroblasts (Werb *et al.* 1989). Fab fragments of the antibody were ineffective, indicating that cross-linking of the receptor is required. Interestingly, adhesion of fibroblasts to native fibronectin also had no effect, but binding to immobilised peptides containing the RGD sequences derived from fibronectin induced collagenase and stromelysin expression, suggesting that degradation products of fibronectin may be the natural inductive ligands. No alteration in cell shape or actin microfilament organisation was detected when metalloproteinase genes were induced so that the two events are mediated through distinct signals via triggering of the fibronectin receptor.

The transcription of proteinase genes is very receptive to a wide array of growth factors and cytokines. For example, TGF-β is a potent inducer of ECM components *in vitro* and *in vivo*. This net accumulation of ECM is achieved by increasing production of these components together with increased synthesis of TIMP and PAI-1 and, at the same time, reducing production of plasminogen activators and metalloproteinases, thus shifting the balance towards ECM synthesis. The reciprocal effect also operates in that cells grown on a substrate of reconstituted basement membrane matrix are observed to downregulate TGF-β_1 gene expression due to suppression of transcription of the promoter (Streuli *et al.* 1993). In contrast, TGF-β_1 promoter activity is strongly induced by the absence of basement membrane when the cells are cultured directly on plastic. This could provide a feedback loop whereby TGF-β_1-induced ECM synthesis is repressed once sufficient production has occurred. In contrast to TGF-β_1, EGF increases production of stromelysin as does PDGF, thus resulting in increased ECM degradation. Since growth factors and cytokines can dramatically alter the physiological state of a cell as can ECM proteins, the question arises as to whether the actions of growth factors and cytokines can, at least in part, be mediated via specific alterations in the integrity or composition of ECM by the co-ordinated transcriptional regulation of proteinases and their inhibitors.

There is accumulating evidence to suggest that invasive phenotype of both normal and transformed cells is associated with unusual production of plasminogen activators and metalloproteinases. For example, melanoma cells are observed to invade across amniotic membrane using a plasminogen activator-dependant cascade and a gelatinase as final lytic enzyme (Stetler-Stevenson *et al.* 1993). The invasive phenotype of Ha-*ras*-transformed rat embryo cells secrete a 92 kDa gelatinase (MMP-9) (Bernhard *et al.* 1994). The contribution of these proteinases to cell invasion raises the possibility that specific proteinase inhibitors could be used to control the spread and metastases of neoplastic cells. Available evidence suggests that this may be a feasible proposition. The addition of exogenous TIMP is observed to inhibit the invasion of melanoma cells in an amniotic membrane invasion assay and, *in vivo*, the coinjection of TIMP with melanoma cells reduces metastases to the lung in experimental animals (Mignatti *et al.* 1986; Schultz *et al.* 1988). In addition, downregulation of TIMP in 3T3 fibroblasts by transfection with a TIMP antisense construct allows these cells to become tumorigenic and metastatic in athymic mice. TIMP, therefore, is a potent protector against cellular invasion and could, indeed, have therapeutic potential.

Trophoblast degradation of extracellular matrix proteins

That trophoblast has proteolytic activity has been recognised for over 50 years. Subsequent studies have shown that explant cultures of chorionic villi would adhere to and then degrade the surrounding ECM proteins on which they were seeded (Fisher *et al.* 1985). Only first trimester villi could do so. Second trimester villi would adhere to similar matrices but did not degrade the substrate, indicating that only very early villous tissues have degradative properties. A later study by the same research group using isolated cells confirmed that it is the cytotrophoblast cells migrating out of the chorionic villi which are responsible for the matrix degradation (Fisher *et al.* 1989). By using ^{3}H-labelled matrix components such as [^{3}H]glucosamine, [^{3}H]proline and [^{3}H]leucine, it was observed that first trimester cytotrophoblast cells released substantial amounts of these into the culture medium from the ECM substrate, indicating that trophoblast can solubilise carbohydrate- as well as protein-containing matrix components, although the protein components were more extensively degraded into lower molecular mass fragments. This activity was greatly reduced in second and third trimester cytotrophoblast. Surprisingly, the choriocarcinoma cell lines BeWo and JAR also had less degradation activity than first trimester trophoblast. Since choriocarcinomas are highly invasive tumours *in vivo*, these tumour cells would be expected to exhibit a correspondingly high level of matrix degrading ability, if indeed the two processes are related.

Trophoblast metalloproteinases

Available evidence indicates that trophoblast degradation of matrix proteins is by the production of appropriate proteinases. Immunohistology has demonstrated the presence of collagenase in extravillous cytotrophoblast cells (Moll and Lane 1990; Fernandez *et al.* 1992). Zymogram studies using SDS-polyacrylamide gels incorporating gelatin by Fisher and her colleagues (1989) have shown that first trimester trophoblast expresses a wide array of cell-associated gelatin-degrading proteinases ranging from 68 to >200 kDa in size. Many of these are no longer present in second and third trimester trophoblast. Similarly, extracts from first trimester placental fibroblasts exhibited only two bands of relative molecular mass of 68 and 75 kDa. Only one proteinase of 90 kDa was secreted into culture supernatant by trophoblast, while placental fibroblasts secreted only the 68 kDa proteinase. All the above proteinase activities were inhibited by 1,10-phenanthroline, suggesting that they belong to the family of metalloproteinases. Thus, it appears that first trimester cytotrophoblast expresses a unique array of metalloproteinases which are different from those produced by late gestation cytotrophoblast or by placental fibroblasts.

Bischof and his colleagues (1991) also observed by gelatin zymography that first trimester culture supernatants exhibited an array of seven bands of digestion ranging from 59 to 230 kDa molecular mass, with three of these (230, 94, 64 kDa) being particularly intense. Only four of these seven bands (230, 128, 94, 65 kDa) were seen in cell lysates. There are, therefore, more proteinases secreted by trophoblast than associated with the cell membrane, a finding which is in contrast to that reported by Fisher *et al.* (1989). Our own results (unpublished) agree with Bischof *et al.* (1991) in that we also find a greater number and more intensely staining bands from trophoblast culture supernatants than from cell lysates. The two most prominent bands in our study are of 92 and 72 kDa molecular mass. When trophoblast cell preparations were first depleted of contaminating bone-marrow-derived cells by reacting with a Mab to the leucocyte common antigen, Bischof *et al.* (1991) found four remaining secreted gelatinases of 197, 94, 64 and 59 kDa which were, thus, considered to be trophoblast-specific products. The homogeneity of the isolated trophoblast cells used is certainly an important point to bear in mind. Besides leucocytes, future studies of a similar nature might consider depleting fibroblasts and endothelial cells, which are both likely contaminants derived from the chorionic villous mesenchyme. The 59 kDa proteinase appeared only when trophoblast cells were cultured on Matrigel or rat-tail collagen and not when cells were plated on agarose or plastic, suggesting that matrix proteins can influence metalloproteinase gene expression.

Trophoblast plasminogen activators and their inhibitors

Besides metalloproteinases, cultured human trophoblast cells have also been demonstrated to secrete the urokinase-type plasminogen activators (uPA) with proteolytic activity (Martin and Arias 1982; Queenan *et al.* 1987). At the same time, inhibitors to PA can also be detected. Using specific rabbit antisera, Feinberg *et al.* (1989) localised both plasminogen activator inhibitor-1 (PAI-1) and -2 (PAI-2) in cultured trophoblast, with PAI-1 being present in the cytoplasm and cell surface membrane while PAI-2 occurs only in the cytoplasm. Northern blot analysis with appropriate cDNA probes confirmed the presence of PAI-1 and PAI-2 mRNA in these trophoblast cells. mRNA levels for both these inhibitors are shown to be depressed approximately 2-fold after treatment of trophoblast cells with the cAMP analogue 8-bromo-cAMP whereas uPA expression is stimulated 2- to 3-fold by a similar treatment, suggesting there could be reciprocal regulation of the activators and its inhibitor by cAMP. Immunohistological staining of placental sections localised PAI-2 only to villous syncytiotrophoblast, suggesting a possible role of this inhibitor in regulating fibrinolysis within the intervillous space. In contrast, PAI-1 is found mainly among the invading population of extravillous cytotrophoblast, which could reflect a role in trophoblast migration. The observation that both inhibitors were produced by trophoblast *in vitro* raises the question of whether the culture conditions employed truly simulate the *in vivo* situation. In our own experience, we have frequently observed products in cultured trophoblast cells which are not present in the equivalent trophoblast populations *in vivo*. We suspect that the culture systems presently used by investigators for trophoblast research tend to drive these cells towards terminal differentiation. However, a recent immunohistological study claims to detect uPA as well as both PAI-1 and PAI-2 in all trophoblast populations (Hofmann *et al.* 1994), although the tissues used are from ectopic rather than uterine pregnancies.

Trophoblast expression of urokinase receptor

As mentioned earlier, binding of a proteinase to its cell surface receptor may be an important means of spatial regulation of its enzymic activity. The existence of uPA receptors (uPAR) on cultured human trophoblast cells has now been demonstrated (Zini *et al.* 1992). These trophoblast uPAR appear to be similar in many respects to that described on other cell types, such as U937 cells, macrophages and endothelial cells. Urokinase binds to trophoblast uPAR with high affinity via its growth factor domain and binding is largely reversible. The apparent molecular mass of the trophoblast uPAR as determined by immunoblotting is similar to that found in other cells, and they are linked to the cell membrane through a PI-PLC sensitive GPI anchor. Trophoblast uPAR are completely saturated with endogenous uPA, which enables these cells in culture to convert plasminogen to plasmin in the absence of an exogenous source of uPA. This phenomenon is usually associated with cultured cells derived from metastatic carcinomas. First trimester trophoblast expresses more uPAR (468 000 per cell) than term trophoblast (153 000 per cell), indicating there is downregulation of these receptors with increased age and/or differentiation of trophoblast. This supports the hypothesis that trophoblast proteolytic activity is a closely regulated process during gestation. At present, it is not clear whether this regulation is intrinsically programmed by the trophoblast cell or is a response to a changing extracellular milieu in the uterus. The pattern of expression of uPAR *in vivo* also suggests that these receptors may mediate invasion. uPAR was detectable in placental bed giant cells in a polarised fashion with increased expression at the migrating edge (Multhaupt *et al.* 1994).

Trophoblast invasion *in vitro*

The demonstration of protease activity in trophoblast, by itself, does not imply that this is necessarily the mechanism utilised by these cells for invasion. However, *in vitro* invasion assays have now been developed to address this point. Yagel *et al.* (1988) used human amnion as a natural basement membrane-containing tissue after stripping off the attached epithelium and measured the migration of radiolabelled trophoblast cells across it. They found that trophoblast cells derived from first trimester chorionic explants exhibited a degree of invasiveness comparable to that of the choriocarcinoma cell line JAR, and of the highly metastatic murine melanoma line B16F10. This trophoblast invasion was prevented by a collagenase inhibitor (HCI), a metalloproteinase inhibitor (1–10 phenanthrolin), a serine proteinase inhibitor (trasylol) and an antibody directed against uPA. In contrast, mersalyl, a mercurial compound known to activate procollagenase, enhanced trophoblast invasion. These observations are in support of the role of proteases in trophoblast migration. In a subsequent study by the same research group (Graham and Lala 1991), conditioned media from first trimester decidual cells were found to suppress trophoblast invasion, thereby indicating that some control is exerted by the uterine environment. With appropriate inhibitory controls, it was concluded that the cytokine, TGF-β and the metalloproteinase inhibitor, TIMP, were the main components in decidual cell supernatants which inhibited trophoblast invasion. Trophoblast cells themselves produce TGF-β so it is possible that endogenously derived cytokine could also influence trophoblast migration. Our own ELISA experiments have confirmed that first trimester trophoblast as well as decidual stromal cells are important sources of TGF-β production (unpublished). Similarly, TIMP may also be endogenously produced by trophoblast since the mRNA is detected in cultured trophoblast and the protein is secreted during trophoblast culture (Yagel *et al.* 1988). TIMP is probably induced by TGF-β so here we may have one mechanism by which a cytokine can influence trophoblast migration via a metalloproteinase inhibitor.

Other investigators have used artificially constructed membranes for their trophoblast invasion assays. The advantage of this approach is that defined matrix proteins can be tested which makes the system more versatile. Librach *et al.* (1991) plated trophoblast cells onto polycarbonate filters with different pore sizes which were coated with a layer of Matrigel. The following findings were noted with first trimester, but not with term trophoblast: (1) Cytotrophoblast seeded as individual cells aggregated into clumps on the surface of the Matrigel. (2) Cells at the periphery of the aggregates elaborated extensive processes which extended outwards as invadopodia. (3) At points of contact with these processes, the Matrigel showed signs of local degradation. These events could be representative of the sequential stages of trophoblast migration *in vivo*. Both inhibitor TIMP and TIMP-2 effectively blocked trophoblast invasion in this assay in a dose-dependent manner. Interestingly, only the matrix disruption was diminished by TIMP and not the formation of cellular aggregates or invadopodia, so it seems that this inhibitor affects mainly the proteolytic activity of trophoblast and not the other two aspects of trophoblast-matrix interaction. Inhibition studies with specific antibodies ascertained that it is the 92 kDa type IV collagenase which is the important mediator of trophoblast invasion. In contrast, specific antibodies to uPA or the addition of exogenous PAI-1 and PAI-2 only resulted in partial inhibition, indicating that the metalloproteinase rather than the serine proteinase enzyme system plays the major role in the final pathway of trophoblast invasion.

10

Cytokines and their receptors in implantation

Introduction

The proliferation, invasion and eventual differentiation of trophoblast cells during implantation is tightly controlled. Such a complex process is normally coordinated by a system of close intercellular signalling mediated by soluble molecules. Cytokines are important examples of these molecules. They are involved in the regulation of cell–cell interactions and tissue remodelling in a variety of normal and pathological conditions. For this reason, reproductive biologists have focussed on these mediators and the role they might play in placental development (Evain-Brion 1992; Rutanen 1993; Giudice 1994; Robertson *et al.* 1994).

General characteristics of cytokines

Cytokines are a broad heterogeneous group of secreted proteins and polypeptides with pleiotropic functions that can act on virtually every nucleated cell of the body. Historically, the field of cytokine research has originated from four independent sources:

(1) *Immunology*. The terms 'lymphokine' and 'monokine' were coined to describe the biologically active proteins secreted by lymphocytes and monocytes respectively. The later observation that many of these proteins acted as communication signals between different populations of leucocytes has led to the general classification of 'interleukin' to encompass these varied proteins.
(2) *Virology*. The 'interferons' were first recognised for their anti-viral activity, but it soon became apparent that these proteins have a wide range of other regulatory actions on cell growth and differentiation.
(3) *Haematology*. The 'colony stimulating factors' which were first noted for their ability to regulate the growth and differentiation of haematopoietic cells are now known to affect other cell types as well.

(4) *Cell biology.* The classical 'growth factors' were proteins originally described that promote growth of a wide variety of cells. It soon became clear that many of these agents also have other functions related to cell behaviour, so that the distinction between them and cytokines is now considered to be arbitrary.

The biological functions of cytokines are difficult to evaluate, especially *in vivo*, because a cell is likely to be exposed to a cocktail of cytokines at any one time resulting in synergistic or antagonistic interactions the sum of which will dictate the final signals transmitted to the cell. Thus, cytokine functions should be considered in the context of a network. Furthermore, many cytokines exhibit activities so diverse as to seem unrelated (ambiguity) and structurally dissimilar cytokines may have similar functions (redundancy). In spite of these difficulties, some general principles shared by the majority of cytokines can, nevertheless, be formulated. Cytokines are single polypeptides or glycoproteins with a molecular mass of around 30 kDa, although some can form higher molecular weight oligomers. Constitutive production is usually low or absent, but is induced by a variety of stimuli acting at the level of transcription or translation. Cytokine production is often transient and the radius of activity usually small. Thus, cytokines tend to act in an autocrine or paracrine manner, unlike endocrine hormones. Cytokines are very powerful and exert their effects at picomolar concentrations by binding to specific, high affinity cell-surface receptors with K_d in the range of 10^{-9} to 10^{-12} M. This results in a cascade of biochemical events within the cell leading to a pattern of gene expression manifested as an altered rate of cell proliferation or cell death, change in cellular differentiation state and/ or influence on cell behaviour such as motility, surface phenotype, extracellular matrix deposition and secretion of other cytokines. In recent years, fresh insights into how the cytokine network operates *in vivo* have come from experiments in mice in which either an appropriate cytokine transgene has been inserted (transgenic mice) or the gene has been rendered inactive ('knock-out' mice) (Taverne 1993), although the picture is still not entirely clear because of the redundancy of so many cytokines.

General features of cytokine receptors

Cytokine receptors are classified into several groups according to their structural characteristics (Sato and Miyajima 1994; Taga and Kishimoto 1995) (Fig. 10.1).

(1) *Class I (haematopoietin) receptor superfamily* includes receptors for most of the interleukins (IL-2 to IL-7, IL-9, IL-11 and IL-15), GM-CSF, G-CSF and LIF. These receptors have a conserved pattern of cysteine residues in their amino-terminal

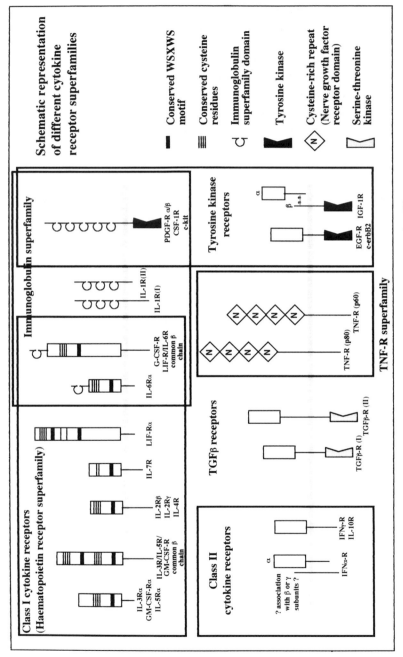

Fig. 10.1. Different cytokine receptor superfamilies.

domain and a Trp-Ser-X-Trp-Ser (WSXWS) motif (where X is any amino acid) in the carboxyl-terminal domain.

(2) *Class II receptor superfamily* includes receptors for the IFNs and IL-10 which possess cysteine residues in their amino-terminal domain analogous to class I receptors, but no WSXWS motif in their carboxyl-terminal domain.

(3) *Immunoglobulin superfamily* (IgSF) is the largest superfamily that includes a variety of cell surface molecules. Of the cytokine receptors, IL-1R (types I and II), CSF-1R, PDGF-R (α and β subunits) and c-*kit* all belong to this group by virtue of the characteristic immunoglobulin domains in their extracellular regions.

(4) *Tyrosine kinase receptor superfamily*, as the name implies, refers to those receptors with intrinsic protein kinase activity. These include receptors for CSF-1, PDGF, EGF, IGF and many others of the 'classical' growth factors. All these receptors share a similar molecular topology in possessing a large glycosylated extracellular ligand-binding domain, a single hydrophobic transmembrane region and a cytoplasmic region that contains a tyrosine kinase catalytic domain.

(5) *Tumour necrosis factor receptor (TNF-R) superfamily* consists of the p60 and p80 TNF-Rs which are characterised by a pattern of three or four cysteine-rich repeats in their extracellular regions not seen in the other receptor types.

(6) *Transforming growth factor β receptor (TGF-βR) superfamily* includes the two major species (receptors I and II) of the TGF-βR, which are unusual in possessing transmembrane serine/threonine kinases. This configuration may partly account for the considerable diversity of TGF-β activity on different cells.

The above classification is not an absolutely rigid one. For example, it can be seen that CSF-1R belongs to the family of tyrosine kinase receptors, but is also a member of the immunoglobulin superfamily because it has the characteristic immunoglobulin domains in its extracellular region. In addition, several cytokine receptors are composed of two or more subunits, such as the IL-2R which is a trimeric receptor consisting of α, β and γ subunits. Of these, the β and γ subunits have the characteristics of a class I receptor and are, therefore, included in this superfamily, but the α subunit remains unclassed. This appears to be a peculiarity of the IL-2R because, in all other receptors, the different subunits tend to belong to the same family. A further point to note in terms of function is that some subunits are shared by several receptors. For example, the high-affinity receptors for GM-CSF, IL-3 and IL-5 are dimeric and consist of a cytokine-specific α subunit and a common β subunit, both of which belong to the class I superfamily of cytokine receptors. While the α subunit is involved in cytokine binding, the common β subunit plays an important part in signal transduction. In addition, the α subunit alone can only bind the relevant cytokine with low affinity, and high-affinity binding is achieved by the combination of the α and β subunits acting together.

Expression of cytokine receptors by cells at the placenta–uterine interphase

Localisation of cytokine receptors would be the first step towards identifying those cell types at the implantation site that are potentially capable of responding to the different cytokines. This section discusses some of these receptors, particularly those where most data are available. The list is by no means comprehensive, but it will serve to illustrate the diversity of cytokine receptors that can be found among the varied cell populations at the placental–uterine interface. Data from our own laboratory are summarised in Tables 10.1–10.4 (Jokhi 1994). No doubt more receptors will be described in the future as the relevant molecular probes or antibodies become available.

CSF-1R

CSF-1R is encoded by the proto-oncogene c-*fms*. The c-*fms* gene, which contains 22 exons and spans a relatively large region of genomic DNA (>30 kDa), has been mapped to the long arm of human chromosome 5, close to the CSF-1 locus (Sherr 1990). It shows a high degree of sequence homology with the gene encoding the platelet-derived growth factor receptor β (PDGF-Rβ) (Yarden *et al*. 1986), with the two genes in close juxtaposition in a tandem head-to-tail array (Roberts *et al*. 1988).

High levels of c-*fms* mRNA have been reported to be present in the whole human placenta, isolated trophoblast cells and choriocarcinoma cell lines with transcripts 3.7–3.9 kb in size (Müller *et al*. 1983; Rettenmier *et al*. 1986; Visvader and Verma 1989; Kauma *et al*. 1991; Pampfer *et al*. 1992; Jokhi *et al*. 1993). Levels of mRNA in the human placenta are observed to increase steadily throughout gestation until term. To date, there are only two publications demonstrating CSF-1R protein in trophoblast by staining with specific antibodies. Pampfer *et al*. (1992) reported that the highest expression of CSF-1R was seen in villous syncytiotrophoblast and that this was maintained throughout gestation. Villous cytotrophoblast, decidual stromal cells and decidual glandular epithelium were also observed to express CSF-1R. Our own study, however, showed a different pattern of CSF-1R expression (Jokhi *et al*. 1993). We found significant staining for this receptor on syncytiotrophoblast only between 8 and 10 weeks gestation. Prior to this period and subsequently until term, there was only weak focal staining. Also, villous cytotrophoblast was always negative, but cytotrophoblast cells of the columns were strongly stained. This expression was initially maintained by the invasive interstitial trophoblast, but was lost deeper

Table 10.1. *Cytokine receptor expression by first trimester trophoblast populations: immunohistology data summary*

Receptor	Villous CT	Villous ST	SC associated with columns	Columns/shell	Interstitial trophoblast	Endovascular trophoblast	Giant cells
CSF-1R (c-*fms*)	−	+/−	−	++	+	+	+/−
GM-CSF-Rα	+	+/−	+	+	+	+	+
c-*kit*	+	−	−	−	−	−	−
EGF-R (c-*erb*B1)	++[a]	++[a]	++	−[b]	−	−	++
c-*erb*B2	−	+/−	−	++	++	++	++
IGF-IR	++	−	−	−[b]	−	−	−
PDGF-Rα	−	−	−	−	−	−	−
PDGF-Rβ	−	−	−	−	−	−	−
IL-2Rα	−	−	−	−	−	−	−
IL-2Rβ	−	−	−	+	+/−	ND	−
IL-6R	−	−	−	−	−	−	−
IL-7R	−	−	−	−	−	−	−
IFNγ-R	+	−	++	++	+	ND	+
TNF-R (p80)	−	−	++	−	−	−	−
Endoglin	−	+	ND	−	−	ND	−

CT, cytotrophoblast; ST, syncytiotrophoblast; SC, multinucleated syncytial cells.

++, strong staining; +, moderate staining; +/−, weak to absent; ND, not determinable.

[a] On 6 week villi, very strong EGF-R expression on villous CT, and weak on villous ST. On 9 week villi, very strong EGF-R expression on villous ST, and weak on villous CT.

[b] Positive on cells in the proximal part of the columns, immediately adjacent to their villous origin.

Table 10.2. *Cytokine receptor expression by first trimester villous mesenchymal cells: Immunohistology data summary*

Receptor	Hofbauer cells	Fibroblasts	Endothelial cells
CSF-1R (c-*fms*)	+	−	−
GM-CSF-Rα	+	−	−
c-*kit*	+	−	−
EGF-R (c-*erb*B1)	−	−	−
c-*erb*B2	−	−	−
IGF-IR	−	−	−
PDGF-Rα	−	+	−
PDGF-Rβ	+	+	−
IL-2Rα	−	−	−
IL-2Rβ	−	−	−
IL-6R	−	−	−
IL-7R	−	−	−
IFNγ-R	+/−	−	ND
TNF-R (p80)	+	−	−
Endoglin	−	−	+

++, strong staining; +, moderate staining; +/−, weak to absent; ND, not determinable.

Table 10.3. *Cytokine receptor expression in term chorionic villi: Immunohistology data summary*

Receptor	Villous[a]	Villous ST	Hofbauer cells	Fibroblasts	Endothelial cells
CSF-1R (c-*fms*)	−	+/−	++	−	−
GM-CSF-Rα	−	+	+	−	−
c-*kit*	−	−	−	−	−
EGF-R (c-*erb*B1)	−	+	−	−	−
c-*erb*B2	−	+	−	−	−
IGF-IR	+	−	−	−	−
PDGF-Rα	−	−	−	+	−
PDGF-Rβ	−	−	−	+	−
IL-2Rα	−	−	−	−	−
IL-2Rβ	−	+/−	−	−	−
IL-6R	−	−	−	−	−
IL-7R	−	−	−	−	−
IFNγ-R	−	−	−	−	++
TNF-R (p80)	−	−	+	−	−
Endoglin	−	++	−	−	++

CT, cytotrophoblast; ST, syncytiotrophoblast.
++, strong staining; +, moderate staining; +/−, weak to absent.
[a]Villous cytotrophoblast layer often difficult to detect by light microscopy at term.

Table 10.4. *Cytokine receptor expression by first trimester maternal decidual cell populations*

Receptor	Large granular lymphocytes	T cells	Macrophages	Stromal cells	Glandular epithelium	Endothelial cells	Arterial media
CSF-1R (c-*fms*)	–	–	++	–	–	–	–
GM-CSF-Rα	–	–	++	–	+	–	–
c-*kit*	–[a]	–	+	–	–	–	–
EGF-R (c-*erb*B1)	–	–	–	+	–	–	–
c-*erb*B2	–	–	–	–	+	–	–
IGF-IR	–	–	–	+	+	ND	–
PDGF-Rα	–	–	–	+	–	–	–
PDGF-Rβ	–	–	–	++	–	–	+
IL-1R (II)	+/–[b]	+[c]	+	NT	NT	NT	NT
IL-2Rα	+/–[d]	+/–[e]	–	–	–	–	–
IL-2Rβ	+	–	–	–	–	–	–
IL-6R	–	–	–	–	–	–	–
IL-7R	–	+[c]	+	–	–	–	–
IFNγ-R	–	–	+	+/–[h]	–	++	–
TNF-R (p80)	+/–[f]	+/–[g]	+/–	+	–	+	–
Endoglin	+/–[i]	–	+	–	–	++	–

++, strong staining; +, moderate staining; +/–, weak to absent; ND, not determinable; NT, not tested by immunochemistry.
[a] Expressed at high levels by the small CD56^{dim} CD16^{+} subset of decidual large granular lymphocytes (LGL) by FACS.
[b] Expressed at low levels by ≈10% of decidual LGL
[c] Expressed by the majority of decidual T cells.
[d] Expressed at low levels by 10–15% of decidual LGL.
[e] Expressed at low levels by 14–15% of decidual T cells.
[f] Expressed at low levels by 4–5% of decidual LGL.
[g] Expressed at low levels by 25–30% of decidual T cells.
[h] Nuclear staining at higher concentrations by immunochemistry.
Expressed at higher concentrations by immunochemistry.
[i] Expressed at low levels by 5–7% of decidual LGL.

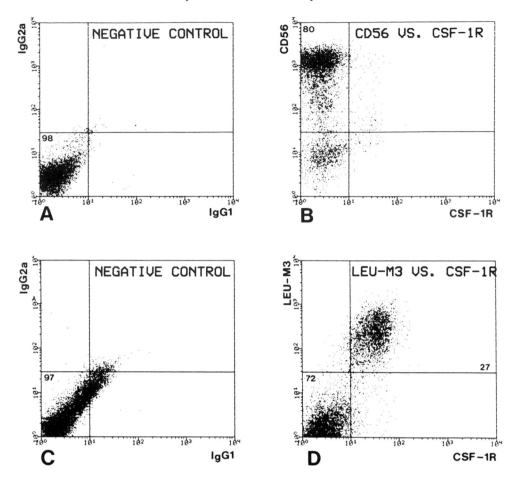

Fig. 10.2. Two-colour flow cytometric analysis of decidual leucocytes. **A, C**. Negative controls. **B**. CD56 (PE) versus CSF-1R (FITC). There is no surface expression of CSF-1R on decidual CD56+ NK cells, which account for 80% of cells in this sample. **D**. CD14 (Leu-M3) (PE) versus CSF-1R (FITC). Twenty-seven per cent of cells in this preparation of decidual leucocytes are CD14+ macrophages which all express CSF-1R.

in the placental bed when these cells differentiate into sessile multinucleated giant cells. Our findings, therefore, suggest that CSF-1R expression is mainly related to the invasive trophoblast phenotype. In decidua, we did not find CSF-1R expression by stromal cells nor by glandular epithelium. Instead, the maternal cells which were seen to express CSF-1R were decidual CD14+ macrophages (Fig. 10.2). Fetal macrophages (Hofbauer cells) in the chorionic villous mesenchyme were also observed to express CSF-1R, only weakly during the first trimester, but the staining intensity became much stronger by term.

Transcription of c-*fms* mRNA in trophoblast cells and in cells of the monocyte/macrophage lineage appears to be initiated by two independent promoters that function in a tissue-specific manner. The one used by trophoblast lies only 350 bp downstream of the 3′ end of the PDGF-Rβ gene (Roberts *et al.* 1988; Visvader and Verma 1989) and it has been suggested that this tandem organisation of the CSF-1R and PDGF-Rβ genes might be a mechanism for their mutually exclusive expression (Roberts *et al.* 1992).

We have also studied CSF-1R expression by isolated trophoblast cells cultured *in vitro* (Jokhi *et al.* 1993). Staining of cytospin preparations on permeabilised cells in suspension revealed an intracellular granular pattern. This could be a reflection of rapid internalisation of the ligand–receptor complex following ligand binding, which has been described by Sherr (1990).

GM-CSF-R

The high-affinity receptor GM-CSF-R is formed by the association of an α and a β subunit, the latter of which is shared by the receptors for IL-3 and IL-5 (Kastelein and Shanafelt 1993). Because of its short cytoplasmic domain, it is still unclear whether the low-affinity α subunit is capable of transducing a functional signal on its own. However, Metcalf *et al.* (1990) have shown that GM-CSF can stimulate proliferation of murine cells transfected with this subunit. It has also been reported that binding of GM-CSF to GM-CSF-Rα alone was sufficient for receptor activation, and this was independent of ligand interaction with GM-CSF-Rβ (Kastelein and Shanafelt 1993). Recently, it has been confirmed that the cytoplasmic domain of the α chain does play a critical role in mediating cell proliferation (Lopez *et al.* 1992; Polotskaya *et al.* 1993).

Although the GM-CSF-Rα subunit was originally cloned from a human placental cDNA library (Gearing *et al.* 1989), there have been no published data on the localisation of this receptor protein in the human placenta or uterine tissues. This is due mainly to the unavailability of appropriate antibodies. We have recently undertaken such a study (Jokhi *et al.* 1994b) using a pool of Mabs to the GM-CSF-Rα subunit generated by Dr Paul Jubinsky of the Dana Farber Cancer Institute in Boston, Massachusetts. Immunohistology showed GM-CSF-Rα to be strongly expressed by villous cytotrophoblast as well as by all the extravillous trophoblast populations, including the cell columns, interstitial trophoblast, endovascular trophoblast and placental bed giant cells. Syncytiotrophoblast in the first trimester did not express this receptor, but staining became much stronger and more uniform at term. This is in agreement with the report by Hampson *et al.* (1993)

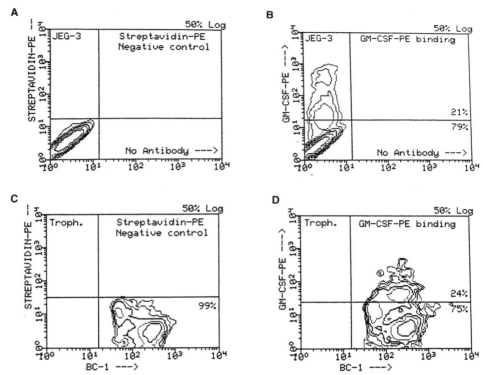

Fig. 10.3. Two-colour flow cytometric analysis of GM-CSF binding by JEG-3 choriocarcinoma cells and normal first trimester trophoblast. **A**. JEG-3-streptavidin (PE), negative control. **B**. Twenty-one per cent of JEG-3 cells are binding GM-CSF (PE). **C**. Normal trophoblast identified by staining with Mab, BC-1 (FITC) with streptavidin (PE), negative control. **D**. Twenty-four per cent of the trophoblast cells are binding GM-CSF (PE).

in which isolated human term syncytiotrophoblast microvillus plasma membrane vesicles was found to bind GM-CSF with low affinity.

That these GM-CSF-Rα are functional is confirmed by flow cytometric demonstration of binding to fluorochrome-conjugated rhGM-CSF (Fig. 10.3) (Loke *et al.* 1992a; Jokhi *et al.* 1994b). Interestingly, only a proportion of trophoblast cells expressing the receptor were seen to bind the cytokine. This suggests that the detection system for cytokine binding was either not sensitive enough or was only able to detect relatively high affinity binding which occurs as a result of the association of the α and β subunits of the receptor. Studies on other systems have shown that the α subunit is often expressed in excess of the β chain (Hallek *et al.* 1992), so it remains to be established whether human trophoblast cells express both subunits equally.

Like CSF-1R, GM-CSF-Rα is expressed also by both decidual and fetal macrophages (Hofbauer cells). This is confirmed by flow cytometry with the macrophage marker CD14. Unlike CSF-1, decidual glandular epithelium also expresses GM-CSF-Rα. In non-pregnant endometrium, this receptor is expressed by glandular epithelium during the secretory phase, but not the proliferative phase of the cycle, implying that receptor expression is hormonally regulated in these cells.

c-kit

Like the receptor for CSF-1 (c-*fms*), c-*kit* is a proto-oncogene product and is a member of the tyrosine kinase superfamily of receptors. The ligand for c-*kit*, known simply as kit ligand (KL), is also called stem cell factor. c-*kit* is known to be expressed by primitive haematopoietic stem cells and by primordial germ cells (Morrison-Graham and Takahashi 1993; Horie *et al.* 1993) where it plays an important role in the proliferation and maturation of these progenitor cells. We have investigated the expression of this receptor in the placenta and decidua using two polyclonal antibodies (Sharkey *et al.* 1994). No c-*kit* expression was detected in any trophoblast populations in any stage of pregnancy. This is in contrast to the mouse placenta, where the labyrinthine trophoblast has been reported to express c-*kit* protein (Horie *et al.* 1992)

As for the CSF-1R and GM-CSF-R, c-*kit* was detected on first trimester fetal Hofbauer cells, although by term this expression was much weaker or absent. In general, c-*kit* expression is usually relatively restricted in adult life so it is rather surprising to find that maternal decidual macrophages express this receptor, especially as peripheral blood monocytes do not. In addition to macrophages, preliminary flow cytometric analysis in our laboratory revealed another c-*kit*[+] cell population in decidua. These are the CD56[dim] subset of decidual NK cells which express the receptor at a level 2–3 times higher than decidual macrophages (Fig. 10.4). c-*kit* expression has been reported on primitive lymphoid precursor cells in the bone marrow and thymus (Godfrey *et al.* 1992), so the CD56[dim] c-*kit*[+] cells might represent precursors of the main CD56[bright] c-*kit*[−] population of decidual NK cells (Chapter 7).

EGF-R and c-erbB2 protein

Both EGF-R and c-*erb*B2 protein are receptors belonging to the tyrosine kinase superfamily of receptors. The epidermal growth factor receptor (EGF-R) is the product of the c-*erb*B1 proto-oncogene, while the other receptor is the product of the homologous c-*erb*B2 proto-oncogene (also known as *neu*, HER-2 and NGL). These two molecules are closely related to each other and have a high

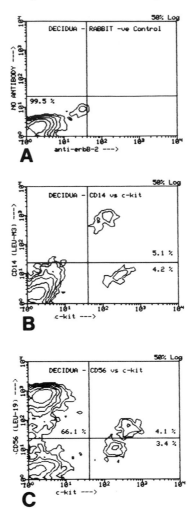

Fig. 10.4. Two-colour flow cytometric analysis of c-*kit* expression on decidual leucocytes. **A**. Rabbit irrelevant antibody used as a negative control. **B**. CD14 (PE) versus c-*kit* (FITC). c-*kit* expression is seen on CD14$^+$ decidual macrophages but there is another non-macrophage population which is also positive. **C**. CD56 (PE) versus c-*kit* (FITC). c-*kit* expression is seen on the CD56^{dim} subset of decidual NK cells at 2-4 times the levels on decidual macrophages.

degree of sequence and structural homology (Coussens *et al.* 1985; Bargmann *et al.* 1986; Yamamoto *et al.* 1986). Both are expressed in various fetal and adult epithelia (Damjanov *et al.* 1986; Press *et al.* 1990) and can be over-expressed in certain types of tumour (Harris and Neal 1987; Singleton and Strickler 1992).

While there have been several studies on localisation of EGF-R in human placenta (Maruo and Mochizuki 1987; Bulmer *et al.* 1989; Maruo *et al.* 1992; Hofmann *et al.* 1992; Filla *et al.* 1993), there has only been one where EGF-R and c-*erb*B2 were investigated together (Mülhauser *et al.* 1993). Even this last report focussed only on trophoblast of the chorionic villi. To date, the publication by Jokhi *et al.* (1994a) is the first to compare EGF-R and c-*erb*B2 expression in all the trophoblast populations. The interesting finding is that these two receptors are expressed in a reciprocal fashion (Fig. 10.5, opposite p. 35). Villous cytotrophoblast expresses EGF-R but, as they migrate off the basement membrane to form cell columns, they lose their EGF-R and express c-*erb*B2 instead. The invasive trophoblast and endovascular trophoblast continue to express c-*erb*B2, but EGF-R expression is reacquired with terminal differentiation into multinucleated placental bed giant cells. This co-expression of EGF-R and c-*erb*B2 is also seen in syncytiotrophoblast which is the end-point in the villous pathway of differentiation.

A similar reciprocal pattern of expression is also seen in the glandular epithelium of the non-pregnant endometrium during different phases of the cycle. In the proliferative phase when there is a high degree of glandular proliferation, there is a correspondingly strong EGF-R expression. During the second half of the cycle with increasing differentiation, there is a reduction of EGF-R expression accompanied by an increase in c-*erb*B2 expression. These changes have also been observed by Press *et al.* (1990) and Jasonni *et al.* (1991). A similar phenomenon also occurs in other epithelia. Damjanov *et al.* (1986) have shown that actively proliferating epithelia such as the ductal cells of the breast express EGF-R. In contrast, maximum c-*erb*B2 expression occurs in many adult epithelia only when the tissue has reached functional maturity, such as in the lactating mammary gland (Dati *et al.* 1990). Similarly, in the adult small intestine, immature enterocytes within the crypts express little or no c-*erb*B2, but as they drop out of the mitotic cycle and differentiate into mature enterocytes, they acquire c-*erb*B2 (Cohen *et al* 1989).

From all these observations, therefore, it may be concluded that the EGF-R is probably involved in the transmission of mitogenic signals while c-*erb*B2 influences differentiated functions. Amplification of c-*erb*B2 occurs in many adenocarcinomas and is reported to correlate with a poor clinical prognosis (Singleton and Strickler 1992). However, a recent study has shown that c-*erb*B2 amplification in breast tumours is not associated with a higher proliferative index (Kreipe et al. 1993). Instead, the poor prognosis is due to the c-*erb*B2 gene inducing high metastatic potential by promoting adhesion and invasion (Yu *et al.* 1992). These findings are highly relevant to human placentation because invasive interstitial trophoblast which strongly expresses c-*erb*B2 is also non-proliferative, but is capable of secreting extracellular matrix for adhesion as well as degradative enzymes for matrix digestion, both of which will facilitate trophoblast migration (Chapter 9).

The simultaneous co-expression of EGF-R and c-*erb*B2 by the two terminally differentiated end cells, villous syncytiotrophoblast and placental bed giant cells, is intriguing. It is tempting to suggest that there could be some form of interaction between these two receptors in these multinucleated cell types. Heterodimerisation between EGF-R and c-*erb*B2 proteins has been demonstrated in other cell systems where it was found that this association altered the basic structure and modified the function of EGF-R (Goldmann *et al.* 1990; Wada *et al.* 1990). Recently, two new members of the erbB family of tyrosine kinase receptors have been identified, c-*erb*B3 and c-*erb*B4, both of which are reported to be able to interact with the EGF-R (Carraway and Cantley 1994). These authors envisage a general model for growth factor signalling whereby receptor dimerisation leading to transphosphorylation of heterologous receptors can modulate the growth regulatory signal by determining which SH2 domain-containing intracellular signalling proteins are recruited to the activated receptor complex.

IGF-IR

Two types of transmembrane receptors, IGF-IR and IGF-IIR mediate binding of the insulin-like growth factors IGF-I and IGF-II. Besides these receptors, IGFs also bind with high affinity to several different soluble IGF binding proteins (IGFBP) found in plasma and other body fluids (LeRoith 1991; Schofield 1992). The major soluble secretory product of the decidualised endometrium is also an IGF binding protein (Bell 1989) (Chapter 3). The IGF-IR is a tyrosine kinase receptor which mediates the activity of both IGF-I and IGF-II, although it binds IGF-I with 15- to 20-fold higher affinity than IGF-II (Germain-Lee *et al.* 1992). The IGF-IIR is a structurally unrelated receptor devoid of tyrosine kinase activity and might not, therefore, participate in IGF-II signal transduction although it does bind IGF-II with high affinity (Kornfeld 1992). This receptor for IGF-II shows gene imprinting in the mouse, with exclusive maternal expression but, surprisingly, is not imprinted in humans (Chapter 4).

We have investigated IGF-IR expression by immunohistology of the placental bed (Jokhi 1994). To our knowledge, no other similar studies have been published. Expression of IGF-IR was found to be restricted to villous cytotrophoblast and to cells in the proximal regions of the cell columns in first trimester chorionic villi, mirroring exactly the distribution of trophoblast with mitotic activity. This strongly suggests that IGF-IR transduces a proliferative signal in the developing placenta. *In vitro* studies have shown that while IGF-I alone is often only a weak stimulator of cell proliferation, it markedly potentiates the activity of other mitogens such as EGF or PDGF (Corps and Brown 1988). It is, therefore, notable that both the IGF-IR and EGF-R are expressed by the same trophoblast population. None of the other trophoblast populations express the IGF-IR.

PDGF-R

The PDGF-R belongs to the tyrosine kinase superfamily of cytokine receptors. It is a 180 kDa dimer composed of an α and/or a β subunit which forms either $\alpha\alpha$, $\alpha\beta$ or $\beta\beta$ receptors. These bind the various isoforms of PDGF and show differential expression in different cell populations (Ross 1989). The α subunit of the receptor can bind to either PDGF-A or PDGF-B isoforms of the cytokine, whereas the β subunit can only bind PDGF-B. Thus, a cell's response is dependent on both its receptor subunit expression and the cytokine isoforms present locally.

An early study reported that cultured trophoblast cells expressed high-affinity PDGF-Rs (Goustin et al. 1985). In contrast we ourselves could not detect either the PDGF-Rα or -β in any trophoblast populations by immunohistology and flow cytometry of isolated cells (Jokhi 1994), although strong staining for PDGF-Rβ and weak staining for PDGF-Rα were noted in villous mesenchymal fibroblasts. Holmgren et al. (1993) also observed no PDGF-Rβ expression by villous cytotrophoblast or syncytiotrophoblast by in situ hybridisation. It is possible that cultured trophoblast cells have acquired PDGF-Rs as a result of the in vitro conditions. More likely the trophoblast cultures used by Goustin et al. (1985), which had been passaged several times, could have been overgrown by PDGF-R-expressing villous mesenchymal cells. Interestingly, Holmgren et al. (1993) observed strong PDGF-Rβ expression by hydatidiform moles and choriocarcinoma cell lines, indicating that this receptor may play a role in aberrant trophoblast behaviour.

In our immunohistological study, we found intense staining for PDGF-Rβ in first trimester decidual stromal cells, and in the media of spiral arteries. Some staining for PDGF-Rα was also detected on decidual stromal cells; in contrast the arterial media was not stained. This would be in accord with the known mitogenic and angiogenic properties of PDGF (Raines et al. 1990). In their in situ hybridisation studies on the implantation site at term, Franklin et al. (1993) noted positive hybridisation by a subset of cells in decidua which they believed to be trophoblast, although it is difficult to be certain from examination of their published photomicrographs.

IL-IR

Two species of IL-1R exist – the type I (~80 kDa) receptor and and the type II (60–68 kDa) receptor (Dinarello 1991) – both belonging to the immunoglobulin superfamily of cytokine receptors. They are distinct gene products and differ from each other in their binding affinities, cell surface expression and kinetics of ligand internalisation and degradation. While both receptors can bind to either the IL-1α or IL-1β isoforms of the cytokine, in general IL-1α binds best to the type I IL-1R and IL-1β to the type II receptor. The type I receptor is expressed constitutively on most cell types and is thought to play a major role in IL-1 signalling. Expression of the type II receptor, in contrast, is more restricted and its role in IL-1 signal transduction has been questioned because of its heavily truncated cytoplasmic domain (Dinarello 1991; Sims *et al.* 1993).

To date, there is only one published immunohistological study on the localisation of type I IL-1R at the implantation site in the first trimester (Simón *et al.* 1994b). This receptor was detected in extravillous trophoblast, villous syncytiotrophoblast and mesenchymal cells, but not in villous cytotrophoblast. In decidua, the receptor was strongly expressed by glandular epithelium, but no mention was made of decidual leucocytes. It would be particularly relevant to determine the expression of IL-1R by these cells because IL-1 has been shown to influence the activation of lymphocytes, including Th2 cells and NK cells where it often acts as a co-stimulator by induction of other cytokines and their receptors (Shirawaka *et al.* 1986). Our own flow cytometric analysis of the type II IL-1R has shown very strong expression by decidual macrophages, and by the majority of T cells. In contrast, only about 10% of the CD56[+] NK cells expressed detectable amounts of this receptor (Jokhi 1994).

IL-2R

The IL-2R complex is known to comprise at least three subunits (α, β and γ) which can be expressed individually or in various combinations resulting in receptors that bind IL-2 with markedly different affinities. Whereas the α subunit alone is capable of binding IL-2 with low affinity, neither the β nor γ subunit alone can do so. However, a combination of the β and γ subunits binds IL-2 with intermediate affinity and can transmit signals in the absence of the α subunit. The high-affinity receptor is formed by all three subunits. The IL-2Rβ and γ, but not the α subunit, are members of the class I superfamily of cytokine receptors. Recent studies have shown that the γ subunit of the IL-2R is a shared component of the receptors for IL-4, IL-7, IL-15 and possibly for other cytokines as well (Nakarai *et al.* 1994; Grabstein *et al.* 1994; Taga and Kishimoto 1995). While expression of the IL-2R by T and B cells is dependent upon antigen stimulation, expression of the IL-2Rβ subunit by NK cells appears to be constitutive (Nagler *et al.* 1989; Nakarai *et al.* 1994).

The expression of IL-2Rβ by first trimester decidual NK cells has been reported by many investigators (K. Nishikawa *et al.* 1991; Starkey 1991; King *et al.* 1992) and we have shown that a small proportion (~10%) of these cells co-express the IL-2Rα. In contrast, IL-2Rα was not detected on the main populations of peripheral blood CD56^{dim} NK cells, suggesting they may lack the high-affinity receptor. Saito *et al.* (1992) have detected very slight expression of IL-2Rα and β on a small population of decidual T cells as well as on peripheral blood T cells. As yet, there have been no studies on IL-2Rγ expression. It would be of interest to know if this subunit is expressed by decidual NK cells because the level of functional response by these cells could be limited by γ chain expression since the β chain is already present in abundance constitutively.

We have not detected IL-2Rα or β on decidual macrophages so this cytokine is unlikely to have an influence on this cell type. Surprisingly, we have observed expression of IL-2Rβ on trophoblast of the cell columns, although this was not seen in the other extravillous trophoblast populations such as interstitial trophoblast and placental bed giant cells (Jokhi 1994). What action IL-2 might exert on trophoblast is unclear since IL-2R expression is generally restricted to lymphoid cells.

IL-6R

Like many interleukin receptors, the IL-6R belongs to the class I superfamily of cytokine receptors. It is expressed by various tissues and is composed of a ligand-specific α subunit and a signal-transducing β subunit (gp130) which is shared with the receptors of other growth factors, such as IL-11, LIF, CNTF and oncostatin (Sato and Mayajima 1994). We recently looked for IL-6Rα expression by cells of the first trimester placenta and in decidua using immunohistology and flow cytometry and found no positive staining cells (Jokhi 1994). We have used two different antibodies, both of which were clearly able to detect IL-6R on the surface of peripheral blood T cells by flow cytometry. We had expected some trophoblast cells to express this receptor because cultured trophoblast cells have been reported to respond to IL-6 by increased secretion of hCG (Nishino *et al.* 1990). It is possible that this *in vitro* effect is mediated by a newly described soluble version of the IL-6R containing the extracellular portion. This soluble receptor can bind to IL-6 and then aggregate with the signal-transducing gp130 chain expressed by appropriate cells to trigger functional activity (Yawata *et al.* 1993).

IL-7R

Because IL-7 has been shown to play an important role in early lymphopoiesis (Goodwin and Namen 1991), we have investigated whether any of the lymphoid cells in decidua express the corresponding receptor (Jokhi 1994). As expected, IL-7R was not detected in any trophoblast populations. However, scattered decidual leucocytes were seen to express this receptor. Flow cytometry by double staining of the cells confirmed that these were mostly decidual T cells and macrophages, while only a very small number of CD56+ NK cells expressed IL-7R. It therefore seems unlikely that this cytokine plays any significant role in decidual NK cell biology.

IFN-γR

Receptors for IFN belong to the class II superfamily of cytokine receptors. Their structural characteristics remain largely undefined. Binding studies with isolated membranes have inferred that human placental tissues express large numbers of IFN-γ receptors (Calderon *et al.* 1988). Since then, Peyman and Hammond (1992) and Peyman *et al.* (1992) have localised these receptors to both villous cytotrophoblast and syncytiotrophoblast in the first trimester and to syncytiotrophoblast at term. Similarly, Paulesu *et al.* (1994) reported the most intense staining for IFN-γR in villous syncytiotrophoblast. However, our own study (Jokhi 1994) is not in agreement with these findings in that we did not detect IFN-γR expression by villous syncytiotrophoblast either in the first trimester or at term. As discussed in Chapter 4, we feel that syncytiotrophoblast is particularly susceptible to non-specific staining, and great care is needed to interpret immunohistological findings. However, we have noted strong staining of all other first trimester trophoblast populations, from villous cytotrophoblast to all extravillous trophoblast, including placental bed giant cells. This supports previous observations that isolated trophoblast cells can respond to IFN-γ but not IFN-α *in vitro* by upregulation of their MHC class I expression (Feinman *et al.* 1987; Grabowska *et al.* 1990b; Chumbley *et al.* 1991). Flow cytometric analysis has shown that the levels of IFN-γR expression by isolated trophoblast cells were very low, suggesting there could be tight regulation of expression of this receptor *in vivo*. In contrast to the lack of IFN-γR on syncytiotrophoblast, there is intense staining of the remnants of the primitive syncytium associated with the cell columns and cytotrophoblast shell which are involved in the early stages of blastocyst implantation (Chapter 4). The reason for this dichotomy in IFN-γR expression is not immediately apparent.

Within uterine decidua, weak IFN-γR staining was seen on scattered cells which were shown to be decidual macrophages by flow cytometry. This again is in accord with functional studies where IFN-γ is shown to have important stimulatory properties for macrophages such as activation, phagocytosis, anti-microbial and tumoricidal activities, modulation of MHC antigen expression and cytokine secretion (Trinchieri and Perussia 1985; Vilcek 1990). The only other cell populations to express the IFN-γR are vascular endothelial cells of both the chorionic villous mesenchyme and the decidua. IFN-γ is reported to have wide effects on endothelial cells, particularly the enhancement of surface expression of various proteins such as MHC antigens, cytokine receptors and adhesion molecules (De Maeyer and De Maeyer-Guignard 1991). Modulation of adhesion molecules on endothelial cells of the decidual spiral arteries could influence their interaction with endovascular trophoblast migrating down the lumen of these vessels (Burrows *et al.* 1994).

TNF-R

Two distinct types of TNF-R have been identified – the p60 and the p80 – both of which specifically bind TNF-α and TNF-β. The extracellular domains of these receptors are very similar in sequence and structure which accounts for their ability to bind these two species of TNF with equal affinity. Their intracellular domains, however, are very different, suggesting that the two types of receptors employ different signal transduction pathways (Vilcek and Lee 1991; Tartaglia and Goeddel 1992). The specific role of each of these receptors is still under debate. While some studies have shown that either the p60 or the p80 TNF-R alone is sufficient for high-affinity binding and full biological activity, others have concluded that the p60 receptor is essential for TNF function in many cell types and the p80 receptor is unable to initiate a variety of responses (Vilcek and Lee 1991). The two receptors have also been shown to mediate different cellular functions when bound to TNF, such as cell cytotoxicity by the p60 receptor and lymphoproliferation by the p80 receptor (Higuchi and Aggarwal 1994). This is not surprising as their intracellular domains differ.

Our recent immunohistological localisation of p80 TNF-R (Jokhi 1994) showed no staining by any of the trophoblast populations at any stage of gestation except for those remnants of the primitive syncytium which also stained strongly for the IFN-γR (Jokhi 1994). Fetal Hofbauer cells in the chorionic villous mesenchyme also expressed p80 TNF-R throughout gestation. In addition, we detected a low level of expression of this receptor on decidual macrophages and on a subset of decidual NK cells and T cells by flow cytometry. Macrophages are known to be major targets of TNF so their expression of the receptors would be expected. Resting T cells do not normally express TNF-R, but they do so after activation when they respond to TNF by proliferation and upregulation of the high-affinity IL-2R. Similarly, NK cells also respond to TNF by increased IL-2R expression and enhanced cytotoxicity of target cells (Vassalli 1992). Yelavarthi and Hunt (1993) have studied the p60 TNF-R and have localised this receptor predominantly to first trimester villous syncytiotrophoblast with little expression seen in villous cytotrophoblast or mesenchyme. The pattern of expression of the p60 TNF-R in the placenta, therefore, appears to be different from that of the p80.

TGF-βR

Although many TGF-β binding proteins have been described, only two have been definitely identified as signalling receptors. These are the 53 kDa type I receptor and the 75 kDa type II receptor, both of which have been shown to be members of a novel transmembrane serine/threonine kinase receptor family (Massagué 1992). These two receptors are believed to co-operate in ligand binding and in initiation of signalling. A third cell surface receptor has also been recognised. This is the type III receptor (betaglycan) which, although not directly involved in signal transduction, is capable of binding TGF-β with high affinity and is thought to present different isoforms of the cytokine selectively to the type I/type II signalling receptor complex. A related molecule similar to this type III receptor is endoglin, which has been demonstrated in macrophages and vascular endothelial cells (López-Casallas *et al.* 1991; Lastres *et al.* 1992). Endoglin is a disulphide-linked homodimer that binds TGF-β_1, but not TGF-β_2. Like betaglycan, it is also thought to play a role in TGF-βR responsiveness by binding and presenting selected TGF-β isoforms to the type I/type II receptor signalling complex.

The type I/type II TGF-βR have been detected in a variety of cell types at the human implantation site (Mitchell and O'Conner-McCourt 1991; Mitchell *et al.* 1991; Graham *et al.* 1992; Selick *et al.* 1994). This is not surprising as these receptors are ubiquitous, making it difficult to arrive at any definitive views regarding their function in implantation. For this reason, we have decided to investigate the expression of the more restricted endoglin (Jokhi 1994). Immunohistology showed endoglin was weakly expressed by first trimester villous syncytiotrophoblast and this expression became much stronger by term. No expression was seen in the other trophoblast populations. A possible interpretation of these findings is that this receptor is predominantly involved in the more differentiated functions of trophoblast, such as placental transport. As expected, both villous capillary endothelial cells and decidual endothelial cells expressed endoglin strongly. Flow cytometry revealed endoglin expression also by decidual macrophages and by a small subset of decidual CD56[+] NK cells. Interestingly, the corresponding CD56[+] NK cells in peripheral blood did not express endoglin. This could be a reflection of the activated state of decidual NK cells.

LIF-R

The LIF-R is a member of the class I receptor superfamily with the conserved WSXWS motif in the extracellular domain. High-affinity binding arises when the ligand–receptor complex interacts with the accessory signal transduction molecule gp130 (Kishimoto *et al.* 1994). In addition to the membrane receptors, soluble LIF-R is described, at least in the mouse (Rathjen *et al.* 1990).

LIF-R mRNA has been detected in human blastocysts (Charnock-Jones *et al.* 1994b), and we have demonstrated abundant LIF-R transcripts in isolated first trimester trophoblast (King *et al.* 1995). It is significant that mRNA encoding LIF itself is not demonstrable in either of these tissues so that maternally derived LIF is likely to be mainly responsible for modulating trophoblast behaviour in a paracrine manner. We have similarly detected LIF-R mRNA in isolated decidual LGL and T cells so these cells are also likely targets for maternal LIF (Jokhi *et al.* 1994d).

VEGF-R

Vascular endothelial growth factor (VEGF) is a recently characterised angiogenic growth factor which causes endothelial cell proliferation and increased vascular permeability (Ferrara *et al.* 1992). Two receptors have been identified: the *fms*-like tyrosine kinase (*flt*) and a kinase domain-containing receptor (KDR) (De Vries *et al.* 1992). Recently, Charnock-Jones *et al.* (1994a) showed expression of *flt* mRNA in the cytotrophoblast shell, cell columns and interstitial trophoblast in the first trimester. This is the first demonstration of *flt* on non-endothelial cells. The BeWo choriocarcinoma cell line also expresses this receptor and was observed to respond to VEGF by tyrosine phosphorylation of mitogen-activated protein (MAP) kinase. This study raises the possibility that VEGF may act on trophoblast and affect growth, differentiation and migration.

Detection of cytokine mRNA

While the presence of mRNA in a cell does not necessarily guarantee that the protein is translated (Chapter 6), it nevertheless identifies those cells which are the most likely source of cytokine production. Furthermore, when a cytokine has been localised to a cell, a corresponding mRNA analysis will distinguish between synthesis and sequestration. A frequently used method for the estimation of levels of mRNA in tissues is by procedures such as Northern blot or dot blot. However, this extraction of total RNA from homogenised tissue does not identify the cellular source of the cytokine, particularly in an organ such as the placenta or the uterus which contains a variety of different cell types. While the technique of *in situ* hybridisation does allow accurate localisation of cytokine transcripts to cells within a tissue, it may not be sufficiently sensitive to detect small amounts of mRNA.

Recent years have seen the development and application of the reverse transcriptase polymerase chain reaction (RT-PCR) to mRNA analysis. This method is becoming increasingly popular because it is rapid and extremely sensitive. The procedure consists of isolating RNA from cells which is then used as a template for reverse transcription to complementary DNA (cDNA). The cDNA, in turn, is used as the template for PCR, using primers selected to amplify a selected cDNA region. Following PCR, the amplified product is analysed by agarose gel electrophoresis and can be identified by its size, which is predicted from knowledge of the cDNA nucleotide sequence. The PCR product can then be further characterised by restriction digestion, hybridisation or nucleotide sequencing. Because of the sensitivity of the technique, it is clear that very highly purified cell preparations are required to avoid detection of mRNA from trace levels of contaminating cells. Furthermore, a rapid method of cell isolation is needed because cytokine mRNA is usually present in cells only in small amounts, has a short half-life and is highly susceptible to degradation (Chapter 5). Some examples of the detection of cytokine mRNA in decidual leucocytes are shown in Fig. 10.6.

Detection of cytokine protein

Immunohistology with appropriate cytokine antibodies on tissue sections can provide data on the *in situ* distribution of cytokine proteins. However, there can be difficulties in the interpretation of such data. As mentioned earlier, this method cannot distinguish between a protein which has been synthesised by the cell or one that has been internalised, unless there is ancillary information on mRNA expression. In addition, cytokines are generally soluble so they can be lost easily

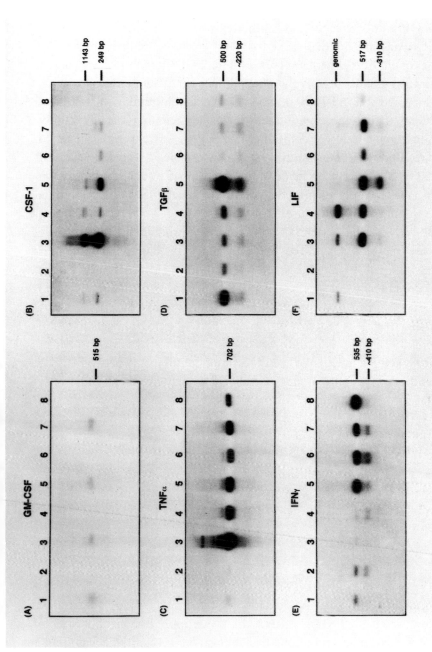

Fig. 10.6. Southern blot autoradiograms of first-round RT-PCR products from decidual NK cells and T cells. mRNA from equal numbers of decidual CD56-bright NK cells (lanes 1, 3, 5 and 7) and decidual CD3+ T cells (lanes 2, 4 ,6 and 8) was reverse transcribed and amplified with primers to: **A**, GM-CSF; **B**, CSF-1; **C**, TNF-α; **D**, TGF-β_1; **E**, IFN-γ; **F**, LIF. The RT-PCR products were then blotted onto a nylon membrane and hybridised with corresponding ^{32}P-labelled cytokine-specific cDNA probes. On all blots controls with yeast tRNA only were present and these were uniformly negative in all cases.

during processing of the tissue. Their antigenic epitopes are also susceptible to modification or destruction by the fixatives used. Thus, false positive or false negative information can be conveyed. Further confusion is caused by different antibodies having dissimilar reactivities. Although possible to some extent if the staining characteristics are optimal, it is frequently very difficult to make any quantitative assessment of the cytokine present. Finally, immunohistology cannot indicate whether the cytokine is actively secreted, in what quantities and to which stimuli it is responsive. For all these reasons, the available immunohistological data on the sources of cytokine production at the implantation site are highly variable and sometimes totally conflicting, making it extremely difficult to document the results in a meaningful way. Nevertheless, for the sake of completeness, an attempt has been made to collate the accumulated information as clearly as possible in order to provide a basis for comparison with new data as they become available in the future.

For the analysis of the dynamics of cytokine production, quantitative measurements are required by testing cellular fluids or culture supernatants derived from relevant cell types. A convenient method of quantitation is by the enzyme-linked immunosorbent assay (ELISA) which is rapid, sensitive and highly specific. To confirm that the cytokine secreted is bioactive, the ELISA can be supplemented with a bioassay using appropriate cytokine sensitive cell lines. The specificity and reproducibility of these methods make them superior to immunohistology as a means of demonstrating cytokine production. The drawback is that these assays are *in vitro* and therefore may not represent exactly the *in vivo* situation.

Cytokine production by placental and uterine cells

Data from our own laboratory on cytokine mRNA expression and cytokine protein production by trophoblast and decidual cells are summarised in Tables 10.5 and 10.6 (Jokhi 1994).

TNF-α

Chen *et al.* (1991) have localised TNF-α transcripts in human first trimester placenta and decidua by *in situ* hybridisation. Of the two villous trophoblast populations, they detected TNF-α mRNA in syncytiotrophoblast but not in cytotrophoblast. Among the extravillous trophoblast, TNF-α mRNA was found in endovascular trophoblast but not in interstitial trophoblast. Within the decidua, only stromal cells were reported to be positive for TNF-α mRNA expression. Our own data on isolated trophoblast and decidual cells using RT-PCR (Jokhi

Table 10.5. *Summary of RT-PCR data on cytokine mRNA expression by trophoblast and lymphocyte populations*

	EGF-R+ villous cytotrophoblast	c-*erb*B2+ extravillous trophoblast	CD56+ CD3- decidual LGL	CD3+ CD56- decidual T cells	CD56^{dim} CD3- peripheral blood NK cells	CD56^{bright} CD3- peripheral blood NK cells	CD3+ CD56- peripheral blood T cells
TNF-α	+	+	+	+	+	+	+
TGF-β$_1$	+	+	+	+	+	+	+
GM-CSF	+/–	+/–	+	–	–	–	–
CSF-1	+	+/–	+	+	–	–	–
IFN-γ	–	–	+	+	–	–	–
IL-2	–	–	+/–	+/–	–	–	–
LIF	–	–	+	+	–	–	–
LIF-R	+	+	+	NT	NT	NT	NT

+, consistently positive; +/–, only occasionally positive; NT, not tested.

Table 10.6. *Cytokine secretion by different cell populations from comparable experiments, as measured by ELISA*

	GM-CSF	CSF-1	EGF	LIF	IL-1β	IL-2	IL-3	TNF-α	IFN-α	IFN-γ	TGF-β$_1$
Whole decidua	911 ± 100	158 ± 29.7	0.4 ± 0.7	50 ± 9.4	186 ± 74.4	<6	<3	219 ± 54.3	<10	<10	279 ± 63.7
Decidual stromal cells	<1.5	38.3 ± 2.6	<0.2	<2	2.9 ± 0.3	<6	<3	2.3 ± 0.6	25 ± 2.5	<10	2286 ± 429
Decidual LGL, untreated	73 ± 17.7	44 ± 19.1	<0.2	<2	18.5 ± 8.7	<6	<3	7.7 ± 5.3	<10	<10	188 ± 47
Decidual LGL + 20 U/ml IL-1β	176 ± 54	29 ± 10.5	<0.2	<2	–	NT	NT	10 ± 4.0	<10	<10	174 ± 51
Decidual LGL + 20 U/ml IL-2	609 ± 121	91 ± 15.8	<0.2	<2	25 ± 11.3	–	<3	42 ± 6.1	<10	12 ± 1.5	157 ± 72
Decidual LGL + 1000 U/ml IFN-α	40 ± 14.9	19 ± 11.2	<0.2	<2	17.6 ± 8.3	<6	NT	15 ± 3.5	–	<10	253 ± 48
Decidual CD3$^+$ T cells	<1.5	2.5 ± 1.0	NT	NT	NT	NT	NT	NT	NT	NT	326
PBL^a	11.0	<2	11.5	<2	43.2	NT	NT	34.8	<10	<10	1769
Trophoblast (laminin)	270 ± 95	2.3 ± 1.5	<0.2	<2	64 ± 41.9	<6	<3	5.2 ± 2.1	<10	<10	393 ± 106
Trophoblast (fibronectin)	NT	3.1 ± 2.0	<0.2	<2	101 ± 54.3	NT	NT	6.8 ± 1.7	<10	<10	460 ± 102
JEG-3 choriocarcinoma cells	<1.5	<2	<0.2	<2	<0.3	<6	<3	<1	<10	<10	207 ± 18.9

All results are given in pg/ml secreted except for CSF-1 (given in U/ml, as the rhCSF-1 standard used to calibrate the ELISA was in U/ml). All results shown are mean values +/-SEM from at least three experiments (except for decidual CD3$^+$ T cells where experiments were tested, and also see note *a* below). NT, not tested.

^{a}Results for PBL are from a single experiment only, except for GM-CSF and CSF-1 ELISAs where three experiments were performed.

et al. 1994d; King *et al.* 1995) are somewhat different, presumably reflecting the relative sensitivities of the two detection systems. We observed abundant TNF-α mRNA in all samples of cytotrophoblast analysed. In addition, transcripts are also present in decidual NK and T cells.

The same authors (Chen *et al.* 1991) have also studied the pattern of TNF-α expression by immunohistology and have localised the protein to both villous cytotrophoblast and syncytiotrophoblast whereas, surprisingly, they did not detect any transcripts in villous cytotrophoblast by *in situ* hybridisation. Endovascular trophoblast and large decidual stromal cells also stained for TNF-α. Our own recent study based on an ELISA assay has shown that isolated first trimester trophoblast cells as well as mixed cell preparations from decidua secrete TNF-α in culture, with the latter producing appreciable quantities of the cytokine (Jokhi 1994). This is consistent with earlier studies demonstrating TNF-α in the supernatant fluid of placental and decidual explants cultured *in vitro* (Jaattela *et al.* 1988; Casey *et al.* 1989). That decidual NK cells contribute to the secretion of TNF-α is demonstrated by the use of purified preparations of these cells in the ELISA assays. Saito *et al.* (1993a) have reported similar findings. However, Vince *et al.* (1992) are of the opinion that macrophages are the major source of TNF-α in decidua. We did not observe any secretion by decidual stromal cell cultures. It would appear, therefore, that the bone marrow derived cells (macrophages and NK cells) are mainly responsible for the TNF-α found in this tissue.

We have tested the effects of IL-2, IL-1β and IFN-α on TNF-α secretion by decidual NK cells and have found that only IL-2 had a significant stimulatory effect (Jokhi 1994). This is a well-recognised response in circulating NK cells which are also known to produce TNF-α (Trinchieri 1989; Perussia 1991).

TGF-β/TGF-α

We have detected TGF-β$_1$ mRNA by RT-PCR in first trimester villous as well as extravillous trophoblast cells (King *et al.* 1995). Abundant transcripts are also seen in decidual NK cells and T cells (Jokhi *et al.* 1994d). Since the TGF-β primers used in our study were specifically designed to detect TGF-β$_1$, expression of other isoforms cannot be excluded. In the mouse, while one *in situ* hybridisation study has localised TGF-β$_1$ mRNA to uterine epithelial cells, GMG cells, macrophages and placental trophoblast (Chen *et al.* 1994), another has claimed that TGF-β$_2$ was the predominant species in uterine epithelium (Cheng *et al.* 1993). Selective expression of different TGF-β isoforms during fetal development has been previously noted although the functional significance of this is not clear (Roberts and Sporn 1990).

The immunohistological data on localisation of the protein are rather conflicting. While Graham *et al.* (1992) reported strong staining of only syncytiotrophoblast and the villous mesenchymal core, Selick *et al.* (1994) described staining of all trophoblast populations, with a gradient of staining from villous cytotrophoblast (strongest) to extravillous trophoblast in the distal portions of the cell columns (weakest). Immunoreactive TGF-β_1 and TGF-β_2 were also detected in decidual stromal cells and in the extracellular matrix by both groups of investigators, but Selick *et al.* noted staining of glandular epithelium whereas Graham *et al.* did not.

Our ELISA studies have demonstrated TGF-β_1 secretion by isolated trophoblast cells as well as by decidual NK cells, T cells and stromal cells (Jokhi 1994), which is consistent with our findings of TGF-β_1 transcripts by RT-PCR (King *et al.* 1995). No significant difference in cytokine secretion is seen between trophoblast cultured on laminin or on fibronectin. Interestingly, JEG-3 choriocarcinoma cells were also shown to secrete TGF-β_1. Of the wide variety of cytokines we have assayed for, TGF-β_1 is the only one found to be secreted by these choriocarcinoma cells in culture. Using a bioassay, Graham and Lala (1991) have similarly detected TGF-β in decidual and trophoblast-conditioned media. It would appear that TGF-β is produced by both placental and uterine cells.

TGF-α also appears to be produced by both sides of the placenta–uterine interface. Lysiak *et al.* (1993) have localised this cytokine to decidual stromal cells as well as to all trophoblast populations throughout gestation. Filla *et al.* (1993), on the other hand, detected TGF-α only in villous cytotrophoblast and not in syncytiotrophoblast, but uterine decidua was also intensely stained. The production of TGF-α by trophoblast appears to be dependent on gestational age as it is detected mainly in first trimester trophoblast, with marked diminution in the second trimester and total absence in the third trimester (Horowitz *et al.* 1993). Studies on rodents have shown that the rat uterine decidua is a major source of TGF-α, producing peak levels on day 8 (Han *et al.* 1987), so this cytokine may have an important role to play in implantation.

CSF-1

Northern blots of human placental and decidual tissues have detected multiple CSF-1 transcripts, with the largest (4.0 kb) species being reported to be the most prominent (Kauma *et al.* 1991; Daiter *et al.* 1992; Saito *et al.* 1993b). However, the *in situ* hybridisation study by Kanzaki *et al.* (1992) on term placenta localised CSF-1 mRNA predominantly to the chorionic villous mesenchyme and not to trophoblast. Our own studies based on RT-PCR showed that the α-form of CSF-1 mRNA was present in all samples of first trimester villous cytotrophoblast, but was absent or difficult to detect in 3 out of 4 samples from extravillous trophoblast (King *et al.* 1995). Earlier in this chapter we have noted that the CSF-1R is not detected in villous cytotrophoblast but only on extravillous trophoblast, so there would appear to be a reciprocal expression of this cytokine and its receptor on the two trophoblast populations. CSF-1 transcripts have also been detected in decidual NK cells and T cells (Saito *et al.* 1993c; Jokhi *et al.* 1994d). This is in agreement with RT-PCR studies demonstrating CSF-1 mRNA in mouse GMG cells, which are the NK-like cells analogous to human CD56[+] NK cells (Croy *et al.* 1991b).

Immunohistological localisation of CSF-1 by Daiter *et al.* (1992) and by Saito *et al.* (1993b) detected the protein in both villous and extravillous cytotrophoblast in first trimester placentae and in uterine glandular epithelium. Saito *et al.* (1993b) found CSF-1 also in decidual stromal cells, macrophages and lymphocytes. These workers demonstrated that CSF-1 was produced by primary cultures of trophoblast and decidual stromal cells, with the latter secreting 2–20 times more CSF-1 than the former. Our own investigation by ELISA has also demonstrated high levels of CSF-1 secretion in cell preparations containing a heterogeneous mixture of freshly isolated decidual cells, indicating that this tissue is a major source of CSF-1 production during pregnancy (Jokhi 1994). A good proportion of this secretion was by decidual stromal cells and NK cells, with little contribution by decidual T cells. Very little secretion of CSF-1 by trophoblast was detected, although the transcripts are present. This could be due to the fact that the majority of the CSF-1 mRNA detected in trophoblast is of the α-form, which encodes a predominantly membrane-bound form of CSF-1. A recent study by Kariya *et al.* (1994) has shown that progesterone significantly enhances the production of CSF-1 by human non-pregnant endometrium in a dose-dependent manner, so this hormone is obviously of prime importance not only in converting non-decidualised into decidualised endometrium but also in regulating the function of decidua once it is formed.

GM-CSF

In contrast to CSF-1, we have found the expression of GM-CSF mRNA by trophoblast cells to be rather inconsistent (King *et al.* 1995). Of the samples analysed from four individuals, two were completely negative while the other two showed the presence of transcripts. In contrast, GM-CSF mRNA was easily detected in all samples of decidual NK cells but not in decidual T cells (Jokhi *et al.* 1994d). A similar RT-PCR study by Saito *et al.* (1993c) also reported GM-CSF mRNA in decidual CD56[+] NK cells.

Data from our ELISA and bioassay studies are in agreement with the expression of GM-CSF transcripts. Appreciable amounts of immunoreactive and bioreactive GM-CSF are produced in maternal decidua. A significant component of this secretion was found to be from decidual CD56$^+$ CD3$^-$ NK cells (Jokhi *et al.* 1994c). Decidual T cells do not secrete this cytokine. Similarly, Saito *et al.* (1993c) detected GM-CSF in culture supernatants of purified first trimester decidual NK cells. Interestingly, peripheral blood NK cells express very little GM-CSF mRNA or protein, suggesting that decidual NK cells may be in an activated state *in vivo*. Our ELISA data show that when decidual NK cells are removed from the uterus, their rate of GM-CSF falls off rapidly after 24–28 hours in culture, implying loss of important *in vivo* regulatory signals. These signals could, at least in part, be provided by decidual stromal cells for we have observed that production of GM-CSF by decidual NK cells was considerably enhanced when they were co-cultured on a substrate of decidual stromal cells.

Addition of IL-2, even the low dose of 20 U/ml, was found to increase considerably GM-CSF secretion by decidual NK cells (Jokhi *et al.* 1994c). Studies on peripheral blood NK cells have also shown that IL-2 stimulates GM-CSF secretion and have implicated the p75 IL-2Rβ rather than the p55 IL-2Rα subunit (Levitt *et al.* 1991; Burdach *et al.* 1991). This is likely to be true also for decidual NK cells as they have been shown to express the IL-2Rβ constitutively. Although having no effects on their own, IFN-α, IL-4 and TGF-β$_1$ were observed to inhibit the IL-2 induced increase in GM-CSF production by decidual NK cells. This is consistent with the finding that IFN-α and IL-4 inhibit the proliferative and lymphokine-activated killer (LAK) responses generated by IL-2 stimulation of peripheral blood NK cells (Sone *et al.* 1988; Spits *et al.* 1988; Nagler *et al.* 1989) as well as IL-2 induced TNF-α expression (Blay *et al.* 1990).

Considerable production of GM-CSF was also seen in trophoblast cultures by ELISA, and immunocytochemical staining has localised this cytokine in the cytoplasm of trophoblast cell smears (Jokhi *et al.* 1994c) in spite of inconsistent mRNA expression. Surprisingly, no immunoreactive or bioreactive GM-CSF was found in the culture supernatants of JEG-3 or JAR choriocarcinoma cells. Whether this loss of GM-CSF production is an *in vitro* artefact resulting from long-term passage of these cells or whether this observation is biologically significant remains to be determined.

IL-2

Although early studies have reported IL-2 mRNA expression in syncytiotrophoblast of term and preterm placenta (Boehm *et al.* 1989) and IL-2-like protein material in human placenta and amnion (Soubiran *et al.* 1987), this has not been confirmed (Haynes *et al.* 1993). This cytokine could not be detected in cultures of first trimester chorionic explants (Main *et al.* 1987) nor in supernatants from purified decidual NK cells (Saito *et al.* 1993c). Our own data are in agreement with these previous *in vitro* studies. We could detect no IL-2 secretion in cell culture supernatants from first trimester trophoblast or decidual cells (Jokhi 1994) nor could we demonstrate IL-2 transcripts in any of these cells even after two rounds of PCR amplification (Jokhi *et al.* 1994d; King *et al.* 1995). It may be concluded that IL-2 is not produced anywhere in the normal implantation site. This is significant in view of the fact that IL-2 can transform decidual NK cells into potent LAK cells which are capable of lysing trophoblast cells *in vitro* (King and Loke 1990). It remains to be determined whether IL-2 is expressed in pathological conditions of pregnancy.

IL-1

The immunohistological data on the localisation of IL-1α and IL-1β are highly conflicting. Paulcsu *et al.* (1991b) detected both forms of IL-1 in villous syncytiotrophoblast only while villous cytotrophoblast and extravillous trophoblast in the cell columns were unreactive. In contrast, later reports by Hu *et al.* (1992) and Simón *et al.* (1994b) demonstrated the cytokine in villous cytotrophoblast and extravillous trophoblast as well as in maternal decidual stromal cells. Even villous mesenchymal cells express this cytokine.

We have recently investigated the secretion of IL-1β on isolated trophoblast and decidual cells by ELISA (Jokhi 1994). Abundant IL-1β was found to be secreted by first trimester mixed decidual cells, much of which is contributed by decidual NK cells rather than stromal cells. Saito *et al.* (1993c), however, could not demonstrate IL-1β secretion by purified decidual NK cells although they detected IL-1β mRNA in a population of decidual mononuclear cells. First trimester trophoblast cultured on either laminin or fibronectin also secrete IL-1β. This is in agreement with early studies which showed IL-1β production by first trimester villous explants and by isolated term trophoblast cells (Main *et al.* 1987). In these studies, production of the cytokine by contaminating cells cannot be entirely excluded, especially as term placental mononuclear phagocytes have been shown to produce abundant IL-1 (Flynn *et al.* 1982). Since both trophoblast and decidual cells express the receptor for IL-1, it is likely that this cytokine functions in an autocrine as well as a paracrine manner.

IL-6

Kameda *et al.* (1990) have demonstrated that bioreactive IL-6 is released into the medium of explant cultures of human placental tissues. Immunohistological staining localised the source of production in syncytiotrophoblast. However, a later study by Kauma *et al.* (1993) concluded that both trophoblast and villous mesenchymal cells are capable of IL-6 production, with trophoblast showing a higher production rate. In contrast, dot blot analysis of IL-6 mRNA expression showed the reverse finding with the steady-state expression being higher in villous mesenchymal cells, suggesting that the synthesis of IL-6 is probably post-transcriptionally regulated. Decidual cells at term also secrete small amounts of IL-6 which can be significantly increased by inflammatory cytokines, such as IL-1 and TNF (Dudley *et al.* 1992).

IFN

IFN-α has been detected in amniotic fluid from normal pregnant women from 16 weeks gestation to term (Lebon *et al.* 1982; Chard *et al.* 1986) and in perfusion studies on human term placenta (Bocci *et al.* 1985). This cytokine has also been localised in first trimester chorionic villous tissue by immunohistology (Howatson *et al.* 1988; Bulmer *et al.* 1990; Paulesu *et al.* 1991a). The most prominent reactivity was described in villous syncytiotrophoblast and in some interstitial trophoblast, but no staining could be seen in villous cytotrophoblast or in trophoblast of the cell columns. Hofbauer cells within the villous mesenchyme also contain IFN-α. In our own ELISA studies on isolated placental and decidual cells (Jokhi 1994), we could detect very low levels of IFN-α secretion only by decidual stromal cells. No other cell types were observed to secrete this cytokine. We therefore conclude that IFN-α is not produced to any great extent in the first trimester by cells at the implantation site. However, at term Chard *et al.* (1986) reported greater concentrations of IFN-α in decidua than in any other normal tissues as measured by a two-site immunoradiometric assay.

Like IFN-α, immunohistological localisation has also detected IFN-γ mainly in villous syncytiotrophoblast (Bulmer *et al.* 1990; Paulesu *et al.* 1991a). The most intense staining is found in the first trimester and becomes almost imperceptible at term (Paulesu *et al.* 1994). In contrast, IFN-α mRNA is found exclusively in first trimester villous cytotrophoblast by *in situ* hybridisation (Haynes *et al.* 1993). In Chapter 4, we mentioned that many placental proteins may be transcribed in the villous cytotrophoblast layer and are then transported to the overlying syncytial layer for storage and eventual secretion. A recent study has shown that IFN-γ, together with IFN-α and IFN-β, are all released by first trimester placental explants cultured *in vitro* and trophoblast cells were proposed as the likely source of these cytokines (Tao and Cao 1993). We ourselves, however, were unable to detect IFN-γ mRNA on isolated trophoblast cells by RT-PCR nor could we demonstrate secretion of this cytokine by ELISA (Jokhi 1994; King *et al.* 1995). The trophoblast cells used in our experiments are derived from villous cytotrophoblast and extravillous trophoblast of the cell columns (see Chapter 5). These are the trophoblast populations which do not contain IFN-γ (Paulesu *et al.* 1994) so it is possible that we do not have the appropriate cell types. However, we (Jokhi *et al.* 1994d) and others (Saito *et al.* 1993c) have detected IFN-γ mRNA in purified decidual NK cells and T cells by RT-PCR although the level of secretion of the protein was very low. This production can be increased by IL-2 *in vitro*.

Recently, mRNA of an IFN very similar to ovine and bovine trophoblast interferons (IFN-τ) has been detected in human trophoblast, particularly in the migrating population (Whaley *et al.* 1994), but what role it plays in implantation is not known.

Kit ligand

Kit ligand (KL) protein has been localised by immunohistology mainly to fetal fibroblasts within the mesenchyme of the larger chorionic villi of first trimester placentae (Jokhi 1994). Although not present in any villous trophoblast populations, KL was found in extravillous trophoblast of the cell columns and in invasive trophoblast. In contrast, an earlier *in situ* hybridisation study detected KL mRNA in both villous cytotrophoblast and extravillous trophoblast (Sharkey *et al.* 1992). A similar observation has been made for MHC class I expression where villous cytotrophoblast expresses mRNA but not the protein (Chapter 6), indicating that, in this cell population, the transcripts are not always translated. Alternatively, it is possible that the monoclonal antibody used in our study does not detect all the isoforms of KL known to be present. At least seven isoforms arising from alternative splicing of the primary transcripts are expressed in the human placenta when analysed by RT-PCR (Sharkey *et al.* 1992, 1994).

Within the decidua, in addition to the invading trophoblast, KL expression was seen in the arterial media of maternal blood vessels. This pattern of expression of KL appears broadly similar to that reported in the mouse where KL is expressed in trophoblast of the ectoplacental cone and in endothelial cells of developing blood vessels at day 7.5 of pregnancy (Motro *et al.* 1991). The local production of KL at the implantation site may influence decidual macrophages or a subset of NK cells which are shown to express the corresponding receptor c-*kit*.

LIF

Using an RNase protection assay to quantitate mRNA levels encoding LIF in human endometrium, Charnock-Jones *et al.* (1994b) detected only low levels in endometrium during the proliferative phase of the cycle, but this increased significantly in the luteal phase. Immunohistology localised the cytokine to glands. This correlates well with the observation in murine pregnancy where LIF mRNA expression in uterine endometrial glands occurs just prior to implantation (Bhatt *et al*. 1991). In a recent RT-PCR study on isolated decidual cells, we have detected LIF mRNA in NK cells and T cells, but not in isolated first trimester trophoblast (Jokhi *et al*. 1994d; King *et al*. 1995). We have also demonstrated the presence of LIF in supernates from cultured decidual cells but, surprisingly, no LIF production was found from purified decidual NK cells in spite of detectable mRNA (Jokhi 1994). It is possible that translation of LIF mRNA to protein does not normally occur in these cells, or if it does, the level of secretion is too low to permit detection by ELISA. Alternatively, the removal of decidual NK cells from their *in vivo* environment could result in the loss of regulatory signals. We have not tested the production of LIF by decidual T cells. Another potential source of LIF production we have not investigated is the decidual glands, because these are important sites of LIF production in mice prior to implantation (Bhatt *et al*. 1991; Stewart *et al*. 1992). The overall conclusion from the available evidence is that LIF is likely to be maternally derived.

EGF

EGF mRNA has been detected in human endometrium and decidua (Haining *et al*. 1991), and Sakakibara *et al*. (1994) have demonstrated the presence of EGF mRNA in decidua by Northern blot analysis and by *in situ* hybridsation with an appropriate cDNA probe. In the latter study no positive hybridisation was seen in non-pregnant endometrium at either the proliferative or the secretory phase. Endometrial cells decidualised *in vitro* by medroxyprogesterone acetate also showed a positive hybridisation band by Northern blot. These results demonstrate that the EGF gene is expressed in decidualised but not in non-decidualised endometrium. EGF proteins have also been localised by immunohistology in human endometrium, decidua and placenta (Hofmann *et al*. 1991, 1992). Staining for EGF was reported to be present in decidual stromal cells and uterine surface epithelium, whilst in the placenta, staining was predominantly in syncytiotrophoblast. The authors themselves acknowledged that the EGF detected may not be due to active synthesis but could be sequestered or internalised. A possible source is maternal blood because EGF is normally present in serum. Surprisingly, in our own study on isolated cells using ELISA, we could not detect EGF in the supernatant of any trophoblast or decidual cells cultured *in vitro* (Jokhi 1994). The ELISA technique is highly sensitive and can detect cytokines down to picogram quantities. We therefore conclude that EGF is not secreted by decidual cells to any great extent *in vitro* even if these cells contain the mRNA or protein *in vivo*. Indeed, it has been proposed that EGF may not be the major physiological ligand for EGF-R *in utero* and that TGF-α is a more likely candidate. TGF-α has considerable sequence homology to EGF, binds to EGF-R with equal affinity to EGF and has similar if not identical biological activities to EGF, both *in vivo* and *in vitro* (Carpenter and Wahl 1990). Both EGF and TGF-α were reported to stimulate uptake of [^{3}H]thymidine by trophoblast cells, indicating similar mitogenic activity of these two cytokines on these cells (Filla *et al.* 1993).

VEGF

The VEGF family is a group of dimeric proteins each consisting of two identical 23 kDa subunits (Gospodarowicz *et al.* 1989). Analysis of cDNA clones predicts five isoforms of 206, 189, 165, 145 and 121 amino acids, arising by alternative splicing of exons 5 to 8 (Houck *et al.* 1991). Four of these isoforms (189, 165, 145 and 121) have been observed in human endometrium and in the placenta (Charnock-Jones *et al.* 1993; Sharkey *et al.* 1993). In the proliferative phase endometrium, VEGF mRNA is localised to the glandular epithelium and to cells of the stroma, while in the luteal phase transcripts are found mainly in glandular cells. In first trimester placenta, faint hybridisation can be seen in syncytiotrophoblast, but the most intense hybridisation occurs in the layer of macrophages situated at the placental–decidual border. Hofbauer cells within the chorionic villous mesenchyme also show positive hybridisation. At term, VEGF mRNA can still be seen in syncytiotrophoblast, but now invading extravillous trophoblast in decidua also contains VEGF transcripts. Hofbauer cells at this stage of pregnancy no longer expresses VEGF mRNA but maternal macrophages continue to do so.

Functional implications

From the preceding sections it can be seen that trophoblast cells express receptors for a variety of cytokines so they are potentially able to respond to these signalling proteins. Furthermore, some of these receptors are expressed differentially in trophoblast sub-populations, suggesting that cytokines may exert their influence on different stages of trophoblast development. In addition to trophoblast, cells in maternal decidua also express cytokine receptors, implying that they are also susceptible to the effects of these molecules. The cytokines themselves appear to be produced by both trophoblast and uterine cells, thereby establishing autocrine and paracrine loops of interactions. Although a complete picture has not yet emerged, these observations should at least provide some preliminary ideas regarding the possible role of cytokines in human implantation.

The colony stimulating factors (CSF-1, GM-CSF, KL)

The observation that CSF-1R is expressed predominantly by invasive trophoblast populations suggests that CSF-1 could be involved with this feature of trophoblast behaviour. This hypothesis is supported by reports that expression of CSF-1R correlates with tumour cell invasiveness (Kacinski *et al.* 1990; Filderman *et al.* 1991). However, *in vitro* studies on trophoblast cells isolated from first trimester and term placenta have claimed that CSF-1 induces differentiation of cytotrophoblast into syncytiotrophoblast, with a concomitant increase in hCG and hPL production (Wegmann 1990; Saito *et al.* 1993d). We have observed that CSF-1 increases [^{3}H]thymidine incorporation slightly by first trimester trophoblast cultured on laminin but not fibronectin (Jokhi 1994), but we are uncertain whether this is indicative of cellular proliferation or whether trophoblast is undergoing endoreduplicative cycles without cytokinesis, as proposed for murine trophoblast by Drake and Head (1994). This latter process would transform invasive trophoblast into multinucleated placental bed giant cells.

Besides trophoblast, decidual macrophages also express CSF-1R. This cytokine is known to have a variety of effects on mononuclear phagocytes, such as supporting their differentiation and survival (Metcalf 1991) or potentiating their functional activities (Sherr 1990). CSF-1 has also been found to alter surface MHC expression on macrophages, an observation which has obvious implications in the regulation of MHC expression by extravillous trophoblast (Vairo and Hamilton 1991). In addition to decidual macrophages, placental macrophages (Hofbauer cells) also express CSF-1R, with a significant increase in expression between early gestation and term. This may reflect an overall maturation of Hofbauer cells and, thus, their functional competence which may have a bearing in the control of transplacental infections (Loke 1982; Loke *et al.* 1982). Homozygous mice with inactivation mutation in the CSF-1 gene (*op/op*) cannot breed. The uteri of these *op/op* animals are completely devoid of macrophages which are usually abundant in either normal or +/*op* heterozygotes (Pollard 1991). This observation suggests that the function of CSF-1 in reproduction could be mediated via its effects on uterine macrophages.

Unlike CSF-1R, GM-CSF-R appears to be expressed by all trophoblast populations. GM-CSF has a modest effect on [^{3}H]thymidine uptake by trophblast as we have shown in culture and, in a later study, we noted that GM-CSF enhanced the survival of primary cultures of first trimester trophoblast *in vitro* (Loke *et al.*

1992a; Jokhi 1994). This is consistent with reports that GM-CSF can inhibit apoptosis and prolong the survival of a variety of cell types (Brach *et al*. 1992; Colotta *et al*. 1992). In the mouse, the effect of GM-CSF on trophoblast proliferation is correlated with gestational age as this cytokine stimulates ectoplacental core trophoblast on day 7.5 of pregnancy, has only an intermediate effect on day 12 trophoblast and no effect at all on day 14 (Wegmann 1990). The fact that GM-CSF-R is expressed by villous syncytiotrophoblast, which is a non-mitotic, terminally differentiated cell type, would suggest that GM-CSF has other functions beside stimulation of trophoblast proliferation. Rat trophoblast cultures have been shown to produce placental lactogen when incubated with GM-CSF (Wegmann 1992) so this cytokine could influence trophoblast synthetic activity. The expression of receptors by the syncytial trophoblast layer is always difficult to interpret because these receptors could be used for transport of molecules from the mother to the fetus rather than to mediate function of the trophoblast itself.

As for CSF-1R, both maternal and placental macrophages also express GM-CSF-R, so these cells are likely to be potential targets for GM-CSF. Indeed, GM-CSF and CSF-1 may act in synergy in dictating macrophage functions (Falk and Vogel 1988). Unlike CSF-1, mice homozygous for a disrupted GM-CSF gene show no major defects in haematopoeisis as reflected in cell populations of the bone marrow, spleen and blood. These animals are also fertile. The only notable changes are observed in the lungs where pathological lesions resembling the human condition of alveolar proteinosis are present (Stanley *et al*. 1994). Therefore, the role of GM-CSF in reproduction remains unconfirmed. Although 'knock-out' mice are often excellent models for cytokine research, there can be problems in interpretation due to species specificity and functional redundancy of some cytokines.

In contrast to CSF-1R and GM-CSF-R, there is no c-*kit* expression by any trophoblast populations at any stage of pregnancy so KL is unlikely to influence placental development, at least directly. This is consistent with the observation that the placentae of *kit*-deficient mice are apparently normal and the animals are fertile (Wordinger *et al*. 1988). The cells that do express c-*kit* are decidual macrophages and fetal Hofbauer cells as well as a small CD56^{dim} subset of decidual NK cells. KL has recently been shown to prevent apoptosis of cultured CD3$^-$ CD56^{bright} NK cells derived from peripheral blood as assessed by DNA fragmentation studies, and this survival is due to induction of expression of the *bcl*-2 protein (Carson *et al*. 1994). Since KL is produced by extravillous trophoblast, the possibility arises that this cytokine could play a role in maintaining decidual macrophage and NK cell viability at the implantation site. Besides the secreted form of KL, the transmembrane form could also be involved in signalling to macrophages and NK cells by a mechanism of cell–cell contact. Evidence for a functional role of the membrane form of KL is seen in *Sl^d* mutants who lack this transmembrane ligand. Germ cells are absent in these animals.

Growth factors (EGF, NDF, PDGF, VEGF, TGF-α, TGF-β, LIF)

The reciprocal pattern of expression of EGF-R and c-*erb*B2 by different trophoblast populations points to the former as a transmitter of mitogenic signals while the latter determines trophoblast differentiation and invasion. However, this could be an over-simplistic interpretation. Maruo *et al.* (1992) found that the primary action of EGF on early first trimester placental explants (<6 weeks) was proliferative, but during the second half of the first trimester EGF stimulated increased hCG and hPL secretion. Kenton and Johnson (1994) have shown that EGF induced the ATP-dependent release of placental alkaline phosphatase by syncytiotrophoblast plasma membrane vesicles. Thus, EGF may have a proliferative or a differentiating function on trophoblast depending on gestational age. This would explain the immunohistological observation that the predominant site of EGF-R expression shifts from the proliferative villous cytotrophoblast to the non-mitotic, terminally differentiated villous syncytiotrophoblast with increasing gestational age. Similarly, c-*erb*B2 may also have a dual function. Candidate ligands for this receptor have recently been identified and are named neu differentiation factor (NDF) and heregulin-α (Peles *et al.* 1992; W. Holmes *et al.* 1992). When tested on breast tumour cell lines, NDF was reported to inhibit proliferation and to induce maturation and phenotypic differentiation of target cells, such as secretion of milk components, whereas heregulin-α caused cells to divide and proliferate. Several NDF-related proteins can be generated by alternative splicing, raising the possibility that different isoforms could fulfil distinct biological functions (Ben-Baruch and Yarden 1994). It is not clear what signals are transmitted into a cell like syncytiotrophoblast or placental bed giant cell that expresses both EGF-R and c-*erb*B2 simultaneously.

Decidual stromal cells also express EGF-R. In many developmental processes, the action of EGF on the surrounding mesenchyme is very important in regulating epithelial morphogenesis (Nilsen-Hamilton 1990). In addition, co-treatment of endometrial stromal cells with EGF and progesterone is observed to stimulate differentiation with increased production of prolactin, laminin and fibronectin (Irwin *et al.* 1991). This interaction between growth factors and hormones is likely to be very important for decidualisation during pregnancy.

Unlike the preceding two growth factor receptors, the IGF-R has a more restricted pattern of expression, being found mainly in the trophoblast population with mitotic activity. This is in accord with the generally accepted view that the

IGF polypeptides are involved in regulation of cellular proliferation and have been implicated in fetal growth and development where their activity is growth-hormone independent (Baker *et al*. 1993). Decidual stromal cells as well as uterine glandular and surface epithelium also express IGF-R. Together with the observation that IGF-I and IGF-II are produced by trophoblast and by decidual cells, it may be proposed that this family of growth factors could play a prominent role in the autocrine and paracrine regulation of trophoblast and decidual growth. The observation that the major secretory product of decidualised endometrium is an IGF-binding protein (Chapter 3) (Bell 1989) would support this conclusion. In mice, the gene encoding IGF-II is maternally imprinted while that of its receptor is paternally imprinted (Chapter 4). The functional implication of this reciprocal expression is not known.

The role of PDGF on trophoblast development is unclear because the data on the expression of the receptors are conflicting. Investigators from Sweden believe that some cytotrophoblast cells express both the cytokine and the receptor, and have proposed an autocrine mechanism of action (Goustin *et al*. 1985). While we would accept that the cytokine itself is probably produced by trophoblast, we do not agree that trophoblast expresses either of the receptors. In our opinion, trophoblast-derived PDGF acts mainly on decidual stromal cells in a paracrine manner, providing an example whereby a growth factor from placenta influences the development of decidual components. The expression of PDGF-Rβ by decidual spiral arterial media could reflect the known angiogenic function of PDGF and its proliferative effect on smooth muscle (Raines *et al*. 1990). Another growth factor with potential influence on decidual arteries is VEGF which is a powerful mitogen for endothelial cells. The surprising observation that the VEGF-R, *flt*, is expressed also by trophoblast cells would indicate that this growth factor can affect other cell types besides endothelial cells. How trophoblast responds to VEGF is unclear. We have cultured isolated first trimester trophoblast cells in the presence of recombinant human VEGF$_{165}$ but observed no enhanced proliferation (Jokhi 1994). However, as *flt* is expressed *in vivo* mainly by the non-mitotic trophoblast populations, proliferation is not a valid end-point to measure. The influence of VEGF on the differentiation of endovascular trophoblast would merit investigation because this trophoblast population replaces endothelial cells over large areas in decidual spiral arteries.

Receptors for TGF-β have been detected in a variety of cell types at the human implantation site and the cytokine itself is demonstrable in decidua. TGF-β has been implicated as an 'immunosuppressive' factor in decidua by modulating the response of maternal leucocytes to trophoblast. In contrast to IFN-γ, TGF-β has been observed to downregulate surface expression of MHC class I antigen (Geiser *et al*. 1993). The cytokine also restricts trophoblast invasion through a reduction in collagenase secretion and induction of tissue inhibitor of metalloproteinases. Recently, TGF-β has been reported to enhance the production of fetal fibronectin by trophoblast (Feinberg *et al*. 1994). All these isolated observations have cumulatively thrust TGF-β forward as potentially a very important cytokine in implantation. In contrast, TGF-α appears to be a stimulator of trophoblast growth *in vitro*, possibly acting via the EGF-R (Filla *et al*. 1993; Lysiak *et al*. 1993).

The leukaemia inhibitory factor (LIF) is a pleiotropic cytokine with the unusual feature of having different functions in embryonic life versus adult life (Gough 1992; Hilton 1992; Metcalf 1992). It has been featured in the 'cross-talk' between the nervous and immune systems (Patterson 1994). In the context of placental development, the most relevant feature of LIF is its ability to prevent differentiation commitment in pluripotential embryonic stem cells, and to stimulate their growth, such as in murine primordial germ cells (Cheng *et al*. 1993). Experiments using transgenic 'knock-out' mice have shown that females lacking a functional LIF gene cannot undergo successful implantation, but their blastocysts are viable and can implant and develop to term when transferred to wild-type pseudopregnant recipients (Stewart *et al*. 1992). Furthermore, post-implantation production of LIF by murine granulated metrial gland (GMG) cells, which are analogous to human decidual NK cells, suggests a continuing role for LIF (Croy *et al*. 1991b). The demonstration of LIF-R mRNA in human trophoblast populations and of LIF mRNA in decidual NK cells and T cells supports the conclusion that maternally derived LIF may be as critical for human trophoblast development as it is in the mouse.

Interleukins and inflammatory cytokines (IL-1, IL-2, IL-6, IL-15, TNF)

As expected, receptors for many interleukins are expressed by decidual leucocytes, indicating that they are potential targets for these cytokines. The established roles for many of these cytokines are the control of growth and development of different leucocyte populations and as mediators of the responses generated by immunological reactions. Because of the large numbers of leucocytes present in decidua, these cytokines could be potentially very important in regulating their activity. Interestingly, trophoblast cells have also been observed to express some interleukin receptors, such as IL-1R and IL-2R, so these cytokines could exhibit a degree of pleiotropism that is wider than hitherto supposed.

IL-1 has been implicated in the process of blastocyst implantation by studies showing secretion of IL-1α and IL-1β by human pre-implantation embryos and correlation of high levels of secretion with successful implantation after *in vitro* fertilisation (Zolti *et al.* 1991; Sheth *et al.* 1991). Furthermore, expression of IL-1R by human endometrial epithelium is reported to peak at the secretory phase of the cycle which is the time when implantation would occur (Simón *et al.* 1993). In mice, embryonic implantation can be blocked by the intraperitoneal administration of IL-1R antagonist (Simón *et al.* 1994a). A role for IL-1 in human placental development is shown by the increase in trophoblast hCG synthesis stimulated by this cytokine (Yagel *et al.* 1989b) and upregulation of CSF-1 production by villous core mesenchymal cells (Harty and Kauma 1992). We have investigated the effects of IL-1β on decidual NK cells *in vitro* and have observed that, while this cytokine did not influence NK cell proliferation, it specifically increased GM-CSF production by these cells. The production of CSF-1, EGF, LIF, IL-2, TNF-α, IFN-α, IFN-γ and TGF-β$_1$ by decidual NK cells was unaffected by IL-1β (Jokhi 1994).

IL-2 is potentially a very important cytokine in implantation because it is a potent mitogenic agent for decidual NK cells (Starkey 1991; K. Nishikawa *et al.* 1991; King *et al.* 1992) and more specifically can transform decidual NK cells into aggressive LAK cells which are capable of lysing first trimester trophoblast *in vitro* in contrast to freshly isolated decidual NK cells which cannot (King and Loke 1990). We have also noted that IL-2, even in low doses, considerably augmented the secretion of GM-CSF by decidual NK cells *in vitro* (Jokhi *et al.* 1994c). However, the significance of these observations to the situation *in vivo* is unclear since IL-2 has not been convincingly demonstrated anywhere in the normal implantation site. This is to be expected as otherwise IL-2 stimulation of decidual NK cells will result in destruction of trophoblast. Perhaps IL-2 is produced only in pathological pregnancies such as infection, where the cytokine is then instrumental in causing the pregnancy failure. The recently described IL-15 is found to share many biological properties with IL-2. Northern blot screening of human tissues revealed that the highest levels of IL-15 mRNA were detected in placenta and skeletal muscle (Grabstein *et al.* 1994). It has been shown that IL-15 requires both the β and γ chains of the IL-2R for binding and signalling (Giri *et al.* 1994). The IL-2Rγ is expressed by the CD56[bright] subset of NK cells in peripheral blood (Ishii *et al.* 1994), although it is not known whether decidual NK cells also express this receptor. However, decidual NK cells as well as extravillous trophoblast do express the IL-2Rβ, so IL-15 may prove to be an important cytokine for implantation *in vivo* especially as IL-2 has not been demonstrated in decidua.

IL-6 has been shown to augment the cytotoxic capability of human peripheral blood NK cells (Luger *et al.* 1989), and also to alter the cell surface phenotype and their adhesion characteristics to extracellular matrix proteins (Rabinowitch *et al.* 1993). However, while we have detected the expression of IL-6R by peripheral blood NK cells, these receptors were not demonstrable in decidual NK cells. These latter cells, therefore, may not respond in a similar way.

The TNF family of cytokines (TNF-α, TNF-β) is grouped among the inflammatory cytokines because of their ability to initiate the cascade of events associated with the inflammatory response. However, the TNFs are extremely pleiotropic factors, a feature attributable to the ubiquity of their receptors, their ability to activate multiple signalling pathways and their ability to induce or suppress the expression of a large number of genes. While they play a beneficial role in normal host resistance to infection and malignant tumours, over-production of TNF can result in chronic wasting conditions or even severe systemic toxicity and death as in septic shock. In the context of implantation, *in vitro* cytotoxicity and growth inhibition studies on trophoblast have led to the suggestion that TNF-α may act to limit the extent of trophoblast invasion into the uterus (Hunt 1989). Jikihara and Handwerger (1994) have shown that TNF-α is the most potent inhibitor of prolactin synthesis and release by human decidual stromal cells *in vitro* compared with other cytokines tested such as IL-1, IL-8 and TGF-β. The role of prolactin in implantation is presently unclear (Chapter 3).

Interferons (IFN-α, IFN-γ)

We have previously reviewed the role of interferons in human placental development (Loke and King 1990). In sheep, the major product of the trophectoderm of pre-implantation embryos is a molecule with significant homology to IFN-α called ovine trophoblast protein-1 (oTP-1). These trophoblast interferons of domestic ruminant species are now termed IFN-τ (Roberts *et al.* 1993), and are believed to be responsible for eliciting maternal recognition of pregnancy by preventing early regression of the corpus luteum (Roberts 1989). In human pregnancy, trophoblast hCG appears to have taken over this role so human placental IFN-α probably does not function in the same way as oTP-1. IFN-α is more likely to influence decidual leucocyte function. This cytokine has been observed to inhibit the proliferation and generation of LAK activity in IL-2 stimulated NK cells (Sone *et al.* 1988), and we have noted that IFN-α inhibited the IL-2 induced increase in GM-CSF secretion by decidual NK cells (Jokhi 1994). These findings suggest that IFN-α could exert a modulatory role on decidual NK cells and, thus, have an important influence on trophoblast–decidual NK cell interaction.

IFN-γ is known to be a powerful upregulator of MHC class I and class II antigen expression by a variety of cell types (Trinchieri and Perussia 1985; Vilcek 1990), including class I expression by trophoblast (Chapter 6), leading to partial protection of trophoblast against lysis by decidual LAK cells (Chapter 8). IFN-γ, therefore, could be a pivotal cytokine in determining trophoblast susceptibility to decidual NK cells. Two other cell populations in decidua express IFN-γR. These are macrophages and endothelial cells. IFN-γ has recognised stimulatory properties for macrophages (Vilcek 1990) and can enhance the expression of various cell surface proteins on endothelial cells such as MHC antigens, cytokine receptors and adhesion molecules (De Maeyer and De Maeyer-Guignard 1991). This latter effect could play an important part in modifying endothelial cells of spiral arteries for interaction with endovascular trophoblast (Chapter 9).

It must not be forgotten that the IFNs, particularly the type I family, were originally recognised because of their anti-viral activity. This may well be their function also on trophoblast. Aboagye-Mathiesen *et al.* (1993) have demonstrated the induction of IFN production by human trophoblast cells *in vitro*. While non-viral inducers induce exclusively IFN-β production, viruses such as Sendai and Newcastle Disease Virus induce a mixture of IFN-αI, IFN-αII1 (omega 1) and IFN-β all of which have physical and anti-viral activities characteristic of the type I IFNs. This Danish group has also reported that virus-induced trophoblast IFN-β has an anti-proliferative effect on mitogen-stimulated peripheral blood lymphocytes and proposed that this could be a mechanism for local control of maternal immune response at the feto-maternal interface (Zdravkovic *et al.* 1994). It should, however, be noted that the lymphoid populations in the human uterus are not the same, phenotypically and functionally, as those in peripheral blood (Chapter 7).

11

Clinical implications of defective implantation

Introduction

In the previous chapters an attempt has been made to describe some of the cellular and molecular events which occur in the placental bed in early pregnancy. It is apparent that much remains to be learnt about how normal placentation in humans is achieved. In particular, it is not clear how placental trophoblast cells interact with the variety of maternal decidual cells present in the uterine lining, and how these interactions result in controlled trophoblast migration and development. However, it is accepted that trophoblast under- or over-invasion has serious clinical consequences (Robertson 1987; Pijnenborg 1994), and many clinical conditions can arise from defective interaction between trophoblast and maternal tissues early in pregnancy. These will be discussed in this chapter.

Infertility

Up to 15% of couples are unable to conceive within one year of attempting pregnancy and, after investigations, up to 20% of these cases are 'unexplained' (Mosher 1985; Page 1989; Azziz 1993). In many of these latter patients the primary cause may be 'poor uterine receptivity', although the age-dependent decrease in fecundity seems most likely to be due to poor oocyte quality (Navot *et al.* 1994). In human *in vitro* fertilisation (IVF) low uterine receptivity is also thought to contribute significantly to pregnancy failure. Until more is known about the presumed window of implantation in humans and what markers can be used to delineate a period of receptivity, little progress can be made. As this is an almost impossible area to investigate in humans because of ethical difficulties, novel approaches need to be sought. Perhaps the paradox that implantation will occur readily at all times at other sites whilst the uterus is only receptive at certain times could be usefully exploited, and a search made for markers of 'resistance' rather than 'receptivity' (Chapter 3).

There are two broad areas which need to be addressed. Firstly, how does the blastocyst attach to the surface epithelium and are signals then transmitted to the trophectoderm to induce the formation of the primitive syncytium which will invade into the underlying stroma? Secondly, what are the properties of primitive syncytium which allow such rapid burrowing of the embryo into the uterus? Until the cytotrophoblast shell pushes through the syncytium at 13–14 days, it is this syncytium which initially contacts stromal cells and maternal leucocytes. That many pregnancies proceed through the attachment phase as far as complete nidation is suggested by the number of biochemical pregnancies reported in both normal pregnancies and in IVF programmes (Chard 1991). In normal fertile couples only 30% of fertilised eggs actually produce viable offspring. Whilst many of these pregnancies may fail due to defects in the embryo, it is also possible that failure of the primitive syncytium to erode into the superficial maternal capillaries is responsible. This process is essential to establish the haemochorial blood supply. It is not known what fetal genes are expressed by the primitive syncytium – in particular, HLA class I genes such as HLA-G, cytokine receptors, proteinases and integrins.

The state of the underlying endometrium must also be relevant, but the relative importance of cyclical changes in glands, stromal cells, vessels and leucocyte populations is unknown. Analyses of biopsies of women with infertility or undergoing donor insemination have shown retarded development in the luteal phase (Li *et al.* 1991, 1993). The abnormalities were mainly confined to reduced secretion from endometrial glands, but alterations in lymphoid populations have also been found (Klentzeris *et al.* 1994). However, IVF programmes have illustrated that the degree of embryo-uterine developmental asynchrony which can be tolerated whilst allowing successful implantation is surprisingly large in humans (at least 6 days) so the importance of retarded endometrial development is questionable (Yaron *et al.* 1994). Indeed, the endometrium may have much less impact on the timing of implantation than the stage of embryonic development.

Once pregnancy has been clinically recognised, many problems can arise from defective trophoblast–maternal interactions. By this stage, the cytotrophoblast shell has formed by pushing through the primitive syncytium. When the shell overlies the opening of a spiral artery, cytotrophoblast moves down the artery to form a plug of endovascular trophoblast. Trophoblast migrating from the shell directly into decidual tissue (interstitial trophoblast) moves to encircle the spiral arteries with eventual medial destruction. By the beginning of the second trimester, trophoblast has penetrated the inner myometrium and become sessile giant cells. As the function of both endovascular trophoblast and interstitial trophoblast is ultimately to regulate the pressure and flow of blood into the developing intervillous space, failure of the normal invasion will have important consequences in the supply of nutrients and oxygen to the fetus.

Miscarriage

Is spontaneous miscarriage one such clinical consequence? About 15% of pregnancies will spontaneously abort in the first trimester, and 1 in 4 women will experience a sporadic early loss (Regan *et al.* 1989). Considerably more pregnancies never even become clinically apparent, although are recognised if sensitive β-hCG assays are used (Wilcox *et al.* 1988; Chard 1991). At least 50% of these losses are due to chromosomal or other genetic abnormalities and a few are due to maternal disease (Boué and Boué 1973; Creasy 1988). However, in a large number of women no cause is found.

Recurrent miscarriage (the loss of three or more consecutive pregnancies) occurs in 1% of women. Epidemiological studies have shown that the single most important factor in determining the risk of miscarriage is the past reproductive performance of the woman (Regan *et al.* 1989). The risk of miscarriage is increased in women who have never had a live birth. Why the outcome of a woman's first pregnancy should have such a profound influence on subsequent reproductive performance is not known (Regan 1992). There is a link between infertility, premature deliveries and neonatal deaths in women with recurrent miscarriage (Strobino *et al.* 1986). Detailed endocrine, genetic and immunological investigations in 500 women with recurrent miscarriage have shown a low incidence of karyotype abnormalities, thyroid disease and diabetes (Clifford *et al.* 1994). The high incidence of subfertility was confirmed (32%). Two abnormal investigation results were found in a significant number of women: polycystic ovaries (56%) and anti-phospholipid antibodies (14%). Polycystic ovaries are associated with hypersecretion of luteinising hormone (LH), but whether high levels of this hormone affect the developing oocyte or interfere with correct priming of the endometrium is unclear.

The presence of anti-phospholipid antibodies in women with reproductive failure is well documented. Recent evidence now suggests that 'anti-phospholipid' autoantibodies are not directed against anionic phospholipids, but are a group of autoantibodies directed against phospholipid-binding plasma proteins such as prothrombin (Roubey 1994). Many studies have shown that women with clinically overt systemic lupus erythematosus (SLE), and women who have anti-phospholipid antibodies detectable in the serum but no clinically overt disease, both have a high incidence of fetal loss. It is thought that the underlying mechanism is thrombosis of the utero-placental vessels leading to poor placental perfusion. An alternative explanation is that some of the antibodies found in the sera of these women with anti-phospholipid syndrome may cross-react with endovascular trophoblast or villous syncytiotrophoblast (McCrae *et al.* 1993). Anti-trophoblast antibodies were found in 20 of 27 such patients, and these were still reactive to trophoblast after adsorption with cardiolipin-containing liposomes. No anti-trophoblast antibodies were found in normal pregnant women (Chapter 8). McCrae *et al.* suggest a spectrum of auto-reactive antibodies occur in women with the anti-phospholipid syndrome, but only some are trophoblast-reactive. This is in keeping with the new view of 'anti-phospholipid' autoantibodies proposed by Roubey (1994) where the antibodies found occur together in different combinations. These observations would explain why many women who have anti-phospholipid antibodies experience normal pregnancies (Picillo *et al.* 1992). Interestingly, the anti-trophoblast antibodies described by McCrae *et al.* inhibited binding of pro-urokinase to trophoblast urokinase receptors, suggesting another pathogenetic mechanism underlying fetal loss. Expression of urokinase plasminogen activator (uPA) by trophoblast is likely to be critical in the invasive process (Chapter 9).

In a group of women who had experienced three or more consecutive spontaneous miscarriages and who had no abnormalities detected after extensive clinical investigations, endometrial biopsies were analysed morphologically and immunohistochemically for cycle-dependent mucin epitopes (Serle *et al.* 1994). The LH surge was used to give a precise chronological date and all biopsies were taken on day LH + 7. Two distinct subgroups were identified: one with normal endometrial differentiation and the other where retarded development was found. The latter group (60% of patients) also showed a reduction in secretory glandular activity indicating a generalised retardation in gland cell function. Therefore, in both women undergoing IVF and women who have recurrent spontaneous fetal losses, a group of women are observed who show defective maturation of the endometrium. Although glandular differentiation has so far been used as the marker of differentiation, the role played by glandular secretions in post-implantation events is obscure (Chapter 3). Nevertheless, this retardation is likely to reflect other less easily quantifiable changes in the endometrium such as alterations in endometrial leucocytes, stromal cell protein production and deposition of the pericellular stromal extracellular matrix. How retarded endometrial maturation affects placentation remains to be clarified.

Despite these recent observations, in the majority of women the underlying cause for their fetal loss remains a mystery. The clinical importance of spontaneous recurrent miscarriage can be appreciated from the number of treatment regimes which have been devised. Many of these treatments are based on the idea that the pregnancy fails due to an 'immune' defect (Hill 1990; Coulam *et al*. 1994). It has been postulated that the maternal immune response to the invading embryo is not adequately 'suppressed' or conversely that an immune response is actually beneficial and needs to be generated to stimulate the production of blocking antibodies. It should now be clear from the preceding chapters that any aetiological theory of miscarriage based on the assumption that a classical T and B immune response to the fetus/placenta fails to be correctly modulated seems unlikely. If this is the case, then what does go wrong?

There are inherent difficulties in establishing a haemochorial placenta. Adaptations are required in the uterine arteries supplying the placenta to increase the blood flow up to 5-fold. This is achieved by the vascular transformation of arteries by interstitial trophoblast which destroys the media, removing the possibility of vasoconstriction. However, in early pregnancy, patency of these arteries (which at this time have most of their media still intact) could lead to very high pressures in the developing intervillous space, and the embryo could be 'blown out'. The formation of loosely cohesive plugs of endovascular trophoblast seems to provide protection from the high maternal blood pressure and high oxygen tension with potentially damaging free radicals (Hustin *et al*. 1990). The absence of a clearly demonstrable continuous maternal blood flow into the intervillous space and the presence of low partial pressures of oxygen found in the placenta during the first trimester reflect this slow seepage of blood filtrate through the trophoblast plugs and shell (Rodesch *et al*. 1992; Hustin 1992).

Obviously, failure of both endovascular and interstitial pathways of extravillous trophoblast differentiation could lead to early pregnancy failure, yet little is known about signals which lead to this divergent differentiation or functional differences in the two invading trophoblast populations. Phenotypic differences between endovascular and interstitial trophoblast have been identified (Burrows *et al*. 1994). Of particular interest is the expression of the neural cell adhesion molecule (NCAM) containing the polysialic acid (PSA) side chain by trophoblast in the vessels and in parts of the shell overlying the arterial opening. The factors inducing NCAM expression on endovascular trophoblast (possibly from maternal serum) and the role of NCAM in maintaining cohesiveness of the plug and in interaction with the maternal endothelium will certainly be interesting areas to explore.

In other cases of early pregnancy failure, interstitial trophoblast may not reach the spiral arteries at all. Then tapping of the arteries would not occur and the blood supply through unmodified spiral arteries would rapidly become inadequate towards the end of the first trimester. Physiological changes in spiral arteries were found to be frequently lacking in spontaneous abortion (Khong *et al*. 1987).

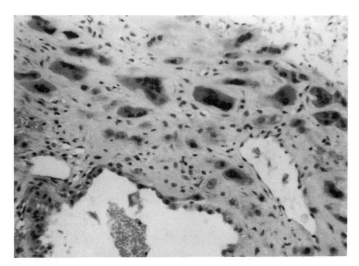

Fig. 11.1. Section of decidua basalis from a woman who had six previous recurrent miscarriages. This pregnancy also failed at 9 weeks gestation. Numerous multinucleated placental bed giant cells are unusually abundant in the decidua. (Obj × 16, H & E)

The failure of trophoblast to invade the media might be reflected by the premature appearance of placental bed giant cells in the decidual stroma. In the case illustrated in Fig. 11.1, of a woman who had had six recurrent miscarriages, the number of multinucleated giant cells in the superficial decidua (when these should normally be very sparse at this site) was remarkable. However, great care must be exercised in investigating the placental bed in spontaneous miscarriage. Once the pregnancy has clinically failed, the secondary changes of inflammation and repair can easily lead to misinterpretation. For example, uterine NK cells rapidly undergo apoptosis when progesterone levels drop either before the onset of menstruation or in a failing pregnancy. These morphological and (presumably functional) changes in the NK cells, therefore, may be the result rather than the cause of the pregnancy failure. Whether defective interactions between NK cells, macrophages and trophoblast can contribute to trophoblast death, premature differentiation into placental bed giant cells and eventual miscarriage remains speculative.

Pre-eclamptic toxaemia (PET) and intra-uterine growth retardation (IUGR)

Whilst the part played by inadequate trophoblast migration in spontaneous miscarriage is still uncertain, poor trophoblast invasion has been much better documented as the primary defect in PET, unexplained still-birth and IUGR

(Pijnenborg 1994). These conditions have been linked with miscarriage as a spectrum of disorders all caused by poor placentation (Khong *et al.* 1987). In the original, now classic, descriptions the absence of trophoblast invasion of the deep myometrial spiral arteries was most convincingly demonstrated in PET but was also present in some cases of IUGR (Brosens *et al.* 1967, 1977, 1992; de Wolf *et al.* 1980; Khong *et al.* 1986; Gerretson *et al.* 1981).

There has been some difficulty in clearly defining PET and IUGR clinically, and the debate in the literature over the importance of vascular changes reflects this diagnostic confusion. Obviously, essential hypertension must not be confused with true PET. Likewise, growth retardation can be due to other diverse causes including viral infection, genetic abnormalities, maternal undernutrition and smoking (Wigglesworth 1989). In addition, the difficulty of examining the anatomy and pathology of the entire uteroplacental vasculature makes the contribution of defective trophoblast migration into vessels in IUGR and PET hard to assess. Attempts to use placental bed biopsies to study the uterine vasculature are particularly problematic. It is difficult for the surgeon to locate the centre of the placental insertion. In addition, both the number of vessels invaded by trophoblast ($\sim$100) and the depth of invasion of each vessel will ultimately determine the blood flow to the intervillous space at each stage of gestation, and this cannot be determined by biopsy (Meekins *et al.* 1994). Nonetheless, it is now widely accepted that PET and many cases of unexplained IUGR and still-birth, are due to inadequate transformation of uterine spiral arteries by trophoblast. These are essentially the same condition, but in PET there is a superimposed maternal systemic syndrome triggered by placental ischaemia which results in widespread endothelial cell activation from unknown placentally derived factors (Friedman *et al.* 1991; Wallenburg and Visser 1994). In both IUGR and PET the broad spectrum of changes found in the feto-placental unit can be explained by the extent and depth of vascular invasion. Although the placenta has a great functional reserve, compensatory growth will vary according to the stage of gestation at which the insult occurs. Thus, if the blood flow is compromised early in pregnancy due to widespread failure of vascular transformation, both fetus and placenta are likely to be small. However, if the blood supply is adequate until the late second to third trimester, the placenta may be able to respond by compensatory hypertrophy and become large relative to the fetus.

The long-term effects of poor uterine arterial perfusion of the intervillous space may be profound. The evidence that health in later life can be influenced by events *in utero* is now strong (Barker 1994). This has given rise to the concept of 'programming', whereby an insult suffered at a critical period of development results in a permanent effect on the structure or function of the organ or tissue (Lucas 1991). Poor growth *in utero* is associated with the development of hypertension and diabetes in later life. This may result from reduction of islet β cells or modifications in vascular development at a critical stage of development.

It has been suggested that the main cause of fetal undernutrition is maternal malnutrition (Barker *et al.* 1993). Whilst this is true at times of famine or in developing countries, it is unlikely to be of major importance in England where most of the epidemiological studies were carried out. Indeed the effects were largely independent of social class (Wigglesworth 1989; Godfrey *et al.* 1991). Other epidemiologists have also questioned the importance of maternal nutritional intake (Paneth and Susser 1995). These authors point out that fetal growth is a 'doubtful surrogate measure' of fetal nutrition. Maternal nutrition is even less likely to relate to 'a baby's nourishment' when one considers that fetal–placental growth depends entirely on the amount of maternal blood delivered via the basal plate uterine arteries. The crucial point is how enough maternal nutrients and oxygen can be delivered to the intervillous space right up to the end of gestation. This again leads back to the uterine arteries and the overwhelming importance of trophoblast–decidual interactions in the first trimester (King and Loke 1994). Since other animal species (even primates) do not require the same degree of vascular adaptation for normal fetal growth *in utero*, the relevance of experimental animal models such as protein-deficient rats and malnourished sheep is open to question.

The relative role of hypoxia compared with maternal nutrients for correct programming also needs addressing. That hypoxia is more important than nutritional factors is suggested by a recent study on the effect of malnutrition *ex utero* in pre-term infants (Lucas and Morley 1994). Early nutritional deficits and poor growth in these pre-term babies did not lead to high blood pressure at 8 years of age, suggesting non-nutritional influences such as hypoxia are more important in programming blood pressure. The pathology of the placenta in idiopathic IUGR and PET is also indicative of a hypoxic insult. The chronic hypoxia is likely to activate vasoactive systems in the fetus such as the renin–angiotensin system which might modulate arterial smooth muscle cell development, and also play a role in the redistribution in blood flow with preservation of blood supply to vital organs such as the brain and heart. This leads to the asymmetric growth retardation which is often a feature of IUGR.

PET and eclampsia are serious complications of pregnancy and are of major obstetric importance in all parts of the world (Douglas and Redman 1994; Wallenburg and Visser 1994). One in 2000 pregnancies are affected and it is the commonest cause of maternal mortality. PET is characterised by high blood pressure, proteinuria and generalised oedema. Without treatment it can lead to grand-mal convulsions (eclampsia) and a wide range of disturbances in many organs. Pregnancy-induced hypertension (140/90 mmHg or an increase of

30/15 mmHg in pregnancy) occurs in the latter half of pregnancy, and this temporal pattern of hypertension distinguishes PET from other hypertensive disorders. It is, however, noteworthy that eclampsia may occur in the absence of hypertension or proteinuria. This is because the underlying pathogenetic mechanism is an endothelial cell disorder which can have diverse clinical consequences. PET only occurs in pregnancy. Furthermore, it is a disease associated with the presence of placental tissue only, as it is common in complete hydatidiform mole where no associated fetus is present.

There are other well recognised risk factors for PET. It is a disease of primigravidas (75% of cases occur in primigravidas of whom 2–6% are affected), particularly those at the extremes of their reproductive life (under 15 years or more than 35 years). However, multigravidas are also at risk, particularly if there is a change in paternity (Robillard *et al.* 1993). The presence of increased placental mass such as in twins, hydrops fetalis and molar tissue is also associated with an increased incidence. The interesting possibility that PET is increased in oocyte-donation pregnancies needs exploring further as in these cases there is no contribution of the maternal genotype to the pregnancy (Serhal and Craft 1987).

Susceptibility to PET does have a large genetic component, but it has been difficult to determine the pattern of inheritance and the relative contribution of maternal and fetal genotype (Cooper *et al.* 1993). Several studies have found that there is a greatly increased risk of this disease in the blood relatives of affected women compared to controls (2–5 times higher). The maternal susceptibility may be under a dominant major gene with moderately low penetrance or be determined by multifactorial inheritance. Paradoxically, though, monozygotic twins show lack of concordance (Thornton and Onwude 1991). This fact and the variable maternal susceptibility have led to the interpretation that a fetal genetic contribution is required. As only the placenta is required for the disease to occur, these fetal genes must be expressed in placental tissues and trophoblast. The association of PET with fetal trisomy 13 and triploidy lends support to the contribution of the fetal genotype (Feinberg *et al.* 1991a). Thus, a particular genotype in the mother and a particular genotype in the fetus (which may be at a different locus) would need to be combined for the condition to appear.

A high rate of recurrent spontaneous miscarriages in two families with a strong familial tendency to PET underlines the notion that defective placentation resulting from failure of normal EVT–decidual interaction is important (Arngrimsson *et al.* 1994). It is not yet apparent how the other clearly identified risk factors such as the high incidence in primigravida can be explained in this genetic model. It is as though in the first encounter between the maternal defence system and trophoblast the invading cells are more vigorously kept in place than in subsequent pregnancies. This could merely reflect that arteries once penetrated are more easily breached a second time. More esoteric explanations are also possible. Perhaps the putative innate decidual NK recognition system is capable of some kind of 'learning' after exposure to paternal antigens. The suggestion that PET is associated with primipaternity rather than primigravidity is therefore of interest (Robillard *et al.* 1994). In addition, as a long period of exposure to semen before conception protects against PET, the possible genes involved need not be specifically expressed by trophoblast but also by semen. Whatever the mechanism, trophoblast does appear to penetrate further into the uterus in second pregnancies with the same paternity.

The likelihood that both fetal (placental) and maternal genotypes contribute to PET is attractive when considering what is known about the underlying pathology. The basic defect is a failure of trophoblast to invade into the maternal spiral arteries. The presence of increased placental bed giant cells in the decidua has also been noted (Gerretson *et al.* 1981). Although difficult to quantitate accurately, this is an important observation because trophoblast giant cells are thought to be static and to have lost the ability to invade and destroy the media. Furthermore, the lack of any interstitial invasion in other primates could explain the failure to obtain a reliable animal model of eclampsia (Ramsey *et al.* 1976; Enders and King 1991). In these animals, an adequate placental blood supply does not depend on trophoblast invasion through the decidua to prime the vessels from outside. These observations suggest that premature differentiation of interstitial trophoblast into placental bed giant cells might be the underlying problem. This leads inevitably to questions of what normally influences the switch from cohesive rounded cells of the columns to isolated interstitial cells and eventually formation of giant cells. Of relevance to this are recent observations on pre-eclamptic pregnancies that have detected phenotypic differences in these placentae from normals. The normal change of trophoblast integrin expression from $\alpha_6\beta_4$ to $\alpha_1\beta_1$ as these cells migrate into decidua is not seen in PET (Zhou *et al.* 1993). This raises the question of whether the integrin switch is developmentally programmed in trophoblast, or whether it is influenced by maternal decidua. A possible scenario is that after interaction of trophoblast with uterine NK cells (? via HLA-G/C), the NK cells are stimulated to produce cytokines which in turn alter the pattern of integrins expressed by the trophoblast. The role of decidua in modulating the inherently invasive properties of trophoblast seems obvious despite views to the contrary.

Besides integrins, there are many phenotypic differences between extravillous trophoblast (EVT) and villous cytotrophoblast and it will be important to discover which of these changes are specifically induced by decidua, and which will occur on any tissue substrate. Decidual stromal cells and their characteristic pericellular rim of extracellular matrix, uterine-specific NK-like cells, and the abundant decidual placental bed macrophages seem the obvious candidates to exert effects on EVT differentiation.

The morphology of trophoblast invasion at ectopic sites (most commonly the Fallopian tube) has not been studied extensively, but would provide information on the role of decidua in altering trophoblast behaviour. There are limited morphological studies addressing this question (Randall *et al.* 1987). Our own unpublished study of tubal pregnancies has found that the characteristic change from cohesive rounded cells of the cell columns and shell to isolated spindly cells does not occur. Instead, the trophoblast invades as a clean front instead of the ragged margin seen in the normal situation in the uterus. In addition, in the tube trophoblast invades readily into both arteries and veins. The characteristic fibrinoid change in smooth muscle media of uterine spiral arteries is not confined to arterial media in the tube but is seen extensively throughout the smooth muscle of the wall. This raises the interesting question of why normally in the uterus only the arterial media is susceptible to the degenerative effects of surrounding trophoblast. Both decidua and myometrium show no such change. In addition, in tubal pregnancies giant cells are not seen, although this could be related to the early stage of gestation of the samples. Immunohistological studies examining the phenotype of EVT in ectopic sites compared with the uterus would be informative. However, a further difficulty in investigating this phenomenon is that there are still very few markers of the extravillous trophoblast differentiation pathway *in vivo* which could be used in *in vitro* assays (Chapter 5). Only the appearance of the terminal stage of class I HLA-positive giant cells is available at present.

It would obviously be an advantage to be able to predict which women are at risk for PET/IUGR. As the vascular invasion by trophoblast takes place in the first half of gestation, this should be possible. However, virtually all screening tests, whether based on biochemical, clinical or other markers, have been of no real value (Lim and Friedman 1993). Direct visualisation by Doppler sonography of the uterine spiral arteries in the placental bed would appear to be the most logical approach as this is where the primary pathology lies and the technique is non-invasive. Technically, though, this has proved difficult because of the complexity of uterine vessels supplying the placenta. Nevertheless, associations are found between pathological Doppler findings in uterine arteries and both reduced fetal growth and PET (Harrington and Campbell 1992; Dornan and Harper 1994). In the non-pregnant uterine artery, a high-resistance waveform with a diastolic notch is found. During normal pregnancy, a low-resistance waveform is created by the trophoblast transformation of uterine arteries with disappearance of the notch (Steel *et al.* 1990; Marsal 1994). Persistent notching after mid-gestation is indicative of poor placentation. This approach seems the one likely to have predictive value as accurate identification of the arteries supplying the placental bed becomes easier. It will also be interesting to see how early the absence of trophoblast invasion into decidual arteries can be detected with the use of transvaginal ultrasound. If it is possible to diagnose abnormal invasion by Doppler sonography before early therapeutic or spontaneous abortion, studies of these tissues can be carried out and compared with normal pregnancies *in vitro*.

PET will lead to maternal death if untreated. In developing countries, maternal mortality from PET is >100 times higher than in Europe. This high death rate in the absence of medical intervention is enigmatic as it is hard to see why genes predisposing to such a lethal condition in women reproducing for the first time could have survived in populations world wide. It could be that PET is both the clinically recognised extreme and a side effect of a good defence against the demands of trophoblast invasion and a growing fetus. Fetal/trophoblast genes which determine vigorous invasive trophoblast will lead to large healthy fetuses and these genes will tend to be selected. However, the downside of this is always the risk of uterine rupture by trophoblast and maternal death (Haig 1993). The evolution of placentation in primates has resulted in humans developing an extremely dangerous mechanism to ensure an adequate supply of nutrients and oxygen from mother to fetus. The newborn human is much larger in relation to its mother than the newborn ape. This may reflect the complex brain development which requires a longer period *in utero*. In primitive societies this large size means many women die in childbirth – a phenomenon rarely seen in other higher primates. To achieve the relatively large size, the fetal genes which enable more efficient tapping of trophoblast into maternal arteries must have been selected for, but always at great risk to the mother of uterine rupture and death from haemorrhage. Maternal genes to counteract this may act either via imprinting of genes in the trophoblast or by ensuring a strong defensive system in the decidua. In a population these maternal genes must be of overwhelming importance as obviously to lose mothers by trophoblast over-penetration means eventual extinction. In contrast, an occasional fetus lost by over-enthusiastic maternal defence does not prevent further pregnancies. Thus, the continuing presence of such a lethal disease as PET can be explained by the requirement to maintain maternal defensive genes in a population.

It seems paradoxical with the increasing world population to suggest that human reproductive strategies are poor compared with many species. Nevertheless, the high incidence of both maternal death and fetal loss compared with other species does indicate that the system is inefficient. Maternal death can occur because the fetus is disproportionately large, by uterine rupture because decidual defences are inefficient, or by PET and its complications when decidual defences work too well. Fetal losses will occur if the trophoblast over-invades or under-invades. Therefore, the balance between trophoblast invasion and maternal defence must be maintained. Unravelling how this is done remains a major challenge in reproductive biology.

References

Aboagye-Mathiesen, G., Toth, F.D., Hager, H., Zdravkovic, M., Petersen, P.M., Villadsen, J.A., Zachar, V. and Ebbesen, P. (1993) Human trophoblast interferons. *Antiviral Research* **22**: 91–105.

Acheson, A., Sunshine, J.L. and Rutishauser, U. (1991) NCAM polysialic acid can regulate both cell–cell and cell–substrate interactions. *Journal of Cell Biology* **114**:143–153.

Adams, J.C. and Watt, F.M. (1989) Fibronectin inhibits the terminal differentiation of human keratinocytes. *Nature* **340**: 307–309.

Adamson, E.D. (1987) Expression of proto–oncogenes in the placenta. *Placenta* **8**: 449–466.

Adinolfi, M. (1992) Fetal cells in the maternal circulation. In: *Prenatal Diagnosis and Screening*, Eds. Brock, D.J., Rodeck, C.D. and Ferguson-Smith, M.A., Churchill Livingstone, Edinburgh, pp. 651–660.

Ahrons, S. (1971) Leucocyte antibodies: occurrence in primigravidae. *Tissue Antigens* **1**: 178–183.

Albelda, S.M. (1993) Role of integrins and other cell adhesion molecules in tumour progression and metastasis. *Laboratory Investigation* **68**: 4–15.

Albelda, S.M. and Buck, C.A. (1990) Integrins and other cell adhesion molecules. *FASEB Journal* **4**: 2868–2880.

Alcaraz, G. and Goridis, C. (1991) Biosynthesis and processing of polysialated NCAM by AtT–20 cells. *European Journal of Cell Biology* **55**: 165–173.

Alexander, C.M. and Werb, Z. (1989) Proteinases and extracellular matrix remodelling. *Current Opinion in Cell Biology* **1**: 974–982.

Alizadeh, M., Legras, C., Semana, G., Le Bouteiller, P., Genetet, B. and Fauchet, R. (1993) Evidence for a polymorphism of HLA-G gene. *Human Immunology* **38**: 206–212.

Allavena, P., Paganin, C., Martin-Padura, I., Peri, G., Gaboli, M., Dejana, E., Marchisio, P.C. and Mantovanni, A. (1991) Molecules and structures involved in the adhesion of natural killer cells to vascular endothelium. *Journal of Experimental Medicine* **173**: 439–448.

Amoroso, E.C. (1968) The evolution of viviparity. *Proceedings of the Royal Society of Medicine* **61**: 1188–1200.

Amso, N.N., Crow, J. and Shaw, R.W. (1994) Comparative immunohistochemical study of oestrogen and progesterone receptors in the Fallopian tube and uterus at different stages of the menstrual cycle and the menopause. *Human Reproduction* **9**: 1027–1037.

237

Antczak, D.F. (1989) Maternal antibody responses in pregnancy. *Current Opinion in Immunology* **1**: 1135–1140.

Antczak, D.F., Poleman, J.C., Stenzler, L.M., Volsen, S.G. and Allen, W.R. (1987) Monoclonal antibodies to equine trophoblast. In: *Trophoblast Research* Vol. 2, Eds. Miller, R.K. and Thiede, H.A., Plenum Press, New York, pp. 199–223.

Aplin, J.D. (1989) Cellular biochemistry of the endometrium. In: *Biology of the Uterus*, Eds. Wynn, R.P. and Jollie, W.P., Plenum Medical, New York, pp. 89–125.

Aplin, J.D. (1991a) Glycans as biochemical markers of human endometrial secretory differentiation. *Journal of Reproduction and Fertility* **91**: 525–541.

Aplin, J.D. (1991b) Implantation, trophoblast differentiation and haemochorial placentation: mechanistic evidence *in vivo* and *in vitro*. *Journal of Cell Science* **99**: 681–692.

Aplin, J.D. (1993) Expression of integrin $\alpha_6\beta_4$ in human trophoblast and its loss from extravillous cells. *Placenta* **14**: 203–215.

Aplin, J.D. and Church, H.J. (1994) Basement membrane–hemidesmosome interactions. In: *Molecular Biology of Desmosomes and Hemidesmosomes*, Eds. Garrod, D.R. and Collins, J., R.G. Landes, Austin, Texas, pp. 87–106.

Ariel, I., Lustig, O., Oyer, C.E., Elkin, M., Gonik, B., Rachmilewitz, J., Biran, H., Goshen, R., De Groot, N. and Hochberg, A. (1994) Relaxation of imprinting in trophoblastic disease. *Gynecology and Oncology* **53**: 212–219.

Ariel, M., Robinson, E., McCarrey, J.R. and Cedar, H. (1995) Gamete-specific methylation correlates with imprinting of the murine *Xist* gene. *Nature Genetics* **9**: 312–315.

Arngrimsson, R., Connor, J.M., Geirsson, R.T., Brennecke, S. and Cooper, D.W. (1994) Is genetic susceptibility for pre–eclampsia and eclampsia associated with implantation failure and fetal demise? *Lancet* **343**: 1643–1644.

Aubry, J.–P., Pochon, S., Graber, P., Jansen, K.U. and Bonnefoy, J.-Y. (1992) CD21 is a ligand for CD23 and regulates IgE production. *Nature* **358**: 505–507.

Azziz, R. (1993) Fertility and infertility. *Current Opinion in Obstetrics and Gynecology* **5**: 225–227.

Bagshawe, K.D. and Lawler, S.D. (1982) Choriocarcinoma. In: *Cancer Epidemiology and Prevention*, Eds. Schottenfeld, D. and Fraumeni, J.F., Saunders, Philadelphia, pp. 909–924.

Bahram, S., Bresnahan, M., Geraghty, D.E. and Spies, T. (1994) A second lineage of mammalian major histocompatibility complex class I genes. *Proceedings of the National Academy of Sciences USA* **91**: 6259–6263.

Baker, J., Liu, J.-P., Robertson, E.J. and Efstratiadis, A. (1993) Role of insulin-like growth factors in embryonic and postnatal growth. *Cell* **75**: 73–82.

Banville, D. and Boie, Y. (1989) Retroviral long terminal repeat is the promoter of the gene encoding the tumour–associated calcium binding protein oncomodulin in the rat. *Journal of Molecular Biology* **207**: 481–490.

Barber, L.D. and Parham, P. (1993) Peptide binding to major histocompatibility complex molecules. *Annual Review of Cell Biology* **9**: 163–206.

Bargmann, C.L., Hung, M.-C. and Weinberg, R.A. (1986) The *neu* oncogene encodes an epidermal growth factor receptor–related protein. *Nature* **319**: 226–230.

Barker, D.J.B. (1994) *Mothers, Babies, and Disease in Later Life*. BMJ Publishing Group, London.

Barker, D.J.B., Gluckman, P.D., Godfrey, K.M., Harding, J.E., Owens, J.A. and Robinson, J.S. (1993) Fetal nutrition and cardiovascular disease in adult life. *Lancet* **341**: 938–941.

Bartl, S., Baltimore, D. and Weissman, I.L. (1994) Molecular evolution of the vertebrate immune system. *Proceedings of the National Academy of Sciences USA* **91**: 10769–10770.

Barton, S.C., Surani, M.A.H. and Norris, M.L. (1984) Role of paternal and maternal genomes in mouse development. *Nature* **311**: 374–376.

Beck, G. and Habicht, G.S. (1991) Primitive cytokines: harbingers of vertebrate defense. *Immunology Today* **12**: 180–183.

Beckman, E.M., Porcell, S.A., Morita, C.T., Behar, S.M., Furlong, S.T. and Brenner, M.B. (1994) Recognition of a lipid antigen by CD1-restricted $\alpha\beta^+$ T cells. *Nature* **372**: 691–694.

Bell, S.C. (1989) Decidualization and insulin-like growth factor (IGF) binding protein: implications for its role in stromal cell differentiation and the decidual cell in haemochorial placentation. *Human Reproduction* **4**: 125–130.

Bell, S.C. and Billington, W.D. (1980) Major anti-paternal alloantibody induced by murine pregnancy is non-complement-fixing IgG1. *Nature* **288**: 387–388.

Ben-Baruch, N. and Yarden, Y. (1994) *Neu* differentiation factors: a family of alternatively spliced neuronal and mesenchymal factors. *Proceedings of the Society for Experimental Biology and Medicine* **206**: 221–227.

Benichou, G., Takizawa, P.A., Olson, C.A., McMillan, M. and Sercarz, E.E. (1992) Donor major histocompatibility complex (MHC) peptides are presented by recipient MHC molecules during graft rejection. *Journal of Experimental Medicine* **175**: 305–308.

Benveniste, R.E., Lieber, M.M., Livingston, D., Sherr, C.J. and Todaro, G. (1974) Infectious C-type virus isolated from a baboon placenta. *Nature* **248**: 17–20.

Bergqvist, A., Ljungberg, O. and Skoog, L. (1993) Immunohistochemical analysis of oestrogen and progesterone receptors in endometriotic tissue and endometrium. *Human Reproduction* **8**: 1915–1922.

Bernhard, E.J., Gruber, S.B. and Muschel, R.J. (1994) Direct evidence linking expression of matrix metalloproteinase 9 (92-kDa gelatinase/collagenase) to the metastatic phenotype in transformed rat embryo cells. *Proceedings of the National Academy of Sciences USA* **91**: 4293–4297.

Bersinger, N.A., Sinosich, M.J., Baber, R., Torode, H. and Saunders, D.M. (1993) Trophoblast–endometrium co-cultures as a means of assessment of endometrial readiness for implantation. *Trophoblast Research* **7**: 211–222.

Bezouška, K., Yuen, C.-T., O'Brien, J., Childs, R.A., Chai, W., Lawson, A.M., Drbal, K., Fišerová, A., Pospišil, M. and Feizi, T. (1994) Oligosaccharide ligands for NKR-P1 protein activate NK cells and cytotoxicity. *Nature* **372**: 150–157.

Bhatt, H., Brunet, L.J. and Stewart, C.L. (1991) Uterine expression of leukemia inhibitory factor coincides with the onset of blastocyst implantation. *Proceedings of the National Academy of Sciences USA* **88**: 11408–11412.

Bierings, M.B., Adriaansen, H.J. and Van Dijk, J.P. (1988) The appearance of transferrin receptors on cultured human cytotrophoblast and *in vitro*-formed syncytiotrophoblast. *Placenta* **9**: 387–396.

Billingham, R.E. (1964) Transplantation immunity and the maternal–fetal relation. *New England Journal of Medicine* **270**: 667–672.

Billington, W.D. (1971) Biology of the trophoblast. *Advances in Reproductive Physiology* **5**: 27–66.

Billington, W.D. (1993) Species diversity in the immunogenetic relationship between mother and fetus: is trophoblast insusceptibility to immunological destruction the only essential common feature for the maintenance of allogeneic pregnancy? *Experimental and Clinical Immunogenetics* **10**: 73–84.

Billington, W.D. and Burrows, F.J. (1986) The rat placenta expresses paternal class I major histocompatibility antigens. *Journal of Reproductive Immunology* **9**: 155–160.

Birchmeier, W. and Birchmeier, C. (1994) Mesenchymal-epithelial transitions. *BioEssays* **16**: 305–307.

Bischof, P., Friedli, E., Martelli, M. and Campana, A. (1991) Expression of extracellular matrix degrading metalloproteinases by cultured human cytotrophoblast cells: effects of cell adhesion and immunopurification. *American Journal of Obstetrics and Gynecology* **165**: 1791–1801.

Bix, M. and Raulet, D. (1992) Functionally conformed free class I heavy chains exist on the surface of β2 microglobulin negative cells. *Journal of Experimental Medicine* **176**: 829–834.

Blay, J.-Y., Branellec, D., Robinet, E., Dugas, B., Gay, F. and Chaouïb, S. (1990) Involvement of cyclic adenosine monophosphate in the interleukin 4 inhibitory effect on interleukin 2-induced lymphokine-activated killer generation. *Journal of Clinical Investigation* **85**: 1909–1913.

Blithe, D.L., Richards, R.G. and Skarulis, M.C. (1991) Free alpha molecules from pregnancy stimulate secretion of prolactin from human decidual cells: a novel function for free alpha in pregnancy. *Endocrinology* **129**: 2257–2259.

Bocci, V., Paulesu, L. and Ricci, M.G. (1985) The physiological interferon response. IV. Production of interferon by the perfused human placenta at term. *Proceedings of the Society of Experimental Biology and Medicine* **180**: 137–143.

Bodmer, J.G., Marsh, S.G.E., Albert, E.D., Bodmer, W.F., Dupont, B., Erlich, H.A., Mach, B., Mayr, W.R., Parham, P., Sasazuki, T., Schreuder, G.M.Th., Strominger, J.L., Svejgaard, A. and Terasaki, P.I. (1994) Nomenclature for factors of the HLA system. *Tissue Antigens* **44**: 1–18.

Boehm, K.D., Kelley, M.F., Ilan, J. and Ilan, J. (1989) The interleukin 2 gene is expressed in the syncytiotrophoblast of the human placenta. *Proceedings of the National Academy of Sciences USA* **86**: 656–660.

Boismenu, R. and Havran, W.L. (1994) Modulation of epithelial cell growth by intraepithelial γδ T cells. *Science* **266**: 1253–1255.

Boller, K., Konig, H., Sauter, M., Mueller-Lantzsch, N., Lower, R. and Kurth, R. (1993) Evidence that HERV-K is the endogenous retrovirus sequence that codes for the human teratocarcinoma-derived retrovirus HTDV. *Virology* **196**: 349–353.

Borén, T. and Falk, P. (1994) *Helicobacter pylori* binds to blood group antigens. *Science & Medicine* **1**: 28–37.

Borrego, F., Pena, J. and Solana, R. (1993) Regulation of CD69 expression on human natural killer cells: differential involvement of protein kinase C and protein tyrosine kinases. *European Journal of Immunology* **23**: 1039–1043.

Boucrat, J., Hakem, R., Gauthier, A., Fauchet, R. and Le Bouteiller, P. (1991) Transfected trophoblast-derived human cells can express a single HLA class I allelic product. *Tissue Antigens* **37**: 84–89.

Boucrat, J., Guillaudeux, T., Alizadeh, M., Boretto, J., Chimini, G., Malecaze, F., Semana, G., Fauchet, R., Pontarotti, P. and Le Bouteiller, P. (1993) HLA-E is the only class I gene that escapes CpG methylation and is transcriptionally active in the trophoblast-derived human cell line JAR. *Immunogenetics* **38**: 117–130.

Boué, J. and Boué, A. (1973) Chromosomal analysis of two consecutive abortuses in each of 43 women. *Humangenetik* **19**: 275–280.

Boyd, J.D. and Hamilton, W.J. (1970) *The Human Placenta*, W. Heffer & Sons, Ltd, Cambridge.

Boyd, M.T., Bax, C.M., Bax, B.E., Bloxam, D.L. and Weiss, R.A. (1993) The human endogenous retrovirus ERV-3 is upregulated in differentiating placental trophoblast cells. *Virology* **196**: 905–909.

Brach, M.A., deVos, S., Gruss, H.-J. and Herrmann, F. (1992) Prolongation of survival of human polymorphonuclear neutrophils by granulocyte-macrophage colony-stimulating factor is caused by inhibition of programmed cell death. *Blood* **80**: 2920–2924.

Brannan, C.I., Dees, E.C., Ingram, R.S. and Tighlman, S.M. (1990) The product of the H19 gene may function as an mRNA. *Molecular Cell Biology* **10**: 28–36.

Brennan, J., Mager, D., Jefferies, W. and Takei, F. (1994) Expression of different members of the Ly-49 gene family defines distinct natural killer cell subsets and cell adhesion properties. *Journal of Experimental Medicine* **180**: 2287–2295.

Brewer, L.M. and McManus, J.P. (1987) Detection of oncomodulin, an oncodevelopmental protein in human placenta and choriocarcinoma cell lines. *Placenta* **8**: 351–363.

Brosens, I., Robertson, W.B. and Dixon, H.G. (1967) The physiological response of the vessels of the placental bed to normal pregnancy. *Journal of Pathology and Bacteriology* **93**: 569–579.

Brosens, I., Dixon, H.G. and Robertson, W.B. (1977) Fetal growth retardation and the arteries of the placental bed. *British Journal of Obstetrics and Gynaecology* **84**: 656–663.

Brosens, I., Robertson, W.B. and Dixon, H.G. (1992) The role of the spiral arteries in the pathogenesis of pre-eclampsia. *Obstetrics and Gynecology Annal* **1**: 177–191.

Buck, C.A. (1992) Immunologlobulin superfamily: structure, function and relationship to other receptor molecules. *Seminars in Cell Biology* **3**: 179–188.

Bulmer, J.N. and Johnson, P.M. (1985) Immunohistological characterization of the decidual leucocytic infiltrate related to endometrial gland epithelium in early human pregnancy. *Immunology* **55**: 35–44.

Bulmer, J.N. and Johnson, P.M. (1986) The T-lymphocyte population in first trimester human decidua does not express the interleukin-2 receptor. *Immunology* **58**: 685–687.

Bulmer, J.N. and Sunderland, C.A. (1983) Bone marrow origin of endometrial granulocytes in the early human placental bed. *Journal of Reproductive Immunology* **5**: 383–387.

Bulmer, J.N. and Sunderland, C.A. (1984) Immunohistological characterisation of lymphoid cell populations in the early human placental bed. *Immunology* **52**: 349–357.

Bulmer, J.N., Wells, M., Bhabra, K. and Johnson, P.M. (1986) Immunohistological characterization of endometrial gland epithelium and extravillous fetal trophoblast in third trimester human placental bed tissues. *British Journal of Obstetrics and Gynaecology* **93**: 823–832.

Bulmer, J.N., Johnson, P.M. and Bulmer, D. (1987) Leukocyte populations in human decidua and endometrium. In: *Immunoregulation and Fetal Survival*, Eds. Gill T.J. and Wegmann, T.G., Oxford University Press, New York, pp. 111–196.

Bulmer, J.N., Morrison, L. and Johnson, P.M. (1988a) Expression of the proliferation markers Ki-67 and transferrin receptor by human trophoblast populations. *Journal of Reproductive Immunology* **14**: 291–302.

Bulmer, J.N., Pace, D. and Ritson, A. (1988b) Immunoregulatory cells in human decidua: morphology, immunohistochemistry and function. *Reproduction, Nutrition, Development* **28**: 1599–1614.

Bulmer, J.N., Thrower, S. and Wells, M. (1989) Expression of epidermal growth factor receptor and transferrin receptor by human trophoblast populations. *American Journal of Reproductive Immunology* **21**: 87–93.

Bulmer, J.N., Morrison, L., Johnson, P.M. and Meager, A. (1990) Immunohistochemical localization of interferons in human placental tissues in normal, ectopic, and molar pregnancy. *American Journal of Reproductive Immunology* **22**: 109–116.

Bulmer, J.N., Morrison, L., Longfellow, M., Ritson, A. and Pace, D. (1991) Granulated lymphocytes in human endometrium: histochemical and immunohistochemical studies. *Human Reproduction* **6**: 791–798.

Burdach, S., Zessack, N., Dilloo, D., Shatsky, M., Thompson, D. and Levitt, L. (1991) Differential regulation of lymphokine production by distinct subunits of the T cell interleukin 2 receptor. *Journal of Clinical Investigation* **87**: 2114–2121.

Burgeson, R.E., Chiquet, M., Deutzmann, R., Ekblom, P., Engel, J., Kleinman, H., Martin, G.R., Meneguzzi, G., Paulsson, M., Sanes, J. *et al.* (1994) A new nomenclature for the laminins. *Matrix Biology* **14**: 209–211.

Burmeister, W.P., Gastinel, L.N., Simister, N.E., Blum, M.L. and Bjorkman, P.J. (1994) Crystal structure at 2.2 Å resolution of the MHC-related neonatal Fc receptor. *Nature* **372**: 336–343.

Burnet, F.M. (1971) "Self-recognition" in colonial marine forms and flowering plants in relation to the evolution of immunity. *Nature* **232**: 230–235.

Burrows, T.D. (1994) Cell–cell and cell–matrix interactions in human placental implantation. PhD Thesis, University of Cambridge.

Burrows, T.D., King, A. and Loke, Y.W. (1993a) Expression of integrins by human trophoblast and differential adhesion to laminin or fibronectin. *Human Reproduction* **8**: 475–484.

Burrows, T.D., King, A. and Loke, Y.W. (1993b) Expression of adhesion molecules by human decidual large granular lymphocytes. *Cellular Immunology* **147**: 81–94.

Burrows, T.D., King, A. and Loke, Y.W. (1994) Expression of adhesion molecules by endovascular trophoblast and decidual endothelial cells: implications for vascular invasion during implantation. *Placenta* **15**: 21–33.

Butcher, E.C. (1991) Leukocyte–endothelial cell recognition: three (or more) steps to specificity and diversity. *Cell* **67**: 1033–1036.

Butterworth, B.H. and Loke, Y.W. (1985) Immunocytochemical identification of cytotrophoblast from other mononuclear cell populations isolated from first trimester human chorionic villi. *Journal of Cell Science* **76**: 189–197.

Calderon, J., Sheehan, K.C.F., Chance, C., Thomas, M.L. and Schreiber, R.D. (1988) Purification and characterization of the human interferon–γ receptor from placenta. *Proceedings of the National Academy of Sciences USA* **85**: 4837–4841.

Campbell, S., Swann, H.R., Seif, M.W., Kimber, S.J. and Aplin, J.D. (1995) Cell adhesion molecules on the oocyte and pre-implantation human embryo. *Human Reproduction* – in press.

Carbone, E., Stuber, G., André, S., Franksson, L., Klein, E., Beretta, A., Siccardi, A.G. and Kärre, K. (1993) Reduced expression of major histocompatibility complex class I free heavy chains and enhanced sensitivity to natural killer cells after incubation of human lymphoid lines with β2-microglobulin. *European Journal of Immunology* **23**: 1752–1756.

Carpenter, G. and Wahl, M.I. (1990) The epidermal growth factor. In: *Peptide Growth Factors and their Receptors I*, Eds. Sporn, M.B. and Roberts, A.B., Springer-Verlag, Berlin, pp. 70–171.

Carraway, K.L. and Cantley, L.C. (1994) A *neu* acquaintance for *erb*B3 and *erb*B4: a role for receptor heterodimerization in growth signaling. *Cell* **78**: 5–8.

Carreno, B.M. and Hansen, T.H. (1994) Exogenous peptide ligand influences the expression of half-life of free HLA class I heavy chains ubiquitously detected at the cell surface. *European Journal of Immunology* **24**: 1285–1292.

Carson, D.D., Wilson, O.F. and Dutt, A. (1990) Glycoconjugate expression and interactions at the cell surface of mouse uterine epithelial cells and periimplantation stage embryos. *Trophoblast Research* **4**: 211–241.

Carson, W.E., Haldar, S., Baiocchi, R.A., Croce, C.M. and Caligiuri, M.A. (1994) The c-*kit* ligand suppresses apoptosis of human natural killer cells through the upregulation of *bcl*-2. *Proceedings of the National Academy of Sciences USA* **91**: 7553–7557.

Casey, M.L., Cox, S.M., Beutler, B., Milewich, L. and MacDonald, P.C. (1989) Cachetin/tumor necrosis factor-α formation in human decidua. *Journal of Clinical Investigation* **83**: 430–436.

Caulfield, J.J., Sargent, I.L., Ferry, B.L., Starkey, P.M. and Redman, C.W.G. (1992) Isolation and characterisation of a subpopulation of human chorionic cytotrophoblast using a monoclonal anti-trophoblast antibody in flow cytometry. *Journal of Reproductive Immunology* **21**: 71–86.

Cella, M., Longo, A., Battista Ferrara, G., Strominger, J.L. and Colonna, M. (1994) NK3-specific Natural Killer cells are selectively inhibited by Bw4-positive HLA alleles with isoleucine 80. *Journal of Experimental Medicine* **180**: 1235–1242.

Cepek, K.L., Parker, C.M., Madara, J.L. and Brenner, M.B. (1993) Integrin $\alpha_E\beta_7$ mediates adhesion of T lymphocytes to epithelial cells. *Journal of Immunology* **150**: 3459–3470.

Cerf-Bensussan, N., Jarry, A., Brousse, N., Lisowska-Grospierre, B., Guy-Grand, D. and Griscelli, C. (1987) A monoclonal antibody (HML-1) defining a novel membrane present on human intestinal lymphocytes. *European Journal of Immunology* **17**: 1279–1285.

Cerf-Bensussan, N., Bègue, B., Gagnon, J. and Meo, T. (1992) The human intraepithelial lymphocyte marker HML-1 is an integrin consisting of a β_7 subunit associated with a distinctive α chain. *European Journal of Immunology* **22**: 273–277.

Chambers, W.H., Adamkiewicz, T. and Houchins, J.P. (1993) Type II integral membrane proteins with characteristics of C-type animal lectins expressed by natural killer (NK) cells. *Glycobiology* **3**: 9–14.

Chandra, S., Liszczak, T., Korol, W. and Jensen, E.M. (1970) Type-C particles in human tissues. I. Electron microscopic study of embryonic tisues *in vivo* and *in vitro*. *International Journal of Cancer* **6**: 40–45.

Chao, H.-S., Myers, S.E. and Handwerger, S. (1993) Endothelin inhibits basal and stimulated release of prolactin by human decidual cells. *Endocrinology* **133**: 505–510.

Chard, T. (1991) Frequency of implantation and early pregnancy loss in natural cycles. *Baillieres Clinical Obstetrics and Gynaecology* **5**: 179–189.

Chard, T. (1993) Placental radar. *Journal of Endocrinology* **138**: 177–179.

Chard, T. and Olajide, F. (1994) Endometrial protein PP14: a new test of endometrial function? *Reproductive Medicine Review* **3**: 43–52.

Chard, T., Craig, P.H., Menabawey, M. and Lee, C. (1986) Alpha interferon in human pregnancy. *British Journal of Obstetrics and Gynaecology* **93**: 1145–1149.

Charnock-Jones, D.S., Sharkey, A.M., Rajput-Williams, J., Burch, D., Schofield, P.J., Fountain, S.A., Boocock, C.A. and Smith, S.K. (1993) Identification and localization of alternatively spliced mRNAs for vascular endothelial growth factor in human uterus and steroid regulation in endometrial carcinoma cell lines. *Biology of Reproduction* **48**: 1120–1128.

Charnock-Jones, D.S., Sharkey, A.M., Boocock, C.A., Ahmed, A., Plevin, R., Ferrara, N. and Smith, S.K. (1994a) Vascular endothelial growth factor receptor localization and activation in human trophoblast and choriocarcinoma cells. *Biology of Reproduction* **51**: 524–530.

Charnock-Jones, D.S., Sharkey, A.M., Fenwick, P. and Smith, S.K. (1994b) Leukaemia inhibitory factor mRNA concentration peaks in human endometrium at the time of implantation and the blastocyst contains mRNA for the receptor at this time. *Journal of Reproduction and Fertility* **101**: 421–426.

Charpin, C., Kopp, F., Pourreau-Schneider, N., Lissitzky, J.C., Lavant, M.N., Martin, P.M. and Toga, M. (1985) Laminin distribution in human decidua and immature placenta. *American Journal of Obstetrics and Gynecology* **151**: 822–826.

Chen, H.-L., Yang, Y., Hu, X.-L., Yelavarthi, K., Fishback, J.L. and Hunt, J.S. (1991) Tumor necrosis factor alpha mRNA and protein are present in human placental and uterine cells at early and late stages of gestation. *American Journal of Pathology* **139**: 327–335.

Chen, H.-L., Yelavarthi, K.K. and Hunt, J.S. (1994) Identification of transforming growth factor-β1 mRNA in virgin and pregnant rat uteri by *in situ* hybridization. *Journal of Reproductive Immunology* **25**: 221–233.

Cheng, H-L., Schneider, S.L., Kane, C.M., Gollnick, S.O., Grande, C., Thompson, D., Pietrzak, E. and Tomasi, T.B. (1993) TGF-β2 gene and protein expression in maternal and fetal tissues at various stages of murine development. *Journal of Reproductive Immunology* **25**: 133–148.

Cherny, R.A. and Findlay, J.K. (1990) Separation and culture of ovine endometrial and stromal cells: evidence of morphological and functional polarity. *Biology of Reproduction* **43**: 241–250.

Chernyshov, V.P., Slukvin, I.I. and Bondarenko, G.I. (1993) Phenotypic characterization of CD7+, CD3+, and CD8+ lymphocytes from first trimester human decidua using two-color flow cytometry. *American Journal of Reproductive Immunology* **29**: 5–16.

Chiquet-Ehrismann, R. (1990) What distinguishes tenascin from fibronectin? *FASEB Journal* **4**: 2598–2604.

Chou, J.Y. (1978a) Human placental cells transformed by tsA mutants of simian virus 40: a model system for the study of placental functions. *Proceedings of the National Academy of Sciences USA* **75**: 1409–1413.

Chou, J.Y. (1978b) Establishment of clonal human placental cells synthesising human choriogonadotropin. *Proceedings of the National Academy of Sciences USA* **75**: 1854–1858.

Christiansen, F.T., Witt, C.S., Ciccone, E., Townend, D., Pende, D., Viale, D., Abraham, L.J., Dawkins, R.L. and Moretta, L. (1993) Human natural killer (NK) alloreactivity and its association with the major histocompatibility complex: ancestral haplotypes encode particular NK-defined haplotypes. *Journal of Experimental Medicine* **178**: 1033–1039.

Christmas, S.E., Bulmer, J.N., Meager, A. and Johnson, P.M. (1990) Phenotypic and functional analysis of human CD3− decidual leucocyte clones. *Immunology* **71**: 182–189.

Christmas, S.E., Brew, R., Deniz, G. and Taylor, J.J. (1993) T-cell receptor heterogeneity of γδ T-cell clones from human female reproductive tissues. *Immunology* **78**: 436–443.

Chumbley, G., Hawley, S., Carter, N.P. and Loke, Y.W. (1991) Human extravillous trophoblast MHC class I expression is resistant to regulation by interferon–α. *Journal of Reproductive Immunology* **20**: 289–296.

Chumbley, G., King, A., Holmes, N. and Loke, Y.W. (1993) In–situ hybridization and Northern blot demonstration of HLA-G mRNA in human trophoblast populations by locus-specific oligonucleotide. *Human Immunology* **37**: 17–22.

Chumbley, G., King, A., Gardner, L., Howlett, S., Holmes, N. and Loke, Y.W. (1994a) Generation of an antibody to HLA-G in transgenic mice and demonstration of the tissue reactivity of this antibody. *Journal of Reproductive Immunology* **27**: 173–186.

Chumbley, G., King, A., Robertson, K., Holmes, N. and Loke, Y.W. (1994b) Resistance of HLA-G and HLA-A2 transfectants to lysis by decidual NK cells. *Cellular Immunology* **155**: 312–322.

Chuong, C.-M. and Chen, H.-M. (1991) Enhanced expression of the neural cells adhesion molecules and tenascin (cytotactin) during wound healing. *American Journal of Pathology* **138**: 427–440.

Cianciolo, G.J., Copeland, T.D., Oroszlan, S. and Snyderman, R. (1985) Inhibition of lymphocyte proliferation by a synthetic peptide homologous to retroviral envelope proteins. *Science* **230**: 453–455.

Ciccone, E., Pende, D., Nanni, L., Di Donato, C., Viale, O., Beretta, A., Vitale, M., Sivori, S., Moretta, A. and Moretta, L. (1994a) General role of HLA class I molecules in the protection of target cells from lysis by NK cells: evidence that the free heavy chains of class I molecules are not sufficient to mediate the protective effect. Abstract of Second Meeting of the Society for Natural Immunity, Taormina, Italy. *Natural Immunity* **13**: 182.

Ciccone, E., Pende, D., Vitale, M., Nanni, L., Di Donato, C., Bottino, C., Morelli, L., Viale, O., Amoroso, A., Moretta, A. and Moretta, L. (1994b) Self class I molecules protect normal cells from lysis mediated by autologous natural killer cells. *European Journal of Immunology* **24**: 1003–1006.

Clark, W.R. (1994) The hole truth about perforin. *Nature* **369**: 16–17.

Clevenger, C.V., Altmann, S.W. and Prystowsky, M.B. (1991) Requirement of nuclear prolactin for interleukin-2-stimulated proliferation and T lymphocytes. *Science* **253**: 77–79.

Clifford, K., Rai, R., Watson, H. and Regan, L. (1994) An informative protocol for the investigation of recurrent miscarriage: preliminary experience of 500 consecutive cases. *Human Reproduction* **9**: 1328–1332.

Clover, L.M., Sargent, I.L., Townsend, A., Tampé, R. and Redman, C.W.G. (1995) Expression of TAP1 by human trophoblast. *European Journal of Immunology* **25**: 543–548.

Coffin, J.M. (1990) Retroviridae and their replication. In: *Virology*, Eds. Fields, B.N. and Knipe, D.M., Raven Press, New York, pp. 1437–1500.

Coffin, J.M. (1992) Superantigens and endogenous retroviruses: a confluence of puzzles. *Science* **255**: 411–413.

Cohen, M., Powers, M., O'Connell, C. and Kato, N. (1985) The nucleotide sequence of the *env* gene from the human provirus ERV3 and isolation and characterisation of an ERV3-specific cDNA. *Virology* **147**: 449–458.

Cohen, J.A., Winer, D.B., More, K.F., Kokai, Y., Williams, W.V., Maguire, H.C., LiVolski, V.A. and Greene, M.I. (1989) Expression pattern of the *neu* (NGL) gene-encoded growth factor receptor protein (p185[neu]) in normal and transformed epithelial tissues of the digestive tract. *Oncogene* **4**: 81–88.

Colbern, G.T., Chiang, M.H. and Main, E.K. (1994) Expression of the nonclassic histocompatibility antigen HLA-G by preeclamptic placenta. *American Journal of Obstetrics and Gynecology* **170**: 1244–1250.

Cole, G.J., Loewy, A. and Glaser, L. (1986) Neuronal cell–cell adhesion depends on interactions of N-CAN with heparin-like molecules. *Nature* **320**: 445–447.

Colombo, M.P., Jaenisch, R. and Wettstein, P.J. (1987) Endogenous retroviruses lead to the expression of a histocompatibility antigen detectable by skin graft rejection. *Proceedings of the National Academy of Sciences USA* **84**: 189–193.

Colonna, M., Brooks, E.G., Falco, M., Battista Ferrara, G. and Strominger, J.L. (1993) Generation of allospecific natural killer cells by stimulation across a polymorphism of HLA-C. *Science* **260**: 1121–1124.

Colotta, F., Re, F., Polentarutti, N., Sozzani, S. and Mantovani, A. (1992) Modulation of granulocyte survival and programmed cell death by cytokines and bacterial products. *Blood* **80**: 2012–2020.

Conneely, O.M., Maxwell, B.L., Toft, D.O., Schrader, W.T. and O'Malley, B.W. (1987) The A and B forms of the progesterone receptor arise by alternate initiation of translation of a unique mRNA. *Biochemical and Biophysical Research Communications* **149**: 493–501.

Contractor, S.F. and Soorana, S.R. (1988) Human placental cells in culture: a panning technique using a trophoblast-specific monoclonal antibody for cell separation. *Journal of Developmental Physiology* **10**: 47–51.

Cooper, D.W., Brennecke, S.P. and Wilton, A.N. (1993) Genetics of pre-eclampsia. *Hypertension in Pregnancy* **12**: 1–23.

Cooper, H.M., Tamura, R.N. and Quaranta, V. (1991) The major laminin receptor of mouse embryonic stem cells is a novel isoform of the $\alpha_6\beta_1$ integrin. *Journal of Cell Biology* **115**: 843–850.

Copeland, E.A., Rinehart, J.J., Lewis, M., Mathes, L., Olsen, R. and Sagane, A. (1983) The mechanism of retrovirus suppression of human T cell proliferation *in vitro*. *Journal of Immunology* **131**: 2017–2020.

Corps, A.N. and Brown, K.D. (1988) Ligand–receptor interactions involved in the stimulation of Swiss 3T3 fibroblasts by insulin-like growth factors and insulin. *Biochemical Journal* **252**: 119–125.

Correa, I. and Raulet, D.H. (1995) Binding of diverse peptides to MHC class I molecules inhibits target cell lysis by activated natural killer cells. *Immunity* **2**: 61–71.

Correa, I., Corral, L. and Raulet, D.H. (1994) Multiple natural killer cell-activating signals are inhibited by major histocompatibility complex class I expression in target cells. *European Journal of Immunology* **24**: 1323–1331.

Coulam, C.B., Clark, D.A., Collins, J., Scott, J.R. and Schlesselman, J.S. (1994) Worldwide collaborative observational study and meta-analysis on allogenic leukocyte immunotherapy for recurrent spontaneous abortion. *American Journal of Reproductive Immunology* **32**: 55–72.

Coulombe, P.A. (1993) The cellular and molecular biology of keratins: beginning a new era. *Current Opinion in Cell Biology* **5**: 17–29.

Coussens, L., Yang-Feng, T.L., Liao, Y.C., Chen, E., Gray, A., McGrath, J., Seeburg, P.H., Livermann, F.A., Schlessinger, J., Francke, U., Levinson, A. and Ullrich, A. (1985) Tyrosine kinase receptor with extensive homology to EGF receptor shares chromosomal location with *Neu* oncogene. *Science* **230**: 1132–1139.

Cowell, T.P. (1969) Implantation and development of mouse eggs transferred to the uteri of non-progestational mice. *Journal of Reproduction and Fertility* **19**: 239–245.

Crane, J.P. and Cheung, S.W. (1988) An embryogenic model to explain cytogenetic inconsistencies observed in chorionic villus versus fetal tissue. *Prenatal Diagnosis* **8**: 119–129.

Creasy, R. (1988) The cytogenetics of spontaneous abortion in humans. In: *Early Pregnancy Loss*, Eds. Beard, R.W. and Sharp, F., Royal College of Obstetricians and Gynaecologists, London, pp. 293–304.

Critchley, H.O.D., Bailey, D.A., Au, C.L., Affandi, B. and Rogers, P.A.W. (1993) Immunohistochemical sex steroid receptor distribution in endometrium from long-term subdermal levonorgestrel users and during the normal menstrual cycle. *Human Reproduction* **8**: 1632–1639.

Croy, B.A. (1994) Granulated metrial gland cells: hypotheses concerning possible functions during murine gestation. *Journal of Reproductive Immunology* **27**: 85–94.

Croy, B.A. and Chapeau, C. (1990) Evaluation of the pregnancy immunotrophism hypothesis by assessment of the reproductive performance of young adult mice of genotype *scid/scid.bg/bg*. *Journal of Reproduction and Fertility* **88**: 231–239.

Croy, B.A. and Kiso, Y. (1993) Granulated metrial gland cells: a natural killer cell subset of the pregnant murine uterus. *Microscopy Research and Technique* **25**: 189–200.

Croy, B.A., Chapeau, C., Reed, N., Stewart, I.J. and Peel, S. (1991a) Is there an essential requirement for bone-marrow-derived cells at the fetomaternal interface during successful pregnancy? A study of pregnancies in immunodeficient mice. In: *Molecular and Cellular Immunobiology of the Maternal Fetal Interface*, Eds. Wegmann, T.G., Gill, T.J. and Nisbet-Brown, E., Oxford University Press, Oxford, pp. 168–188.

Croy, B.A., Guilbert, L.J., Browne, M.A., Gough, N.M., Stinchcomb, D.T., Reed, N. and Wegmann, T.G. (1991b) Characterization of cytokine production by the metrial gland and granulated metrial gland cells. *Journal of Reproductive Immunology* **19**: 149–166.

Croy, B.A., Yu, Z.-M. and King, G.J. (1994) A review of the natural killer cell lineage in the uterus of the mouse and of the pig. *Journal of Animal Science* **72**: 9–15.

Daiter, E., Pampfer, S., Yeung, Y.G., Barad, D., Stanley, E.R. and Pollard, J.W. (1992) Expression of colony-stimulating factor-1 in the human uterus and placenta. *Journal of Clinical Endocrinology and Metabolism* **74**: 850–858.

Dalton, A.J., Hellman, A., Kalter, S.S. and Helmke, R.J. (1974) Ultrastructural comparison of placental virus with several type-C oncogenic viruses. *Journal of the National Cancer Institute* **52**: 1379–1381.

Damjanov, I., Mildner, B. and Knowles, B.B. (1986) Immunohistological localization of the epidermal growth factor receptor in normal human tissues. *Laboratory Investigation* **55**: 588–592.

Damsky, C.H., Fitzgerald, M.L. and Fisher, S.J. (1992) Distribution patterns of extracellular matrix components and adhesion receptors are intricately modulated during 1st trimester cytotrophoblast differentiation along the invasion pathway, *in vivo*. *Journal of Clinical Investigation* **89**: 210–222.

Damsky, C., Sutherland, A. and Fisher, S. (1993) Extracellular matrix 5: adhesive interactions in early mammalian embryogenesis, implantation and placentation. *FASEB Journal* **7**: 1320–1329.

Damsky, C.H., Librach, C., Lim, K.-H., Fitzgerald, M.L., McMaster, M.T., Janatpour, M., Zhou, Y., Logan, S.K. and Fisher, S.J. (1994) Integrin switching regulates normal trophoblast invasion. *Development* **120**: 3657–3666.

Daniels, B.F., Karlhofer, F.M., Seaman, W.E. and Yokoyama, W.M. (1994a) A natural killer cell receptor specific for a major histocompatibility complex class I molecule. *Journal of Experimental Medicine* **180**: 687–692.

Daniels, B., Yokoyama, W. and Seaman, W.E. (1994b) Evidence that Ly-49 recognizes carbohydrate structures on H-2D^d. Abstract of Second Meeting of the Society for Natural Immunity, Taormina, Italy. *Natural Immunity* **13**: 192–193.

Dati, C., Antoniotti, S., Taverna, S., Perroteau, I. and DeBortoli, M. (1990) Inhibition of c-*erb*B-2 oncogene expression by estrogens in human breast cancer cells. *Oncogene* **5**: 1001–1006.

Davis, M. and Brown, C.M. (1985) Anti-trophoblast antibody responses during normal human pregnancy. *Journal of Reproductive Immunology* **7**: 285–297.

DeChiara, T.M., Robertson, E.J. and Efstratiadis, A. (1991) Parental imprinting of the mouse insulin-like growth factor II gene. *Cell* **64**: 849–859.

Dedhar, S. (1990) Integrins and tumor invasion. *BioEssays* **12**: 583–590.

De-Groot, N. and Hochberg, A. (1993) Gene imprinting during placental and embryonic development. *Molecular Reproduction and Development* **36**: 390–406.

Dejana, E., Martin-Padura, I., Lauri, D., Bernasconi, S., Bani, M.R., Garofalo, A., Giavazzi, R., Magnani, J., Mantovani, A. and Menard, S. (1992) Endothelial leukocyte adhesion molecule-1-dependent adhesion of colon carcinoma cells to vascular endothelium is inhibited by an antibody to Lewis fucosylated Type I carbohydrate chain. *Laboratory Investigation* **66**: 324–330.

Delfino, D.V., Patrene, K.D., DeLeo, A.B., DeLeo, R., Herberman, R.B. and Boggs, S.S. (1994) Role of CD44 in the development of natural killer cells from precursors in long-term cultures of mouse bone marrow. *Journal of Immunology* **152**: 5171–5179.

De Maeyer, E. and De Maeyer-Guignard, J. (1991) Interferons. In: *The Cytokine Handbook*, Ed. Thomson, A., Academic Press, London, pp. 215–240.

De Maria, R., Faiks, S., Silvestri, M., Frati, L., Pallone, F., Santoni, A. and Testi, R. (1993) Continuous *in vivo* activation and transient hyporesponsiveness to TcR/CD3 triggering of human gut lamina propria lymphocytes. *European Journal of Immunology* **23**: 3104–3108.

Deniz, G., Christmas, S.E., Brew, R. and Johnson, P.M. (1994) Phenotypic and functional cellular differences between human CD3⁻ decidual and peripheral blood leukocytes. *Journal of Immunology* **152**: 4255–4261.

Denker, H.W. (1990) Trophoblast-endometrial interactions at embryo implantation: a cell biological paradox. *Trophoblast Research* **4**: 3–29.

De Sousa, M., De Silva, M.T. and Kupiec-Weglinski, J.W. (1990) Collagen, the circulation and positioning of lymphocytes: a unifying clue? *Scandinavian Journal of Immunology* **31**: 249–256.

De Vries, C., Escobedo, A., Ueno, H., Houck, K., Ferrara, N. and Williams, L.T. (1992) The *fms*-like tyrosine kinase, a receptor for vascular endothelial growth factor. *Science* **255**: 989–991.

DeWit, T.F.R., Vloemans, S., Van Den Elsen, P.J., Haworth, A. and Stern, P.L. (1990) Differential expression of the HLA class I multigene family by human embryonal carcinoma and choriocarcinoma cell lines. *Journal of Immunology* **144**: 1080–1087.

de Wolf, F., Brosens, I. and Renaer, M. (1980) Fetal growth retardation and the maternal arterial supply of the human placenta in the absence of sustained hypertension. *British Journal of Obstetrics and Gynaecology* **87**: 678–685.

Diamond, M.S. and Springer, T.A. (1994) The dynamic regulation of integrin adhesiveness. *Current Biology* **4**: 506–517.

Dietl, J., Ruck, P., Marzusch, K., Horny, H.-P., Kaiserling, E. and Handgretinger, R. (1992) Uterine granular lymphocytes are activated natural killer cells expressing VLA-1. *Immunology Today* **13**: 236.

Dinarello, C.A. (1991) Interleukin-1 and interleukin-1 antagonism. *Blood* **77**: 1627–1652.

Dirksen, E.R. and Levy, J.A. (1977) Virus-like particles in placentas from normal individuals and patients with systemic lupus erythematosus. *Journal of the National Cancer Institute* **59**: 1187–1192.

Donaldson, W.L., Oriol, J.G., Pelkaus, C.L. and Antczak, D.F. (1994) Paternal and maternal major histocompatibility complex class I antigens are expressed co-dominantly by equine trophoblast. *Placenta* **15**: 123–135.

Dorman, P.J. and Searle, R.F. (1988) Alloantigen presenting capacity of human decidual tissue. *Journal of Reproductive Immunology* **13**: 101–112.

Dornan, J.C. and Harper, A. (1994) Where are we with Doppler? *British Journal of Obstetrics and Gynaecology* **101**: 190–191.

Douglas, G.C. and King, B.F. (1989) Isolation of pure villous cytotrophoblasts from term human placenta using immunomagnetic microspheres. *Journal of Immunological Methods* **119**: 259–268.

Douglas, K.A. and Redman, C.W.G. (1994) Eclampsia in the United Kingdom. *British Medical Journal* **309**: 1395–1399.

Drake, B.L. and Head, J.R. (1990) Murine trophoblast cells are not killed by tumor necrosis factor-α. *Journal of Reproductive Immunology* **17**: 93–99.

Drake, B.L. and Head, J.R. (1994) GM-CSF and CSF-1 stimulate DNA synthesis but not cell proliferation in short-term cultures of mid-gestation murine trophoblast. *Journal of Reproductive Immunology* **26**: 41–56.

Drake, B.L. and Loke, Y.W. (1991) Isolation of endothelial cells from human first trimester decidua using immunomagnetic beads. *Human Reproduction* **6**: 1156–1159.

Drezen, J.-M., Barra, J., Babinet, C. and Morello, D. (1994) MHC class I genes are not imprinted in the mouse placenta. *Immunogenetics* **40**: 62–65.

Dudley, D.J., Trautman, M.S., Araneo, B.A., Edwin, S.S. and Mitchell, M.D. (1992) Decidual cell biosynthesis of interleukin-6: regulation by inflammatory cytokines. *Journal of Clinical Endocrinology and Metabolism* **74**: 884–889.

Du Pasquier, L. (1993) Evolution of the immune system. In: *Fundamental Immunology*, Ed. Paul, W.E., Raven Press, New York, pp. 199–233.

Dustin, M.L. and Springer, T.A. (1991) Role of lymphocyte adhesion receptors in transient interactions and cell locomotion. *Annual Review of Immunology* **9**: 27–66.

Earl, U., Estlin, C. and Bulmer, J. (1990) Fibronectin and laminin in the early human placenta. *Placenta* **11**: 223–231.

Eck, M.J., Atwell, S.K., Shoelson, S.E. and Harrison, S.C. (1994) Structure of the regulatory domains of the src-family of tyrosine kinase Lck. *Nature* **368**: 764–769.

Edvardsen, K., Chen, W., Rucklidge, G., Walsh, F.S., Obrink, B. and Bock, E. (1993) Transmembrane neural cell-adhesion molecule (NCAM), but not glycosyl-phosphatidylinositol-anchored NCAM, down-regulates secretion of matrix metalloproteinases. *Proceedings of the National Academy of Sciences USA* **90**: 11463–11467.

Ejima, Y., Sasaki, M.S., Kameko, A. and Tanooka, H. (1988) Types, rates, origin and expressivity of chromosome mutations involving 13q14 in retinoblastoma patients. *Human Genetics* **79**: 118–123.

Ellis, S.A., Strachan, T., Palmer, M.S. and McMichael, A.J. (1989) Complete nucleotide sequence of a unique HLA class I C locus product expressed on the human choriocarcinoma cell line BeWo. *Journal of Immunology* **142**: 3281–3285.

Ellis, S.A., Palmer, M.S. and McMichael, A.J. (1990) Human trophoblast and the choriocarcinoma cell line BeWo express a truncated HLA class I molecule. *Journal of Immunology* **144**: 731–735.

Enders, A.C. (1993) Overview of the morphology of implantation in primates. In: *In Vitro Fertilization and Embryo Transfer in Primates*, Eds. Wolf, D.P., Stouffer, R.L. and Brenner, R.M., Springer Verlag, pp. 145–157.

Enders, A.C. and King, B.F. (1991) Early stages of trophoblastic invasion of the maternal vascular system during implantation in the macaque and baboon. *American Journal of Anatomy* **192**: 329–346.

Enders, A.C. and Liu, I.K.M. (1991) Trophoblast–uterine interactions during equine chorionic girdle cell maturation, migration, and transformation. *American Journal of Anatomy* **192**: 366–381.

Enders, A.C., Lantz, K.C. and Schlafke, S. (1989) Differentiation of trophoblast of the baboon blastocyst. *Anatomical Record* **225**: 329–340.

Erickson, H.P. (1993) Tenascin-C, tenascin-R and tenascin-X: a family of talented proteins in search of functions. *Current Opinion in Cell Biology* **5**: 869–876.

Erickson, H.P. and Bourdon, M.A. (1989) Tenascin: an extracellular matrix protein prominent in specialised embryonic tissues and tumours. *Annual Review of Cell Biology* **5**: 71–92.

Evain-Brion, D. (1992) Growth factors and trophoblast differentiation: a review. *Trophoblast Research* **6**: 1–18.

Faber, M., Wewer, U.M., Berthelsen, J.G., Liotta, L.A. and Albrechtsen, R. (1986) Laminin production by human endometrial stromal cells relates to the cyclic and pathologic state of the endometrium. *American Journal of Pathology* **124**: 384–391.

Falk, K., Rotzschke, O., Grahovac, B., Schendel, D., Stevanic, S., Gnau, V., Jung, G., Strominger, J.L. and Rammensee, H-G. (1993) Allele-specific peptide ligand motifs of HLA-C molecules. *Proceedings of the National Academy of Sciences USA* **90**: 12005–12009.

Falk, L.A. and Vogel, S.N. (1988) Granulocyte-macrophage colony-stimulating factor (GM-CSF) and macrophage colony-stimulating factor (CSF-1) synergize to stimulate progenitor cells with high proliferative potential. *Journal of Leukocyte Biology* **44**: 455–464.

Feinberg, R.F., Kao, L.-C., Haimowitz, J.E., Queenan, J.T., Wun, T.-C., Strauss, J.F. and Kliman, H.J. (1989) Plasminogen activator inhibitor types 1 and 2 in human trophoblasts: PAI-1 is an immunocytochemical marker of invading trophoblasts. *Laboratory Investigation* **61**: 20–26.

Feinberg, R.F., Kliman, H.J. and Cohen, A.W. (1991a) Preeclampsia, trisomy 13 and the placental bed. *Obstetrics and Gynecology* **78**: 505–508.

Feinberg, R.F., Kliman, H.J. and Lockwood, C.J. (1991b) Is oncofetal fibronectin a trophoblast glue for human implantation? *American Journal of Pathology* **138**: 537–543.

Feinberg, R.F., Kliman, H.J. and Wang, C.-L. (1994) Transforming growth factor-beta stimulates trophoblast oncofetal fibronectin synthesis *in vitro*: implications for trophoblast implantation *in vivo*. *Journal of Clinical Endocrinology and Metabolism* **78**: 1241–1248.

Feinman, M.A., Kliman, H.J. and Main, E.K. (1987) HLA antigen expression and induction by γ interferon in cultured human trophoblasts. *American Journal of Obstetrics and Gynecology* **157**: 1429–1434.

Feizi, T. (1985) Demonstration by monoclonal antibodies that carbohydrate structures of glycoproteins and glycolipids are onco–developmental antigens. *Nature* **314**: 53–57.

Feldman, D. (1975) An electron microscopic study of virus particles in rhesus monkey placenta. *Proceedings of the National Academy of Sciences USA* **72**: 118–121.

Fell, H.B. (1976) The development of organ culture. In: *Organ Culture in Biomedical Research*, Eds. Balls, M. and Monnickendam, M.A., Cambridge University Press, Cambridge, pp. 1–13.

Fernandez, P.L., Merino, M.J., Nogales, F.F., Charonis, A.S., Stetler-Stevenson, W. and Liotta, L. (1992) Immunohistochemical profile of basement membrane proteins and 72 kilodalton type IV collagenase in the implantation placental site: an integrated view. *Laboratory Investigation* **66**: 572–579.

Ferrara, N., Houck, K., Jakeman, L. and Leung, D.W. (1992) Molecular and biological properties of the vascular endothelial growth factor family of proteins. *Endocrinology Review* **13**: 18–32.

Ferry, B.L., Starkey, P.M., Sargent, I.L., Watt, G.M.O., Jackson, M. and Redman, C.W.G. (1990) Cell populations in the human early pregnancy decidua: natural killer activity and response to interleukin-2 of CD56-positive large granular lymphocytes. *Immunology* **70**: 446–452.

Ferry, B.L., Sargent, I.L., Starkey, P.M. and Redman, C.W.G. (1991) Cytotoxic activity against trophoblast and choriocarcinoma cells of large granular lymphocytes from early pregnancy decidua. *Cellular Immunology* **132**: 140–149.

Feuchter-Murthy, A.E., Freeman, J.D. and Mager, D.L. (1993) Splicing of a human endogenous retrovirus to a novel phospholipase A2 related gene. *Nucleic Acids Research* **21**: 135–143.

ffrench-Constant, C. and Hynes, R.O. (1988) Patterns of fibronectin gene expression and splicing during cell migration in chicken embryos. *Development* **104**: 369–382.

ffrench-Constant, C., Van de Water, L., Dvorak, H.F. and Hynes, R.O. (1989) Reappearance of an embryonic form of fibronectin splicing during wound healing in adult rat. *Journal of Cell Biology* **109**: 903–914.

Filderman, A.E., Bruckno, A., Kacinski, B. and Remold, H. (1991) Macrophage-colony stimulating factor (CSF-1) enhances invasiveness in CSF-1 receptor-positive lung cell lines. *Journal of Cellular Biochemistry* Suppl. **15FB**: 27 (abstract).

Filla, M.S., Zhang, C.X. and Kaul, K.L. (1993) A potential transforming growth factor alpha/epidermal growth factor receptor autocrine circuit in placental cytotrophoblasts. *Cell Growth and Differentiation* **4**: 387–393.

Finberg, R.W., White, W. and Nicholson-Weller, A. (1992) Decay-accelerating factor expression on either effector or target cells inhibits cytotoxicity by human natural killer cells. *Journal of Immunology* **149**: 2055–2060.

Findlay, J.K. (1986) Angiogenesis in reproductive tissues. *Journal of Endocrinology* **111**: 357–366.

Finn, C.A. (1994) The adaptive significance of menstruation. *Human Reproduction* **9**: 1202–1207.

Fisher, S.J., Leitch, M.S., Kantor, M.S., Basbaum, C.B. and Kramer, R.H. (1985) Degradation of extracellular matrix by trophoblastic cells of first trimester human placentas. *Journal of Cellular Biochemistry* **27**: 31–41.

Fisher, S.J., Cui, T.-Y., Zhang, L., Hartman, L., Grahl, K., Guo-Yang, Z., Tarpey, J. and Damsky, C.H. (1989) Adhesive and degradative properties of human placental cytotrophoblast cells *in vitro*. *Journal of Cell Biology* **109**: 891–902.

Fleming, S. (1991) Cell adhesion and epithelial differentiation. *Journal of Pathology* **164**: 95–100.

Flynn, A., Finke, J.H. and Hilfiker, H.L. (1982) Placental mononuclear phagocytes as a source of interleukin–1. *Science* **218**: 475–476.

Fowler, A.K., Reed, C.D., Todaro, G.J. and Hellman, A. (1972) Activation of C-type RNA virus markers in mouse uterine tissue. *Proceedings of the National Academy of Sciences USA* **69**: 2254–2257.

Fox, H. (1970) Effect of hypoxia on trophoblast in organ culture: a morphologic and autoradiographic study. *American Journal of Obstetrics and Gynecology* **107**: 1058–1064.

Franceschi, C., Cossarizza, A., Monti, D. and Ottaviani, E. (1991) Cytotoxicity and immunocyte markers in cells from the freshwater snail *Planorbarius corneus* (L.) (*Gastropoda pulmonata*): implications for the evolution of natural killer cells. *European Journal of Immunology* **21**: 489–493.

Franklin, G.C., Holmgren, L., Donovan, M., Adam, G.I.A., Walsh, C., Pfeifer-Ohlsson, S. and Ohlsson, R. (1993) Expression and control of PDGF stimulatory loops in the developing placenta. *Trophoblast Research* **7**: 287–303.

Freedman, A.S., Rhynhart, K., Nojima, Y., Svahn, J., Eliseo, L., Benjamin, C.D., Morimoto, C. and Vivier, E. (1993) Stimulation of protein tyrosine phosphorylation in human B cells after ligation of the β_1 integrin VLA-4. *Journal of Immunology* **150**: 1645–1652.

Friedman, S.A., Taylor, R.N. and Roberts, J.M. (1991) Pathophysiology of pre-eclampsia. *Clinical Perinatology* **18**: 661–682.

Fuchs, E. (1993) Epidermal differentiation and keratin gene expression. *Journal of Cell Science* Suppl. **17**: 197–208.

Fujii, T., Ishitani, A. and Geraghty, D.E. (1994) A soluble form of the HLA-G antigen is encoded by a messenger ribonucleic acid containing intron 4. *Journal of Immunology* **153**: 5516–5524.

Fuller, E.G., Highison, G.J., Tibbitts, F.D. and Fuller, B.D. (1994) Migration of intravascular trophoblast cells in uterine arteries of the golden hamster: a scanning electron microscopic study. *Journal of Morphology* **220**: 307–313.

Furmanski, P. (1994) A pregnant possibility: crossing fetal tolerance. *American Journal of Pathology* **145**: 1247–1252.

Gallery, E.D.M., Rowe, J., Schrieber, L. and Jackson, C.J. (1991) Isolation and purification of microvascular endothelium from human decidual tissue in the late phase of pregnancy. *American Journal of Obstetrics and Gynecology* **165**: 191–196.

Garcia, C.F., Weiss, L.M., Lowder, J., Kormoroske, C., Link, M.P., Levy, R. and Warnke, R.A. (1987) Quantitation and estimation of lymphocyte subsets in tissue sections: comparison with flow cytometry. *American Journal of Clinical Pathology* **87**: 470–477.

Garcia, E., Bouchard, P., de Brux, J., Berdah, J., Frydman, R., Schaison, G., Milgrom, E. and Perrot-Applanat, M. (1988) Use of immunocytochemistry of progesterone and estrogen receptors for endometrial dating. *Journal of Clinical Endocrinology and Metabolism* **67**: 80–87.

Gearing, D., King, J.A., Gough, N.M. and Nicola, N. (1989) Expression cloning of a receptor for human granulocyte-macrophage colony-stimulating factor. *EMBO Journal* **8**: 3667–3676.

Geiser, A.G., Letterio, J.J., Kulkarni, A.B., Karlsson, S., Roberts, A.B. and Sporn, M.B. (1993) Transforming growth factor beta 1 (TGF-beta 1) controls expression of major histocompatibility genes in the postnatal mouse: aberrant histocompatibility antigen expression in the pathogenesis of the TGF-beta null mouse phenotype. *Proceedings of the National Academy of Sciences USA* **90**: 9944–9948.

Genbacev, O., Schubach, S.A. and Miller, R.K. (1992) Villous culture of first trimester human placenta: model to study extravillous trophoblast (EVT) differentiation. *Placenta* **13**: 439–461.

Genbacev, O., DeMesy Jensen, K., Schubach Powlin, S. and Miller, R.K. (1993) *In vitro* differentiation and ultrastructure of human extravillous trophoblast (EVT) cells. *Placenta* **14**: 463–475.

Geraghty, D.E. (1993) Structure of the HLA class I region and expression of its resident genes. *Current Opinion in Immunology* **5**: 3–7.

Geraghty, D.E., Koller, B.H. and Orr, H.T. (1987) A human major histocompatibility complex class I gene that encodes a protein with a shortened cytoplasmic segment. *Proceedings of the National Academy of Sciences USA* **84**: 9145–9149.

Geraghty, D.E., Pei, J., Lipsky, B., Hansen, J.A., Taillon-Miller, P., Bronson, S.K. and Chaplin, D.D. (1992) Cloning and physical mapping of the HLA class I region spanning the HLA-E-to-HLA-F interval by using yeast artificial chromosomes. *Proceedings of the National Academy of Sciences USA* **89**: 2669–2673.

Germain-Lee, E.L., Janicot, M., Lammers, R., Ullrich, A. and Casella, S.J. (1992) Expression of the type I insulin-like growth factor with low affinity for insulin-like growth factor II. *Biochemical Journal* **281**: 413–417.

Gerretson, G., Huisjes, H.J. and Elema, J.D. (1981) Morphological changes of the spiral arteries in the placental bed in relation to pre-eclampsia and fetal growth retardation. *British Journal of Obstetrics and Gynaecology* **88**: 876–881.

Giacomini, P., Tosi, S., Murgia, C., Nobili, F., Gaetani, S., Gambari, R., Nicotra, M.R., Simoni, G., Maggi, F. and Natali, P.G. (1994) First-trimester human trophoblast is class II major histocompatibility complex mRNA[+]/antigen[-]. *Human Immunology* **39**: 281–289.

Giannoukakis, N., Deal, C., Paquette, J., Goodyear, C.G. and Polychronakos, C. (1993) Parental genomic imprinting of the human IGF2 gene. *Nature Genetics* **4**: 98–101.

Giblin, P.A., Leahy, D.J., Mennone, J. and Kavathas, P.B. (1994) The role of charge and multiple faces of the CD8α/α homodimer in binding to major histocompatibility complex class I molecules: support for a bivalent model. *Proceedings of the National Academy of Sciences USA* **91**: 1716–1720.

Giri, J.G., Ahdieh, M., Eisenman, J., Shanebeck, K., Grabstein, K., Kumaki, S., Namen, A., Park, L.S., Cosman, D. and Anderson, D. (1994) Utilization of the β and γ chains of the IL-2 receptor by the novel cytokine IL-15. *EMBO Journal* **13**: 2822–2830.

Giudice, L.C. (1994) Growth factors and growth modulators in human uterine endometrium: their potential relevance to reproductive medicine. *Fertility and Sterility* **61**: 1–17.

Glasser, S.R., Mulholland, J., Mani, S.K., Julian, J., Munir, I., Lampelo, S. and Soares, M.J. (1991) Blastocyst endometrial relationships: reciprocal interactions between uterine epithelial and stromal cells and blastocysts. *Trophoblast Research* **5**: 229–280.

Göbel, T.W.F., Chen, C.-L.H., Shrimpf, J., Grossi, C.E., Bernot, A., Bucy, R.P., Auffray, C. and Cooper, M.D. (1994) Characterization of avian natural killer cells and their intracellular CD3 protein complex. *European Journal of Immunology* **24**: 1685–1691.

Godfrey, D.I., Zlotnik, A. and Suda, T. (1992) Phenotypic and functional characterization of c-*kit* expression during intrathymic T cell development. *Journal of Immunology* **149**: 2281–2285.

Godfrey, K.M., Redman, C.W.G., Barker, D.J.P. and Osmond, C. (1991) The effect of maternal anaemia and iron deficiency on the ratio of fetal weight to placental weight. *British Journal of Obstetrics and Gynaecology* **98**: 886–891.

Goldmann, R., Ben-Levy, R., Peles, E. and Yarden, Y. (1990) Heterodimerization of the *erb*B-1 and *erb*B-2 receptors in human breast carcinoma cells: a mechanism for receptor transregulation. *Biochemistry* **29**: 11024–11028.

Goodger, A.M. and Rogers, P.A.W. (1994) Endometrial endothelial cell proliferation during the menstrual cycle. *Human Reproduction* **9**: 399–405.

Goodglick, L. and Braun, J. (1994) Revenge of the microbes. Superantigens of the T and B cell lineage. *American Journal of Pathology* **144**: 623–636.

Goodman, S.L., Risse, G. and von der Mark, K. (1989) The E8 subfragment of laminin promotes locomotion of myoblasts over extracellular matrix. *Journal of Cell Biology* **109**: 799–809.

Goodwin, R.G. and Namen, A.E. (1991) Interleukin-7. In: *The Cytokine Handbook*, Ed. Thomson, A., Academic Press, London, pp.191–200.

Goridis, C. and Brunet, J.-F. (1992) NCAM: structural diversity, function and regulation of expression. *Seminars in Cell Biology* **3**: 189–197.

Goshen, R., Ben-Rafael, Z., Gonik, B., Lustig, O., Tannos, V., de-Groot, N. and Hochberg, A.A. (1994) The role of genomic imprinting in implantation. *Fertility and Sterility* **62**: 903–910.

Gospodarowicz, D., Abraham, J.A. and Schilling, J. (1989) Isolation and characterization of a vascular endothelial cell mitogen produced by pituitary-derived folliculo-stellate cells. *Proceedings of the National Academy of Sciences USA* **86**: 7311–7315.

Gough, N.M. (1992) Molecular genetics of leukemia inhibitory factor (LIF) and its receptor. *Growth Factors* **7**: 175–179.

Goustin, A.S., Betscholtz, C., Pfeifer–Ohlsson, S., Persson, H., Rydnert, J., Bywater, M., Holmgren, G., Heldin, C.-H., Westermark, B. and Ohlsson, R. (1985) Coexpression of the *sis* and *myc* proto-oncogenes in developing human placenta suggests a role for autocrine control of trophoblast growth. *Cell* **41**: 301–312.

Grabowska, A. (1989) Placental antigenicity and maternal immunoregulation in human and murine pregnancy. PhD thesis, University of Cambridge.

Grabowska, A., Carter, N. and Loke, Y.W. (1990a) Human trophoblast cells in culture express an unusual major histocompatibility complex class I-like antigen. *American Journal of Reproductive Immunology* **23**: 10–18.

Grabowska, A., Chumbley, G., Carter, N. and Loke, Y.W. (1990b) Interferon–γ enhances mRNA and surface expression of class I-like antigen on human extravillous trophoblast. *Placenta* **11**: 301–308.

Grabstein, K.H., Eisenman, J., Shanebeck, K., Rauch, C., Srinivasan, S., Fung, V., Beers, C., Richardson, J., Schoenborn, M.A., Ahdieh, M., Johnson, L., Alderson, M.R., Watson, J.D., Anderson, D.M. and Giri, J.G. (1994) Cloning of a T cell growth factor that interacts with the β chain of the interleukin-2 receptor. *Science* **264**: 965–968.

Graham, C.H. and Lala, P.K. (1991) Mechanism of control of trophoblast invasion *in situ*. *Journal of Cellular Physiology* **148**: 228–234.

Graham, C.H. and Lala, P.K. (1992) Mechanisms of placental invasion of the uterus and their control. *Biochemistry and Cell Biology* **70**: 867–874.

Graham, C.H., Lysiak, J.J., McCrae, K.R. and Lala, P.K. (1992) Localization of transforming growth factor-β at the human fetal–maternal interface: role in trophoblast growth and differentiation. *Biology of Reproduction* **46**: 561–572.

Graham, C.H., Hawley, T.S., Hawley, R.G., MacDougall, J.R., Kerbel, R.S., Khoo, N. and Lala, P.K. (1993) Establishment and characterization of first trimester human trophoblast cells with extended lifespan. *Experimental and Cellular Research* **206**: 204–211.

Graham, R.A., Li, T.C., Cooke, I.D. and Aplin, J.D. (1994) Keratan sulphate as a secretory product of human endometrium: cyclic expression in normal women. *Human Reproduction* **9**: 926–930.

Grinnell, F. (1992) Wound repair, keratinocyte activation and integrin modulation. *Journal of Cell Science* **101**: 1–5.

Grinnell, F. (1994) Fibroblasts, myofibroblasts and wound contraction. *Journal of Cell Biology* **124**: 401–404.

Guan, J.-L., Trevithick, J.E. and Hynes, R.O. (1991) Fibronectin/integrin interaction induces tyrosine phosphorylation of a 120 kDa protein. *Cell Regulation* **2**: 951–964.

Guillemot, F., Caspary, T., Tilghman, S.M., Copeland, N.G., Gilbert, D.J., Jenkins, N.A., Anderson, D.J., Joyner, A.L., Rossant, J. and Nagy, A. (1995) Genomic imprinting of *Mash2*, a mouse gene required for trophoblast development. *Nature Genetics* **9**: 235–242.

Güssow, D., Rein, R.S., Meijer, I., de Hoog, W., Seemann, G.H.A., Hochstenbach, F.M. and Ploegh, H.L. (1987) Isolation, expression and the primary structure of HLA-Cw1 and HLA-Cw2 genes: evolutionary aspects. *Immunogenetics* **25**: 313–322.

Guy-Grand, D., Vanden Broecke, C., Briottet, C., Malassis-Seris, M., Selz, F. and Vassalli, P. (1992) Different expression of the recombination activity gene RAG-1 in various populations of thymocytes, peripheral T cells and gut thymus-independent intraepithelial lymphocytes suggests two pathways of T cell receptor rearrangements. *European Journal of Immunology* **22**: 505–510.

Haas, W. (1993) Gamma/delta cells. *Annual Reviews in Immunology* **11**: 637–685.

Hackett, J., Bosma, G.C., Bosma, M.J., Bennett, M. and Kumar, V. (1986) Transplantable progenitors of natural killer cells are distinct from those of T and B lymphocytes. *Proceedings of the National Academy of Sciences USA* **83**: 3427–3431.

Haig, D. (1993) Genetic conflicts in human pregnancy. *Quarterly Review of Biology* **68**: 495–532.

Haining, R.E.B., Schofield, J.P., Jones, D.S., Rajput-Williams, J. and Smith, S.K. (1991) Identification of mRNA for epidermal growth factor and transforming growth factor-α present in low copy number in human endometrium and decidua using reverse transcriptase–polymerase chain reaction. *Journal of Molecular Endocrinology* **6**: 207–214.

Hall, D.E., Reichardt, L.F., Crowley, E., Holley, B., Moezzi, M., Sonnenberg, A. and Damsky, C.H. (1990) The $\alpha_6\beta_1$ integrin heterodimers mediate cell attachment to distinct sites on laminin. *Journal of Cell Biology* **110**: 2175–2184.

Hall, J.G. (1990) Genomic imprinting: review and relevance to human diseases. *American Journal of Human Genetics* **46**: 857–873.

Hallek, M., Lepisto, E.M., Slattery, K.E., Griffin, J.D. and Ernst, T.J. (1992) Interferon-γ increases the expression of the gene encoding the β subunit of the granulocyte-macrophage colony-stimulating factor receptor. *Blood* **7**: 1736–1742.

Halstensen T.S. and Brandtzaeg, P. (1994) Phenotypic characteristics of human intraepithelial lymphocytes. In: *Mucosal Immunology: Intraepithelial Lymphocytes*, Eds. Kiyono, H. and McGhee, J.R., Raven Press, New York, pp.147–161.

Hamann, J., Fiebig, H. and Strauss, M. (1993) Expression cloning of the early activation antigen CD69, a type II integral membrane protein with a C-type lectin domain. *Journal of Immunology* **150**: 4920–4927.

Hamperl, H. (1955) The granular endometrial stromal cells: a new cell type. *Journal of Pathology and Bacteriology* **69**: 358–359.

Hamperl, H. and Hellweg, G. (1958) Granular endometrial stromal cells. *Obstetrics and Gynecology* **11**: 379–387.

Hampson, J., McLaughlin, P.J. and Johnson, P.M. (1993) Low-affinity receptors for tumor necrosis factor-α, interferon-γ and granulocyte-macrophage colony-stimulating factor are expressed on human placental syncytiotrophoblast. *Immunology* **79**: 485–490.

Han, V.K.M., Hunter, E.S., Pratt, R.M., Zendegui, J.G. and Lee, D.C. (1987) Expression of rat transforming growth factor alpha mRNA during development occurs predominantly in the maternal decidua. *Molecular and Cellular Biology* **7**: 2335–2343.

Handwerger, S. and Brar, A. (1992) Placental lactogen, placental growth hormone, and decidual prolactin. *Seminars in Reproductive Endocrinology* **10**: 106–115.

Handwerger, S., Richards, R.G. and Markoff, E. (1992) The physiology of decidual prolactin and other decidual protein hormones. *Trends in Endocrinological Metabolism* **3**: 91–95.

Handwerger, S., Richards, R.G. and Myers, S.E. (1993) Autocrine/paracrine regulation of decidual prolactin. In: *Trophoblast Cells: Pathways for Maternal–Embryonic Communication*, Eds. Soares, M.J., Handwerger, S. and Talamantes, F., Springer-Verlag, Berlin, pp. 134–150.

Hardy, R.R. and Hayakawa, K. (1994) CD5 B cells, a fetal B cell lineage. *Advances in Immunology* **55**: 297–339.

Harrington, K. and Campbell, S. (1992) Doppler ultrasound in prenatal prediction and diagnosis. *Current Opinion in Obstetrics and Gynecology* **4**: 264–272.

Harris, A.L. and Neal, D.E. (1987) Epidermal growth factor and its receptor in human cancer. In: *Growth Factors and Oncogenes in Breast Cancer*, Ed. Sloyser, M., Ellis Horwood, Chichester, pp. 60–86.

Harris, D.T., Cianciolo, G.J., Snyderman, R., Argav, S. and Koren, H.S. (1987) Inhibition of human natural killer cell activity by a synthetic peptide homologous to a conserved retroviral region in the retroviral protein p15E. *Journal of Immunology* **138**: 889–894.

Harrison, G.A., Humphrey, K.E., Jakobsen, I.B. and Cooper, D.W. (1993) A 14 bp deletion polymorphism in the HLA-G gene. *Human Molecular Genetics* **2**: 2200.

Harrison, K.B. (1989) X-chromosome inactivation in the human cytotrophoblast. *Cytogenetics and Cell Genetics* **52**: 37–41.

Harty, J.R. and Kauma, S.W. (1992) Interleukin-1β stimulates colony-stimulating factor-1 production in placental villous core mesenchymal cells. *Journal of Clinical Endocrinology and Metabolism* **75**: 947–950.

Hashimoto, K., Azuma, C., Koyama, M., Ohashi, K., Kamiura, S., Nobunaga, T., Kimura, T., Tokugawa, Y., Kanai, T. and Saji, F. (1995) Loss of imprinting in choriocarcinoma. *Nature Genetics* **9**: 109–110.

Haurum, J.S., Arsequell, G., Lellouch, A.C., Wong, S.Y.C., Dwek, R.A., McMichael, A.J. and Elliott, T. (1994) Recognition of carbohydrate by major histocompatibility complex class I-restricted, glycopeptide-specific cytotoxic T lymphocytes. *Journal of Experimental Medicine* **180**: 739–744.

Havran, W.L. and Allison, J.P. (1990) Origin of Thy-1+ dendritic epidermal cells of adult mice from fetal thymic precursors. *Nature* **344**: 68–70.

Hawes, C.S., Suskin, H.A., Petropoulos, A., Latham, S.E. and Mueller, U.W. (1994) A morphologic study of trophoblast isolated from peripheral blood of pregnant women. *American Journal of Obstetrics and Gynecology* **170**: 1297–1300.

Hay, E.D. (1991) Collagen and other matrix glycoproteins in embryogenesis. In: *Cell Biology of Extracellular Matrix*, Ed. Hay, E.D., Plenum Press, New York, pp. 419–462.

Hayakawa, S., Saito, S., Nemoto, N., Chishima, F., Akiyama, K., Shiraishi, H., Hayakawa, J., Karasaki-Suzuki, M., Fujii, K.T., Ichijo, M., Sakurai, I. and Satoh, K. (1994) Expression of recombinase-activating genes (RAG-1 and 2) in human decidual mononuclear cells. *Journal of Immunology* **153**: 4934–4939.

Haynes, M.K., Jackson, L.G., Tuan, R.S., Shepley, K.J. and Smith, B.J. (1993) Cytokine production in first trimester chorionic villi: detection of mRNAs and protein products *in situ*. *Cellular Immunology* **151**: 300–308.

Hedrick, S.M. (1992) Dawn of the hunt for nonclassical MHC function. *Cell* **70**: 177–180.

Hellman, A. and Fowler, A.K. (1971) Hormone-activated expression of the C-type RNA tumour virus genome. *Nature* **233**: 142–144.

Hellman, A., Weislow, O.S., Twardzik, D.R. and Fowler, A.K. (1979) Type C retrovirus activation and possible functions in the normal and tumour-bearing host. *Cancer Research* **39**: 2902–2907.

Hemler, M.E. (1991) Structures and functions of VLA proteins and related integrins. In: *Receptors for Extracellular Matrix*, Eds. McDonald, J.A. and Mecham, R.P., Academic Press, San Diego, pp. 256–287.

Henkart, P.A. and Sitkovsky, M.V. (1994) Two ways to kill target cells. *Current Biology* **4**: 923–925.

Herzenberg, L.A., Kantor, A.B. and Herzenberg, L.A. (1992) Layered evolution in the immune system: a model for the ontogeny and development of multiple lymphocyte lineages. *Annals of the New York Academy of Sciences* **651**: 1–9.

Hey, N.A., Graham, R.A., Seif, M.W. and Aplin, J.D. (1994) The polymorphic epithelial mucin MUC1 in human endometrium is hormonally regulated with maximal expression in the implantation phase. *Journal of Clinical Endocrinology and Metabolism* **78**: 337–342.

Heyborne, K.D., Cranfill, R.L., Carding, S.R., Born, W.K. and O'Brien, R.L. (1992) Characterization of γδ T lymphocytes at the maternal-fetal interface. *Journal of Immunology* **149**: 2872–2878.

Heyborne, K., Fu, Y.-X., Nelson, A., Farr, A., O'Brien, R. and Born, W. (1994) Recognition of trophoblasts by γδ T cells. *Journal of Immunology* **153**: 2918–2926.

Higuchi, M. and Aggarwal, B.B. (1994) Differential role of two types of the TNF receptor in TNF-induced cytotoxicity, DNA fragmentation, and differentiation. *Journal of Immunology* **152**: 4017–4025.

Hill, J.A. (1990) Immunological mechanisms of pregnancy maintenance and failure: a critique of theories and therapy. *American Journal of Reproductive Immunology* **22**: 33–41.

Hilton, D.J. (1992) LIF: lots of interesting functions. *TIBS* **17**: 72–76.

Hirsch, M.S., Kelly, G.P., Chapin, D.S., Fuller, T.C. and Black, P.H. (1978) Immunity to antigens associated with primate C-type oncoviruses in pregnant women. *Science* **199**: 1337–1340.

Hofmann, G.E., Scott, R.T., Bergh, P.A. and Deligdisch, L. (1991) Immunohistochemical localization of epidermal growth factor in human endometrium, decidua and placenta. *Journal of Clinical Endocrinology and Metabolism* **6**: 107–114.

Hofmann, G.E., Drews, M.R., Scott, R.T., Navot, D., Heller, D. and Deligdisch, L. (1992) Epidermal growth factor and its receptor in human implantation trophoblast: immunohistochemical evidence for autocrine/paracrine function. *Journal of Clinical Endocrinology and Metabolism* **74**: 981–988.

Hofmann, G.E., Glatstein, I., Schatz, F., Heller, D. and Deligdisch, L. (1994) Immunohistochemical localization of urokinase-type plasminogen activator and the plasminogen activator inhibitors 1 and 2 in early human implantation sites. *American Journal of Obstetrics and Gynecology* **170**: 671–676.

Holmes, C.H., Simpson, K.L., Okada, H., Okada, N., Wainwright, S.D., Purcell, D.F.J. and Houlihan, J.M. (1992) Complement regulatory proteins at the feto-maternal interface during human placental development: distribution of CD59 by comparison with membrane cofactor protein (CD46) and decay accelerating factor (CD55). *European Journal of Immunology* **22**: 1579–1585.

Holmes, W.E., Sliwkowski, M.X., Akita, R.S., Henzel, W.J., Lee, J., Park, J.W., Yansura, D., Abadi, N., Raab, H., Lewis, G.D., Shepard, H.M., Kuang, W.-J., Wood, W.I., Goeddel, D.V. and Vandlen, R.L. (1992) Identification of heregulin, a specific activator of p185^{erbB2}. *Science* **256**: 1205–1210.

Holmgren, L., Flam, F., Larsson, E. and Ohlsson, R. (1993) Successive activation of the platelet–derived growth factor β receptor and the platelet-derived growth factor B genes correlates with the genesis of human choriocarcinoma. *Cancer Research* **53**: 2927–2931.

Horie, K., Fujita, J., Takakura, K., Kanzaki, H., Kaneko, Y., Iwai, M., Nakayama, H. and Mori, T. (1992) Expression of c-*kit* during placental development. *Biology of Reproduction* **47**: 614–620.

Horie, K., Fujita, J., Kanzaki, H., Suginami, H., Iwai, M., Nakayama, H. and Mori, T. (1993) The expression of c-*kit* protein in human adult and fetal tissues. *Human Reproduction* **8**: 1955–1962.

Horowitz, G.M., Scott, R.T., Drews, M.R., Navot, D. and Hofmann, G.E. (1993) Immunohistochemical localization of transforming growth factor-alpha in human endometrium, decidua, and trophoblast. *Journal of Clinical Endocrinology and Metabolism* **76**: 786–792.

Horuzsko, A., Tomlinson, P.D., Strachan, T. and Mellor, A.L. (1994) Transcription of HLA-G transgenes commences shortly after implantation during embryonic development in mice. *Immunology* **83**: 324–328.

Hoshina, M., Boothby, M. and Boime, I. (1982) Cytological localization of chorionic gonadotropin α and placental lactogen mRNAs during development of the human placenta. *Journal of Cell Biology* **93**: 190–198.

Houck, K.A., Ferrara, N., Winer, J., Cachianes, G., Li, B. and Leung, D.W. (1991) The vascular endothelial growth factor family: identification of a fourth molecular species and characterization of alternative splicing of RNA. *Molecular Endocrinology* **5**: 1806–1814.

Houlihan, J.M., Biro, P.A., Fergar-Payne, A., Simpson, K.L. and Holmes, C.H. (1992) Evidence for the expression of non-HLA-A,-B,-C class I genes in the human fetal liver. *Journal of Immunology* **149**: 668–675.

Howatson, A.G., Farquharson, M., Meager, A., McNicol, A.M. and Foulis, A.K. (1988) Localization of α-interferon in the human feto-placental unit. *Journal of Endocrinology* **119**: 531–534.

Howcroft, T.K., Strebel, K., Martin, M.A. and Singer, D.S. (1993) Repression of MHC class I gene promoter activity by two-exon Tat of HIV. *Science* **260**: 1320–1322.

Hsi, B.-L., Hunt, J.S. and Atkinson, J.P. (1991) Differential expression of complement regulatory protein on subpopulations of human trophoblast cells. *Journal of Reproductive Immunology* **19**: 209–223.

Hu, X.-L., Yang, Y. and Hunt, J.S. (1992) Differential distribution of interleukin-α and interleukin-1β proteins in human placentas. *Journal of Reproductive Immunology* **22**: 257–268.

Huang, A.Y.C., Golumbek, P., Ahmadzadeh, M., Jaffee, E., Pardoll, D. and Levitsky, H. (1994) Role of bone marrow-derived cells in presenting MHC class I-restricted tumor antigens. *Science* **264**: 961–964.

Huang, J.R., Tseng, L., Bischof, P. and Janne, O.A. (1987) Regulation of prolactin production by progestin, estrogen and relaxin in human endometrial stromal cells. *Endocrinology* **121**: 2011–2017.

Hummell, D.S., Dooley, J.S., Khan, A.S. and Lawton, A.R. (1993) Coordinate transcriptional control of murine endogenous retrovirus and Ig genes during B cell differentiation. *Journal of Immunology* **151**: 3131–3139.

Humphreys, T. and Reinherz, E.L. (1994) Invertebrate immune recognition, natural immunity and the evolution of positive selection. *Immunology Today* **15**: 316–320.

Humphries, M.J., Mould, A.P. and Yamada, K.M. (1991) Matrix receptors in cell migration. In: *Receptors for Extracellular Matrix*, Eds. McDonald, J.A. and Mecham, R.P., Academic Press, San Diego, pp. 195–236.

Hunt, J.S. (1989) Cytokine networks in the uteroplacental unit: macrophages as pivotal regulatory cells. *Journal of Reproductive Immunology* **16**: 1–17.

Hunt, J.S., Fishback, J.L., Chumbley, G. and Loke, Y.W. (1990) Identification of class I MHC mRNA in human first trimester trophoblast cells by in-situ hybridisation. *Journal of Immunology* **144**: 4420–4425.

Husmann, M., Pietsch, T., Fleischer, B., Weisgerber, C. and Bitter-Suermann, D. (1989) Embryonic neural cell adhesion molecules on human natural killer cells. *European Journal of Immunology* **19**: 1761–1763.

Hustin, J. (1992) The maternotrophoblastic interface: uteroplacental blood flow. In: *The First Twelve Weeks of Gestation*, Eds. Barnea, E.R., Hustin J., and Jauniaux, E., Springer-Verlag, Berlin, pp. 97–110.

Hustin, J., Jauniaux, E. and Schaaps, J.P. (1990) Histological study of the materno-embryonic interface in spontaneous abortion. *Placenta* **11**: 477–486.

Hynes, R.O. (1992) Integrins – versatility, modulation, and signaling in cell adhesion. *Cell* **69**: 11–25.

Hynes, R.O. (1994) The impact of molecular biology on models for cell adhesion. *BioEssays* **16**: 663–669.

Hynes, R.O. and Lander, A.D. (1992) Contact and adhesive specificities in the associations, migrations, and targeting of cells and axons. *Cell* **68**: 303–322.

Ikuta, K., Kina, T., MacNeil, I., Uchida, N., Peault, B., Chien, Y.-H. and Weissman, I.L. (1990) A developmental switch in thymic lymphocyte maturation potential occurs at the level of hematopoietic stem cells. *Cell* **62**: 863–874.

Imamura, M., Phillips, P.E. and Mellors, R.C. (1976) The occurrence and frequency of type C virus-like particles in placentas from patients with systemic lupus erythematosus and from normal subjects. *American Journal of Pathology* **83**: 383–389.

Inoue, M., Sasagawa, T., Saito, J., Shimizu, H., Ueda, G., Tanizawa, O. and Nakayama, M. (1987) Expression of blood group antigens A, B, H, Lewis-a, and Lewis-b in fetal, normal and malignant tissues of the uterine endometrium. *Cancer* **60**: 2985–2993.

Inoue, M., Nakayama, M. and Tanizawa, O. (1990) Altered expression of Lewis blood group and related antigens in fetal, normal adult and malignant tissues of the uterine endometrium. *Virchows Archiv A: Pathological Anatomy and Histopathology* **416**: 221–228.

Irwin, J.C., Kirk, D., King, R.J.B., Quigley, M.M. and Gwatkin, R.B.L. (1989) Hormonal regulation of human endometrial stromal cells in culture: an *in vitro* model for decidualisation. *Fertility and Sterility* **52**: 761–768.

Irwin, J.C., Utian, W.H. and Eckert, R.L. (1991) Sex steroids and growth factors differentially regulate the growth and differentiation of cultured human endometrial stromal cells. *Endocrinology* **129**: 2385–2392.

Ishii, N., Takeshita, T., Kimura, Y., Tada, K., Kondo, M., Nakamura, M. and Sugamura, K. (1994) Expression of the IL-2 receptor γ-chain on various populations in human peripheral blood. *International Immunology* **6**: 1273–1277.

Ishimara, T. (1971) A study of synthesis and secretion of HCG in trophoblastic culture. *Acta Obstetrica et Gynaecologica Japonica* **18**: 172–180.

Ishitani, A. and Geraghty, D.E. (1992) Alternative splicing of HLA-G transcripts yields proteins with primary structures resembling both class I and class II antigens. *Proceedings of the National Academy of Sciences USA* **89**: 1–5.

Jaattela, M., Kuusela, P. and Saksela, E. (1988) Demonstration of tumor necrosis factor in human amniotic fluids and supernatants of placental and decidual tissues. *Laboratory Investigation* **58**: 48–52.

Jalall, G.R., Underwood, J.L. and Mowbray, J.F. (1989) IgG on normal human placenta is bound both to antigen and Fc receptors. *Transplantation Proceedings* **21**: 572–574.

Janeway, C.A. (1992) The immune system evolved to discriminate infectious nonself from noninfectious self. *Immunology Today* **13**: 11–16.

Jasonni, V.M., Bulletti, C., Balducci, M., Naldi, S., Martinelli, G., Galassi, A. and Flamigni, C. (1991) The effect of progestin on factors influencing growth and invasion of endometrial carcinoma. *Annals of the New York Academy of Sciences* **622**: 463–468.

Jerabek, L.B., Mellors, R.C., Elkon, K.B. and Mellors, J.W. (1984) Detection and immunochemical characterization of a primate type C retrovirus-related p30 protein in normal human placentas. *Proceedings of the National Academy of Sciences USA* **81**: 6501–6505.

Jikihara, H. and Handwerger, S. (1994) Tumor necrosis factor-alpha inhibits the synthesis and release of human decidual prolactin. *Endocrinology* **134**: 353–357.

Jinno, Y., Yun, K., Nishikawa, K., Kubota, T., Ogawa, O., Reeve, A.E. and Niikawa, N. (1994) Mosaic and polymorphic imprinting of the WT1 gene in humans. *Nature Genetics* **6**: 305–309.

Johnson, P.M. and Bulmer, J.N. (1984) Uterine gland epithelium in human pregnancy often does not express detectable maternal MHC antigens but does express fetal trophoblast antigens. *Journal of Immunology* **132**: 1608–1610.

Johnson, P.M., Lyden, T.W. and Mwenda, J.M. (1990) Endogenous retroviral expression in the human placenta. *American Journal of Reproductive Immunology* **23**: 115–120.

Jokhi, P.P. (1994) Cytokines and their receptors in human placental implantation. PhD thesis, University of Cambridge.

Jokhi, P.P., Chumbley, G., Gardner, L., King, A. and Loke, Y.W. (1993) Expression of the colony stimulating factor-1 receptor (c-*fms* product) by cells at the human uteroplacental interface. *Laboratory Investigation* **68**: 308–320.

Jokhi, P.P., King, A. and Loke, Y.W. (1994a) Reciprocal expression of epidermal growth factor receptor (EGF-R) and c-*erb*B2 by non-invasive and invasive human trophoblast populations. *Cytokine* **6**: 433–442.

Jokhi, P.P., King, A., Jubinsky, P. and Loke, Y.W. (1994b) Demonstration of the low affinity α-subunit of the granulocyte-macrophage colony-stimulating factor receptor (GM-CSF-Rα) on human trophoblast and uterine cells. *Journal of Reproductive Immunology* **26**: 147–164.

Jokhi, P.P., King, A., Sharkey, A.M., Smith, S.K. and Loke, Y.W. (1994c) Production of GM-CSF by human trophoblast cells and by decidual large granular lymphocytes. *Human Reproduction* **9**: 1660–1669.

Jokhi, P.P., King, A., Sharkey, A.M., Smith, S.K. and Loke, Y.W. (1994d) Screening for cytokine mRNAs in purified human decidual lymphocyte populations by the reverse-transcriptase polymerase chain reaction (RT-PCR). *Journal of Immunology* **153**: 4427–4435.

Jones, J.I., Gockerman, A., Busby, W.H., Wright, G. and Clemmons, D.R. (1993) Insulin-like growth factor binding protein 1 stimulates cell migration and binds to the $\alpha_5\beta_1$ integrin by means of its arg-gly-asp sequence. *Proceedings of the National Academy of Sciences USA* **90**: 10553–10557.

Joyce, S., Tabaczewski, P., Angeletti, R.H., Nathenson, S.G. and Stroynowski, I. (1994) A nonpolymorphic major histocompatibility complex class Ib molecule binds a large array of diverse self-peptides. *Journal of Experimental Medicine* **179**: 579–588.

Juliano, R.L. and Haskill, S. (1993) Signal transduction from extracellular matrix. *Journal of Cell Biology* **120**: 577–585.

Jung, L.K.L., Haynes, B.F., Nakamura, S., Pahwas, S. and Fu, S.M. (1990) Expression of early activation antigen (CD69) during human thymic development. *Clinical and Experimental Immunology* **81**: 466–474.

Kacinski, B.M., Carter, D., Mittal, K., Yee, D.L., Scata, K.A., Donfrio, L., Chambers, S.K., Wang, K.-I., Yang-Feng, T., Rohrschneider, L.R. and Rothwell, V.M. (1990) Ovarian adenocarcinomas express *fms*-complementary transcripts and *fms* antigen, often with co–expression of CSF-1. *American Journal of Pathology* **137**: 135–147.

Kägi, D., Ledermann, B., Bürki, K., Seiler, P., Odermatt, B., Olsen, K.J., Podack, E.R., Zinkernagel, R.M. and Hengartner, H. (1994) Cytotoxicity mediated by T cells and natural killer cells is greatly impaired in perforin-deficient mice. *Nature* **369**: 31–37.

Kaiserman-Abramof, I.R. and Padykula, H.A. (1989) Angiogenesis in the postovulatory primate endometrium: the coiled arteriolar system. *Anatomical Record* **224**: 479–489.

Kajino, T., McIntyre, J.A., Faulk, W.P., Deng, S.C. and Billington, W.D. (1988) Antibodies to trophoblast in normal pregnant and secondary aborting women. *Journal of Reproductive Immunology* **14**: 267–282.

Kallapur, S.G. and Akeson, R.A. (1992) The neural cell adhesion molecule (NCAM) heparin binding domain binds to cell surface heparan sulfate proteoglycans. *Journal of Neuroscience Research* **33**: 538–548.

Kalter, S.S. (1983) Viral expression in the trophoblast. In: *Biology of Trophoblast*, Eds. Loke, Y.W. and Whyte, A., Elsevier, Amsterdam, pp. 627–662.

Kalter, S.S., Helmke, R.J., Heberling, R.L., Panigel, M., Fowler, A.K., Strickland, J.E. and Hellman, A.J. (1973) C-type particles in normal human placentas. *Journal of the National Cancer Institute* **50**: 1081–1083.

Kalter, S.S., Heberling, R.L., Smith, G.C. and Helmke, R.J. (1975) C-type viruses in chimpanzee (*Pan* sp.) placentas. *Journal of the National Cancer Institute* **55**: 735–736.

Kämäräinen, M., Riittinen, L., Seppälä, M., Palotie, A. and Andersson, L.C. (1994) Progesterone-associated endometrial protein: a constitutive marker of human erythroid precursors. *Blood* **84**: 467–473.

Kamat, B.R. and Isaacson, P.G. (1987) The immunocytochemical distribution of leukocytic subpopulations in human endometrium. *American Journal of Pathology* **127**: 66–73.

Kameda, T., Matsuzaki, N., Sawai, K., Okada, T., Saji, F., Matsuda, T., Hirano, T., Kishimoto, T. and Tanizawa, O. (1990) Production of interleukin-6 by normal human trophoblast. *Placenta* **11**: 205–217.

Kanbour-Shakir, A., Kunz, H.W. and Gill, T.J. (1993) Differential genomic imprinting of major histocompatibility complex class I antigens in the placenta of the rat. *Biology of Reproduction* **48**: 977–986.

Kanzaki, H., Yui, J., Iwai, M., Imai, K., Kariya, M., Hatayama, H., Mori, T., Guilbert, L.J. and Wegmann, T.G. (1992) The expression and localization of mRNA for colony-stimulating factor (CSF)-1 in human term placenta. *Human Reproduction* **7**: 563–567.

Kariya, M., Kanzaki, H., Hanamura, T., Imai, K., Narukawa, S., Inoue, T., Hatayama, H. and Mori, T. (1994) Progesterone-dependent secretion of macrophage colony-stimulating factor by human endometrial stromal cells of non-pregnant uterus in culture. *Journal of Clinical Endocrinology and Metabolism* **79**: 86–90.

Karlhofer, F.M., Ribando, R.K. and Yokoyama, W.M. (1992) MHC class I alloantigen specificity of Ly-49$^+$ IL-2-activated natural killer cells. *Nature* **358**: 66–70.

Karlhofer, F.M., Hunziker, R., Reichlin, A., Margulies, D.H. and Yokoyama, W.M. (1994) Host MHC class I molecules modulate *in vivo* expression of a NK cell receptor. *Journal of Immunology* **153**: 2407–2416.

Kärre, K. (1993) Natural killer cells and the MHC class I pathway of peptide presentation. *Seminars in Immunology* **5**: 127–145.

Kärre, K. (1995) Express yourself or die: peptides, MHC molecules, and NK cells. *Science* **267**: 978–979.

Kastelein, R.A. and Shanafelt, A.B. (1993) GM-CSF receptor: interactions and activation. *Oncogene* **8**: 231–236.

Kastner, P., Krust, A., Turcotte, B., Stropp, U., Tora, L., Gronemeyer, H. and Chambon, P. (1990) Two distinct estrogen-regulated promoters generate transcripts encoding the two functionally different human progesterone receptor forms A and B. *EMBO Journal* **9**: 1603–1614.

Kato, N., Pfeifer-Ohlsson, S., Kato, M., Larsson, E., Rydnert, J., Ohlsson, R. and Cohen, M. (1987) Tissue-specific expression of human provirus ERV3 mRNA in human placenta: two of the three ERV3 mRNAs contain human cellular sequences. *Journal of Virology* **61**: 2182–2191.

Kato, N., Larsson, E. and Cohen, M. (1988) Absence of expression of a human endogenous retrovirus is correlated with choriocarcinoma. *International Journal of Cancer* **41**: 380–385.

Kaufman, D.S., Schoon, R.A. and Leibson, P.J. (1993) MHC class I expression on tumor targets inhibits natural killer cell-mediated cytotoxicity without interfering with target recognition. *Journal of Immunology* **150**: 1429–1436.

Kaufmann, P. and Burton, G. (1994) Anatomy and genesis of the placenta. In: *Physiology of Reproduction*, 2nd edition, Eds. Knobil, E. and Neill, J.D., Raven Press, New York, pp. 441–483.

Kauma, S.W., Aukerman, S.L., Eierman, D. and Turner, T. (1991) Colony-stimulating factor-1 and c-*fms* expression in human endometrial tissues and placenta during the menstrual cycle and early pregnancy. *Journal of Clinical Endocrinology and Metabolism* **73**: 746–751.

Kauma, S.W., Herman, K., Wang, Y. and Walsh, S.W. (1993) Differential mRNA expression and production of interleukin-6 in placental trophoblast and villous core compartments. *American Journal of Reproductive Immunology* **30**: 131–135.

Kazzaz, B.A. (1972) Specific endometrial granular cells: a semiquantitative study. *European Journal of Obstetrics and Gynecology* **3**: 77–84.

Kelly, P.A., Dijiane, J., Postel-Vinay, M.C. and Edery, M. (1991) The prolactin/growth hormone receptor family. *Endocrinology Review* **12**: 235–251.

Kenton, P. and Johnson, P.M. (1994) Growth factor-induced release of placental alkaline phosphatase from human syncytiotrophoblast membranes. *Journal of Reproduction and Fertility* **100**: 71–76.

Khong, T.Y., De Wolf, F., Robertson, W.B. and Brosens, I. (1986) Inadequate maternal vascular response to placentation in pregnancies complicated by pre-eclampsia and by small-for-gestational age infants. *British Journal of Obstetrics and Gynaecology* **93**: 1049–1059.

Khong, T.Y., Liddell, H.S. and Robertson, W.B. (1987) Defective haemochorial placentation as a cause of miscarriage: a preliminary study. *British Journal of Obstetrics and Gynaecology* **94**: 649–655.

Kim, L.T. and Grinnell, F. (1990) Activation of keratinocytes during wound healing (abstract). *Journal of Cell Biology* **111**: 149a.

Kim, M., Duty, L., Herberman, R. and Gorelik, E. (1994) Divergent effects of H-2K and H-2D genes on sensitivity of BL6 melanoma cells to NK cells or TNF-mediated cytotoxicity. *Cellular Immunology* **155**: 358–371.

King, A. and Loke, Y.W. (1988) Differential expression of blood group related carbohydrate antigens by trophoblast subpopulations. *Placenta* **9**: 513–521.

King, A. and Loke, Y.W. (1990) Human trophoblast and JEG choriocarcinoma cells are sensitive to lysis by IL-2 stimulated decidual NK cells. *Cellular Immunology* **129**: 435–448.

King, A. and Loke, Y.W. (1991) On the nature and function of human uterine granular lymphocytes. *Immunology Today* **12**: 432–435.

King, A. and Loke, Y.W. (1993) Effect of IFN-γ and IFN-α on killing of human trophoblast by decidual LAK cells. *Journal of Reproductive Immunology* **23**: 51–62.

King, A. and Loke, Y.W. (1994) Unexplained fetal growth retardation: what is the cause? *Archives of Disease in Childhood* **70**: F225–F227.

King, A., Birkby, C. and Loke, Y.W. (1989a) Early human decidual cells exhibit NK activity against K562 cell line but not against first trimester trophoblast. *Cellular Immunology* **118**: 337–344.

King, A., Wellings, V., Gardner, L. and Loke, Y.W. (1989b) Immunocytochemical characterisation of the unusual large granular lymphocytes in human endometrium throughout the menstrual cycle. *Human Immunology* **24**: 195–205.

King, A., Balendran, N., Wooding, P., Carter, N.P. and Loke, Y.W. (1991) CD3⁻ leukocytes present in the human uterus during early placentation: phenotypic and morphologic characterization of the CD56⁺⁺ population. *Developmental Immunology* **1**: 169–190.

King, A., Wheeler, R., Carter, N.P., Francis, D.P. and Loke, Y.W. (1992) The response of human decidual leukocytes to IL-2. *Cellular Immunology* **140**: 409–421.

King, A., Wooding, P., Gardner, L. and Loke, Y.W. (1993) Expression of perforin, granzyme A and TIA-1 by human uterine CD56⁺ cells implies they are activated and capable of effector functions. *Human Reproduction* **8**: 2061–2067.

King, A., Jokhi, P.P., Smith, S., Sharkey, A. and Loke, Y.W. (1995) Screening for cytokine mRNA expression in purified human villous and extravillous trophoblast populations using the reverse-transcriptase polymerase chain reaction (RT-PCR). *Cytokine* **7**: 364–371.

Kirby, D.R.S. (1960) Development of mouse eggs beneath the kidney capsule. *Nature* **187**: 707–708.

Kirby, D.R.S. (1970) The extra-uterine mouse egg as an experimental model. *Advances in the Biosciences* **4**: 255–273.

Kirk, D. and Irwin, J.C. (1980) Normal human endometrium in cell culture. *Methods in Cell Biology* **21B**: 51–77.

Kirszenbaum, M., Moreau, P., Gluckman, E., Dausset, J. and Carosella, E. (1994) An alternatively spliced form of HLA-G mRNA in human trophoblasts and evidence for the presence of HLA-G transcript in adult lymphocytes. *Proceedings of the National Academy of Sciences USA* **91**: 4209–4213.

Kishimoto, T., Taga, T. and Akira, S. (1994) Cytokine signal transduction. *Cell* **76**: 253–262.

Kiso, Y., McBey, B.-A., Mason, L. and Croy, B.A. (1992) Histological assessment of the mouse uterus from birth to puberty for the appearance of LGL-1⁺ natural killer cells. *Biology of Reproduction* **47**: 227–232.

Klagsbrun, M. and D'Amore, P.A. (1991) Regulators of angiogenesis. *Annual Review of Physiology* **53**: 217–239.

Klein, J. (1991) Of HLA, tryps and selection: an essay on coevolution of MHC and parasites. *Human Immunology* **30**: 247–258.

Klein, J. and O'hUigin, C. (1994) The conundrum of nonclassical major histocompatibility complex genes. *Proceedings of the National Academy of Sciences USA* **91**: 6251–6252.

Kleiner, D.E. and Stetler-Stevenson, W.G. (1993) Structural biochemistry and activation of matrix metalloproteinases. *Current Opinion in Cell Biology* **5**: 891–897.

Kleinman, H.K. and Weeks, B.S. (1989) Laminin: structure, functions and receptors. *Current Opinion in Cell Biology* **1**: 964–967.

Klentzeris, L.D., Bulmer, J.N., Warren, M.A., Morrison, L., Li, T.C. and Cooke, I.D. (1992) Endometrial lymphoid tissue in the timed endometrial biopsy: morphometric and immunohistochemical aspects. *American Journal of Obstetrics and Gynecology* **167**: 667–674.

Klentzeris, L.D., Bulmer, J.N., Warren, M.A., Morrison, L., Li, T.C. and Cooke, I.D. (1994) Lymphoid tissue in the endometrium of women with unexplained infertility: morphometric and immunohistochemical aspects. *Human Reproduction* **9**: 646–652.

Kliman, H.J. (1994) Trophoblast infiltration. *Reproductive Medicine Review* **3**: 137–157.

Kliman, H.J., Nestler, J.E., Sermasi, E., Sanger, J.M. and Strauss, J.F. (1986) Purification, characterisation and *in vitro* differentiation of cytotrophoblasts from human term placentae. *Endocrinology* **118**: 1567–1582.

Kliman, H.J., Feinberg, R.F. and Haimowitz, J.E. (1990) Interactions between human term trophoblasts and endometrium *in vitro*. In: *Placental Communications: Biochemical, Morphological and Cellular Aspects*, Eds. Cedard, L., Alst, E., Challier J.-C., Chaouat, G. and Malassiné, A., Colloque INSERM/John Libbey Eurotext Ltd, **199**, pp. 3–9.

Klingemann, H.-G. and Fred, R.K. (1991) Involvement of fibronectin and its receptor in human lymphocyte proliferation. *Journal of Leukocyte Biology* **50**: 464–470.

Knapp, L.W., O'Guin, W.M. and Sawyer, R.H. (1983) Drug-induced alterations of cytokeratin organization in cultured epithelial cells. *Science* **219**: 501–503.

Koller, B.H., Sidwell, B., DeMars, R. and Orr, H.T. (1984) Isolation of HLA locus-specific DNA probes from the 3′-untranslated region. *Proceedings of the National Academy of Sciences USA* **81**: 5175–5178.

Korhonen, M., Ylänne, J., Laitinen, L., Cooper, H.M., Quaranta, V. and Virtanen, I. (1991) Distribution of α_1–α_6 integrin subunits in human developing and term placenta. *Laboratory Investigation* **65**: 347–356.

Kornberg, L.J., Earp, H.S., Turner, C.E., Prockop, C. and Juliano, R.L. (1991) Signal transduction by integrins: increased protein tyrosine phosphorylation caused by clustering of β_1 integrins. *Proceedings of the National Academy of Sciences USA* **88**: 8392–8396.

Kornfeld, S. (1992) Structure and function of the mannose 6-phosphate/insulin-like growth factor II receptors. *Annual Review of Biochemistry* **61**: 307–330.

Kovats, S., Main, E.K., Librach, C., Stubblebine, M., Fisher, S.J. and DeMars, R. (1990) A Class I antigen, HLA-G, expressed in human trophoblasts. *Science* **248**: 220–223.

Kreipe, H., Feist, H., Fischer, L., Felgner, J., Heidorn, K., Mettler, L. and Parwaresch, R. (1993) Amplification of c-*myc* but not of c-*erb*B2 is associated with high proliferative capacity in breast cancer. *Cancer Research* **53**: 1956–1961.

Kroemer, G., Cuende, E. and Martinez, C. (1993) Compartmentalization of the peripheral immune system. *Advances in Immunology* **53**: 157–216.

Krog, L. and Bock, E. (1992) Glycosylation of neural cell adhesion molecules of the immunoglobulin superfamily. *Acta Pathologica, Microbiologica et Immunologica Scandinavica* **100** (Suppl. 27): 53–70.

Kubota, Y., Kleinman, H.K., Martin, G.R. and Lawley, T.J. (1988) Role of laminin and basement membrane in the morphological differentiation of human endothelial cells into capillary-like structures. *Journal of Cell Biology* **107**: 1589–1598.

Kühn, K. and Eble, J. (1994) The structural basis of integrin-ligand interactions. *Trends in Cell Biology* **4**: 256–261.

Kung, H.-J., Boerkoel, C. and Carter, T.H. (1991) Retroviral mutagenesis of cellular oncogenes: a review with insights into the mechanisms of insertional activation. In: *Retroviral Insertion and Oncogene Activation*, Eds. Kung, H.-J. and Voght, P.K., Current Topics in Microbiology and Immunology, Springer-Verlag, Berlin, pp.1–25.

Laffón, A., Garcia-Vicuna, R., Humbria, A., Postigo, A.A., Corbi, A.L., de Landazuri, M.O. and Sanchez-Madrid, F. (1991) Upregulated expression and function of VLA-4 fibronectin receptors on human activated T cells in rheumatoid arthritis. *Journal of Clinical Investigation* **88**: 546–552.

Lam, K.-P. and Stall, A.M. (1994) Major histocompatibility complex class II expression distinguishes two distinct B cell developmental pathways during ontogeny. *Journal of Experimental Medicine* **180**: 507–516.

Lanier, L.L. and Phillips, J.H. (1992) Natural killer cells. *Current Opinion in Immunology* **4**: 38–42.

Lanier, L.L., Le, A.M., Civin, C.I., Loken, M.R. and Phillips, J.H. (1986) The relationship of CD16 (Leu-11) and Leu-19 (NKH-1) antigen expression on human peripheral blood NK cells and cytotoxic T lymphocytes. *Journal of Immunology* **136**: 4480–4486.

Lanier, L.L., Testi, R., Bindl, J. and Phillips, J.H. (1989) Identity of Leu-19 (CD56) leukocyte differentiation antigen and neural cell adhesion molecule. *Journal of Experimental Medicine* **169**: 2233–2238.

Lanier, L.L., Chang, C., Spits, H. and Phillips, J.H. (1992a) Expression of cytoplasmic CD3ε proteins in activated human adult natural killer (NK) cells and CD3γ,δ,ε complexes in fetal NK cells. *Journal of Immunology* **149**: 1876–1880.

Lanier, L.L., Spits, H. and Phillips, J.H. (1992b) The developmental relationship between NK cells and T cells. *Immunology Today* **13**: 392–395.

Lanier, L.L., Chang, C. and Phillips, J.H. (1994) A disulfide-linked homodimer of the C-type lectin superfamily expressed by a subset of NK and T lymphocytes. *Journal of Immunology* **153**: 2417–2428.

Larsson, E., Kato, H. and Cohen, M. (1989) Human endogenous proviruses. *Current Topics in Microbiology and Immunology* **148**: 115–132.

Lasky, L.A. (1992) Selectins: interpreters of cell-specific carbohydrate information during inflammation. *Science* **258**: 964–969.

Lastres, P., Bellon, T., Cabanas, C., Sánchez-Madrid, F., Acevedo, A., Gougos, A., Letarte, M. and Bernabeu, C. (1992) Regulated expression on human macrophages of endoglin, an Arg-Gly-Asp-containing surface antigen. *European Journal of Immunology* **22**: 393–397.

Lawler, S.D. and Fisher, R.A. (1993) The contribution of the paternal genome: hydatidiform mole and choriocarcinoma. In: *The Human Placenta*, Eds. Redman, C.W.G., Sargent, I.L. and Starkey, P.M., Blackwell Scientific, Oxford, pp. 82–112.

Lawler, S.D., Pickthall, V.J., Fisher, R.A., Povey, S., Evans, M.W. and Szulman, A.E. (1979) Genetic studies of complete and partial hydatidiform moles. *Lancet* ii: 580.

Laybourn, K.A., Hiserodt, J.C. and Varani, J. (1989) Laminin receptor expression on murine tumor cells: correlation with sensitivity to natural cell-mediated cytotoxicity. *International Journal of Cancer* **43**: 737–742.

Lebon, P., Girard, S., Thepot, F. and Chany, C. (1982) The presence of γ-interferon in human amniotic fluid. *Journal of General Virology* **59**: 393–396.

Le Bouteiller, P. (1994) HLA class I chromosomal region, genes, and products: facts and questions. *Critical Reviews in Immunology* **14**: 89–129.

Le Bouteiller, P., Boucrat, J., Fauchet, R. and Pontarotti, P. (1991) Transfected HLA class I genes in JAR human cell line escape the negative *cis*-regulatory control exerted on endogenous class I genes. In: *Cellular and Molecular Biology of the Materno-Fetal Relationship*, Eds. Chaouat, G. and Mowbray, J., Colloque INSERM, John Libbey Eurotext Ltd, **212**: pp. 41–49.

Lee, C.S., Meeusen, E., Gogolin-Ewens, K. and Brandon, M.R. (1992) Quantitative and qualitative changes in the intraepithelial lymphocyte population in the uterus of nonpregnant and pregnant sheep. *American Journal of Reproductive Immunology* **28**: 90–96.

Lee, M.-C. and Damjanov, I. (1985) Pregnancy-related changes in the human endometrium revealed by lectin histochemistry. *Histochemistry* **82**: 275–280.

Legan, P.K., Collins, J.E. and Garrod, D.R. (1992) The molecular biology of desmosomes and hemidesmosomes: *'What's in a name?'* *BioEssays* **14**: 385–393.

LeRoith, D. (ed.) (1991) *Insulin-like Growth Factors: Molecular and Cellular Aspects*, CRC Press, Boca Raton.

Lessey, B.A. (1994) The use of integrins for the assessment of uterine receptivity. *Fertility and Sterility* **61**: 812–814.

Lessey, B.A., Killam, A.P., Metzger, D.A., Haney, A.F., Greene, G.L. and McCarty, K.S. (1988) Immunohistochemical analysis of human uterine estrogen and progesterone receptors throughout the menstrual cycle. *Journal of Clinical Endocrinology and Metabolism* **67**: 334–340.

Lessey, B.A., Damjanovich, L., Coutifaris, C., Castelbaum, A., Albelda, S.M. and Buck, C.A. (1992) Integrin adhesion molecules in the human endometrium. *Journal of Clinical Investigation* **90**: 188–195.

Lessey, B.A., Castelbaum, A.J., Buck, C.A., Lei, Y., Yowell, C.W. and Sun, J. (1994a) Further characterization of endometrial integrins during the menstrual cycle and in pregnancy. *Fertility and Sterility* **62**: 497–506.

Lessey, B.A., Castelbaum, A.J., Sawin, S.W., Buck, C.A., Schinnar, R., Bilker, W. and Strom, B.L. (1994b) Aberrant integrin expression in the endometrium of women with endometriosis. *Journal of Clinical Endocrinology and Metabolism* **79**: 643–649.

Levesque, J.-P., Hatzfeld, A. and Hatzfeld, J. (1991) Mitogenic properties of major extracellular proteins. *Immunology Today* **12**: 258–262.

Levitt, L.J., Nagler, A., Lee, F., Abrams, J., Shatsky, M. and Thompson, D. (1991) Production of granulocyte/macrophage colony-stimulating factor by human natural killer cells: modulation by the p75 subunit of interleukin 2 receptor and by the CD2 receptor. *Journal of Clinical Investigation* **88**: 67–75.

Li, T.-C., Dockery, P. and Cooke, I.D. (1991) Endometrial development in the luteal phase of women with various types of infertility: comparison with women of normal fertility. *Human Reproduction* **6**: 325–330.

Li, T.-C., Klentzeris, L., Barratt, C., Warren, M.A., Cooke, S. and Cooke, I.D. (1993) A study of endometrial morphology in women who failed to conceive in a donor insemination programme. *British Journal of Obstetrics and Gynaecology* **100**: 935–938.

Librach, C.L., Werb, Z., Fitzgerald, M.L., Chiu, K., Corwin, N.M., Esteves, R.A., Grobelny, D., Galardy, R., Damsky, C.H. and Fisher, S.J. (1991) 92-kD type-IV collagenase mediates invasion of human cytotrophoblasts. *Journal of Cell Biology* **113**: 437–449.

Lim, K.-H. and Friedman, S.A. (1993) Hypertension in pregnancy. *Current Opinion in Obstetrics and Gynecology* **5**: 40–49.

Lin, C.Q. and Bissell, M.J. (1993) Multifaceted regulation of cell differentiation by extracellular matrix. *FASEB Journal* **7**: 737–734.

Lin, P.Y., Joag, S.V., Young, J.D.-E., Ching, Y.-S., Soong, Y.-K., and Kuo, T.-T. (1991) Expression of perforin by natural killer cells within first trimester endometrium in humans. *Biology of Reproduction* **45**: 698–703.

Lindenbaum, E.S., Langer, N. and Beach, D. (1991) Isolation and culture of human decidual capillary endothelial cells in serum-free medium supplemented with human uterine angiogenic factor. *Acta Anatomica* **140**: 273–279.

Lindenberg, S., Kimber, S. and Hamberger, L. (1990) Embryo-endometrium interaction. In: *Ovulation to Implantation*, Eds. Evers, J.H.L. and Heineman, M.J., Elsevier Science Publishers BV (Biomedical Division), Amsterdam, pp. 285–295.

Linder, D., McCaw, B.K. and Hecht, F. (1975) Parthenogenetic origin of benign ovarian teratomas. *New England Journal of Medicine* **292**: 63–66.

Lindeskog, M., Medstrand, P. and Blomberg, J. (1993) Sequence variation of human endogenous retrovirus ERV9-related elements in an *env* region corresponding to an immunosuppressive peptide: transcription in normal and neoplastic cells. *Journal of Virology* **67**: 1122–1126.

Litwin, V., Gumperz, J., Parham, P., Phillips, J.H. and Lanier, L.L. (1993) Specificity of HLA class I antigen recognition by human NK clones: evidence for clonal heterogeneity, protection by self and non-self alleles, and influence of the target cell type. *Journal of Experimental Medicine* **178**: 1321–1336.

Litwin, V., Gumperz, J., Parham, P., Phillips, J.H. and Lanier, L.L. (1994) NKB1: A natural killer cell receptor involved in the recognition of polymorphic HLA-B molecules. *Journal of Experimental Medicine* **180**: 537–543.

Liu, C.-C., Parr, E.L. and Young, J.D-E. (1994) Granulated lymphoid cells of the pregnant uterus: morphological and functional features. *International Review of Cytology* **153**: 105–136.

Liu, H.C. and Tseng, L. (1979) Estradiol metabolism in isolated human endometrial epithelial glands and stromal cells. *Endocrinology* **104**: 1674–1681.

Ljunggren, H.-G. and Kärre, K. (1990) In search of the 'missing self': MHC molecules and NK cell recognition. *Immunology Today* **11**: 237–244.

Logan, S.K., Fisher, S.J. and Damsky, C.H. (1992) Human placental cells transformed with temperature-sensitive simian virus 40 are immortalised and mimic the phenotype of invasive cytotrophoblasts at both permissive and nonpermissive temperatures. *Cancer Research* **52**: 6001–6009.

Loke, Y.W. (1978) *Immunology and Immunopathology of the Human Foetal-Maternal Interaction*, Elsevier/North-Holland, Amsterdam.

Loke, Y.W. (1982) Transmission of parasites across the placenta. In: *Advances in Parasitology* 21, Eds. Lumsden, W.H.R., Baker, J.R. and Muller, R., Academic Press, London, pp. 155–228.

Loke, Y.W. (1983) Human trophoblast in culture. In: *Biology of Trophoblast*, Eds. Loke, Y.W. and Whyte, A., Elsevier/North-Holland, Amsterdam, pp. 663–701.

Loke, Y.W. (1988) Immunocytochemical characterisation of human trophoblast. In: *Placental Protein Hormones*, Eds. Mochizuki, M. and Hussa, R., Excerpta Medica, Elsevier Science Publishers, Amsterdam, pp. 19–31.

Loke, Y.W. (1990) New developments in human trophoblast cell culture. In: *Placental Communications: Biochemical, Morphological and Cellular Aspects*, Eds. Cedard, L., Alsat, E., Challier, J.-C., Chaouat, G. and Malassine, A., John Libbey Eurotext Ltd. **199**, pp. 10–16.

Loke, Y.W. and Burland, K. (1988) Human trophoblast cells cultured in modified medium and supported by extracellular matrix. *Placenta* **9**: 173–182.

Loke, Y.W. and Butterworth, B.H. (1987) Heterogeneity of human trophoblast populations. In: *Immunoregulation and Fetal Survival*, Eds. Gill, T.J. and Wegmann, T.G., Oxford University Press, New York, pp. 197–209.

Loke, Y.W. and Day, S. (1984) Monoclonal antibody to human cytotrophoblast. *American Journal of Reproductive Immunology* **5**: 106–108.

Loke, Y.W. and Hussa, R.O. (1987) Trophoblast cell culture. *Trophoblast Research* **2**: 461–464.

Loke, Y.W. and King, A. (1990) Interferon and human placental development. *Placenta* **11**: 291–299.

Loke, Y.W. and King, A. (1991) Recent developments in the human maternal-fetal immune interaction. *Current Opinion in Immunology* **3**: 762–766.

Loke, Y.W., Eremin, O., Ashby, J. and Day, S. (1982) Characterization of the phagocytic cells isolated from the human placenta. *Journal of the Reticuloendothelial Society* **31**: 317–324.

Loke, Y.W., Gardner, L. and Grabowska, A. (1989a) Isolation of human extravillous trophoblast cells by attachment to laminin-coated magnetic beads. *Placenta* **10**: 407–415.

Loke, Y.W., Gardner, L., Burland, K. and King, A. (1989b) Laminin in human trophoblast-decidua interaction. *Human Reproduction* **4**: 457–463.

Loke, Y.W., King, A., Gardner, L. and Carter, N.P. (1992a) Evidence for the expression of GM-CSF receptors by human first trimester extravillous trophoblast and its response to this cytokine. *Journal of Reproductive Immunology* **22**: 77–81.

Loke, Y.W., Hsi, B.-L., Bulmer, J.N., Grivaux, C., Hawley, S., Gardner, L., King, A. and Carter, N.P. (1992b) Evaluation of a monoclonal antibody, BC-1, which identifies an antigen expressed on the surface membrane of human extravillous trophoblast. *American Journal of Reproductive Immunology* **27**: 77–81.

Loke, Y.W., King, A. and Chumbley, G. (1993) Human trophoblast-uterine immunological interactions. In: *Proceedings of Serono Symposium. Trophoblast Cells: Pathways for Maternal Embryonic Communication*, Eds. Soares, M.J., Handwerger, S. and Talamantes, F., Springer-Verlag, Berlin, pp. 151–159.

Lopez, A.F., Elliott, M.J., Woodcock, J. and Vadas, M.A. (1992) GM-CSF, IL-3 and IL-5: cross-competition on human haematopoietic cells. *Immunology Today* **13**: 495–500.

López-Cabrera, M., Santis, A.G., Fernández-Ruiz, E., Blacher, R., Esch, F., Sánchez-Mateos, P. and Sánchez-Madrid, F. (1993) Molecular cloning, expression and chromosomal localization of the human earliest lymphocyte activation antigen AIM/CD69, a new member of the C-type animal lectin superfamily of signal-ransmitting receptors. *Journal of Experimental Medicine* **178**: 537–547.

López-Casallas, F., Cheifetz, S., Doody, J., Andres, J.L., Lane, W.S. and Massagué, J. (1991) Structure and function of the membrane proteoglycan betaglycan, a component of the TGF-β receptor system. *Cell* **67**: 785–795.

Lotz, M.M., Burdsal, C.A., Erickson, H.P. and McClay, D.R. (1989) Cell adhesion to fibronectin and tenascin: quantitative measurements of initial binding and subsequent strengthening response. *Journal of Cell Biology* **109**: 1795–1805.

Lower, R., Boller, K., Hasenmaier, B., Korbmacher, C., Muller-Lantzsch, N., Lower, J. and Kurth, R. (1993) Identification of human endogenous retroviruses with complex mRNA expression and particle formation. *Proceedings of the National Academy of Sciences USA* **90**: 4480–4484.

Lowin, B., Hahne, M., Mattmann, C. and Tschopp, J. (1994) Cytolytic T-cell cytotoxicity is mediated through perforin and Fas lytic pathways. *Nature* **370**: 650–652.

Lucas, A. (1991) Programming by early nutrition in man. In: *The Childhood Environment and Adult Disease*, Eds. Buck, G.R. and Whelan, J., Ciba Foundation Symposium 156, John Wiley, Chichester, pp. 38–55.

Lucas, A. and Morley, R. (1994) Does early nutrition in infants born before term programme later blood pressure? *British Medical Journal* **309**: 304–308.

Luger, T.A., Krutmann, J., Kirnbauer, R., Urbanski, A., Schwarz, T., Klappacher, G., Köck, A., Micksche, M., Malejczyk, J., Schauer, E., May, L.T. and Sehgal, P.B. (1989) IFN-β$_2$/IL-6 augments the activity of human natural killer cells. *Journal of Immunology* **143**: 1206–1209.

Lyden, T.W., Johnson, P.M., Mwenda, J.M. and Rote, N.S. (1994) Ultrastructural characterization of endogenous retroviral particles isolated from normal human placentas. *Biology of Reproduction* **51**: 152–157.

Lyon, M.F. (1993) Epigenetic inheritance in mammals. *Trends in Genetics* **9**: 123–128.

Lysiak, J.J., Han, V.K. and Lala, P.K. (1993) Localization of transforming growth factor alpha in the human placenta and decidua: role in trophoblast growth. *Biology of Reproduction* **49**: 885–894.

MacLaughlin, D.T., Santoro, N.F., Baner, H.H., Lawrence, D. and Richardson, G.S. (1986) Two-dimensional gel electrophoresis of endometrial proteins in human uterine fluids: qualitative and quantitative analysis. *Biology of Reproduction* **34**: 579–585.

Madri, J.A., Pratt, B.M. and Yannariello-Brown, J. (1988) Matrix-driven cell size change modulates aortic endothelial cell proliferation and sheet migration. *American Journal of Pathology* **132**: 18–27.

Maeda, S., Mellors, R.C., Mellors, J.W., Jerabek, L.B. and Zervoudakis, I.A. (1983) Immunohistologic detection of antigen related to primate type C retrovirus p30 in normal human placenta. *American Journal of Pathology* **112**: 347–356..

Mager, D.L. and Freeman, J.D. (1987) Human endogenous retrovirus like genome with type C *pol* sequence and *gag* sequence related to human T-cell lymphotropic viruses. *Journal of Virology* **61**: 4060–4066.

Main, E.K., Strizki, J. and Sochet, P. (1987) Placental production of immunoregulatory factors: trophoblast is a source of interleukin-1. In: *Trophoblast Research* Vol. 2, Eds. Miller, R.K. and Thiede, H.A., Plenum Press, New York, pp.149–160.

Malnati, M.S., Peruzzi, M., Parker, K.C., Biddison, W.E., Ciccone, E., Moretta, A. and Long, E.O. (1995) Peptide specificity in the recognition of MHC class I by natural killer cell clones. *Science* **267**: 1016–1018.

Manaseki, S. and Searle, R.F. (1989) Natural killer (NK) cell activity of first trimester human decidua. *Cellular Immunology* **121**: 166–173.

Marathias, K., Pinto, C., Rodberg, G., Preffer, F., Wong, J. and Kradin, R. (1994) The T cell antigen receptor CD3 : CD4 molecular complex is diminished on the surface of pulmonary lymphocytes. *American Journal of Pathology* **145**: 1219–1227.

Marsal, K. (1994) Role of Doppler sonography in fetal/maternal medicine. *Current Opinion in Obstetrics and Gynecology* **6**: 36–44.

Marshall, R.J. and Jones, D.B. (1988) An immunohistochemical study of lymphoid tissue in human endometrium. *International Journal of Gynecological Pathology* **7**: 225–235.

Martelli, M., Campana, A. and Bischof, P. (1993) Secretion of matrix metalloproteinases by human endometrial cells in vitro. *Journal of Reproduction and Fertility* **98**: 67–76.

Martin, O. and Arias, F. (1982) Plasminogen activator production by trophoblast cells *in vitro*: effect of steroid hormones and protein synthesis inhibitors. *American Journal of Obstetrics and Gynecology* **142**: 402–409.

Maruo, T. and Mochizuki, M. (1987) Immunohistochemical localization of epidermal growth factor receptor and *myc* oncogene product in human placenta: implication for trophoblast proliferation and differentiation. *American Journal of Obstetrics and Gynecology* **156**: 721–727.

Maruo, T., Matsuo, H., Murata, K. and Mochizuki, M. (1992) Gestational age-dependent dual action of epidermal growth factor on human placenta early in gestation. *Journal of Clinical Endocrinology and Metabolism* **75**: 1362–1367.

Maslar, I.A. (1988) The progestational endometrium. *Seminars in Reproductive Endocrinology* **6**: 115–128.

Massagué, J. (1992) Receptors for the TGF-β family. *Cell* **69**: 1067–1070.

Matrisian, L.M. (1992) The matrix-degrading metalloproteinases. *BioEssays* **14**: 455–463.

Maudsley, D.J. and Pound, J.D. (1991) Modulation of MHC antigen expression by viruses and oncogenes. *Immunology Today* **12**: 429–431.

Mayadas, T.N., Johnson, R.C., Rayburn, H., Hynes, R.O. and Wagner, D.D. (1993) Leukocyte rolling and extravasation are severely compromised in P selectin-deficient mice. *Cell* **74**: 541–554.

Mazur, M.T., Duncan, D.A. and Younger, J.B. (1989) Endometrial biopsy in the cycle of conception: histologic and lectin histochemical evaluation. *Fertility and Sterility* **51**: 764–769.

McCoy, J.P. and Chambers, W.H. (1991) Carbohydrates in the functions of natural killer cells. *Glycobiology* **1**: 321–328.

McCrae, K.R., DeMichele, A.M., Pandhi, P., Balsai, M.J., Samuels, P., Graham, C., Lala, P.K. and Cines, D.B. (1993) Detection of antitrophoblast antibodies in the sera of patients with anticardiolipin antibodies and fetal loss. *Blood* **2**: 2730–2741.

McGrath, J. and Solter, D. (1984) Completion of mouse embryogenesis requires both the maternal and paternal genomes. *Cell* **37**: 179–183.

Medawar, P.B. (1953) Some immunological and endocrinological problems raised by the evolution of viviparity in vertebrates. In: *Evolution 7*. Society for Experimental Biology, Academic Press, New York, pp. 320–338.

Meekins, J.W., Pijnenborg, R., Hanssens, M., McFadyen, I.R. and van Asshe, A. (1994) A study of placental bed spiral arteries and trophoblast invasion in normal and severe pre-eclamptic pregnancies. *British Journal of Obstetrics and Gynaecology* **101**: 669–674.

Mercurio, A.M. (1990) Laminin: multiple forms, multiple receptors. *Current Opinion in Cell Biology* **2**: 845–849.

Mercurio, A.M. and Shaw, L.M. (1991) Laminin binding proteins. *BioEssays* **13**: 469–473.

Metcalf, D. (1991) Control of granulocytes and macrophages: molecular, cellular and clinical aspects. *Science* **254**: 529–533.

Metcalf, D. (1992) Leukemia inhibitory factor: a puzzling polyfunctional regulator. *Growth Factors* **7**: 169–173.

Metcalf, D., Nicola, N.A., Gearing, D.P. and Gough, N.M. (1990) Low-affinity placenta-derived receptors for human granulocyte-macrophage colony-stimulating factor can deliver a proliferative signal to murine hemopoietic cells. *Proceedings of the National Academy of Sciences USA* **87**: 4670–4674.

Mignatti, P., Robbins, E. and Rifkin, D.B. (1986) Tumor invasion through the human amniotic membrane: requirement for a proteinase cascade. *Cell* **47**: 487–498.

Millar, D.A. and Ratcliffe, N.A. (1994) Invertebrates. In: *Immunology: A Comparative Approach*, Ed. Turner, R.J., John Wiley, Chichester, pp. 29–68.

Mincheva-Nilsson, L., Hammarström, S. and Hammarström, M.-L. (1992) Human decidual leukocytes from early pregnancy contain high numbers of γδ+ cells and show selective down-regulation of alloreactivity. *Journal of Immunology* **149**: 2203–2211.

Mincheva-Nilsson, L., Baranov, V., Yeung, M.M.-W., Hammarström, S. and Hammarström, M.-L. (1994) Immunomorphologic studies of human decidua-associated lymphoid cells in normal early pregnancy. *Journal of Immunology* **152**: 2020–2032.

Mitchell, E.J. and O'Conner-McCourt, M.D. (1991) A transforming growth factor-β (TGFβ) receptor from human placenta exhibits a greater affinity for TGFβ$_2$ than for TGFβ$_1$. *Biochemistry* **30**: 4350–4356.

Mitchell, E.J., Fitzgibbon, L. and O'Conner-McCourt, M.D. (1991) Subtypes of betaglycan and of type I and type II transforming growth factor-β (TGFβ) receptors and different affinities for TGFβ$_1$ and TGFβ$_2$ are exhibited by human placental trophoblast cells. *Journal of Cellular Physiology* **150**: 334–343.

Miyake, S., Yagita, H., Muryama, T., Hashimoto, H., Miyasaka, N. and Okumura, K. (1993) Beta-1 integrin-mediated interaction with extracellular matrix proteins regulates cytokine gene expression in synovial fluid cells of rheumatoid arthritis patients. *Journal of Experimental Medicine* **177**: 863–868.

Moll, U.M. and Lane, B.L. (1990) Proteolytic activity of first trimester human placenta: localisation of interstitial collagenase in villous and extravillous trophoblast. *Histochemistry* **94**: 555–560.

Moore, T. and Haig, D. (1991) Genomic imprinting in mammalian development: a parental tug-of-war. *Trends in Genetics* **7**: 45–49.

Morales, P., Corell, A., Martinez-Laso, J., Martin-Villa, J.M., Varela, P., Paz-Artal, E., Allende, L-M. and Arnaiz-Villena, A. (1993) Three new HLA-G alleles and their linkage disequilibria with HLA-A. *Immunogenetics* **38**: 323–331.

More, I.A.R. (1987) The normal human endometrium. In: *Haines and Taylor's Obstetrical and Gynaecological Pathology*, 3rd edition, Ed. Fox, H., Vol.1, Churchill Livingstone, Edinburgh, pp. 302–319.

Moretta, A., Vitale, M., Bottino, C., Orengo, A.M., Morelli, L., Augugliaro, R., Barbaresi, M., Ciccone, E. and Moretta, L. (1993) p58 molecules as putative receptors for major histocompatibility complex (MHC) class I molecules in human natural killer (NK) cells: anti-p58 antibodies reconstitute lysis of MHC class I-protected cells in NK clones displaying different specificities. *Journal of Experimental Medicine* **178**: 597–604.

Moretta, A., Vitale, M., Sivori, S., Bottino, C., Morelli, L., Augugliaro, R., Barbaresi, M., Pende, D., Ciccone, E., Lopez-Botet, M. and Moretta, L. (1994a) Human natural killer cell receptors for HLA-class I molecules. Evidence that the Kp43 (CD94) molecule functions as receptor for HLA-B alleles. *Journal of Experimental Medicine* **180**: 545–555.

Moretta, L., Ciccone, E., Mingari, M.C., Biassoni, R. and Moretta, A. (1994b) Human natural killer cells: origin, clonality, specificity and receptors. *Advances in Immunology* **55**: 341–380.

Morii, T., Nishikawa, K., Saito, S., Enomoto, M., Ito, E., Kurai, N., Shimoyama, T., Ichijo, M. and Narita, N. (1993) T-cell receptors are expressed but down-regulated on intradecidual T lymphocytes. *American Journal of Reproductive Immunology* **29**: 1–4.

Morris, H., Edwards, J., Tiltman, A. and Emms, M. (1985) Endometrial lymphoid tissue: an immunohistological study. *Journal of Clinical Pathology* **38**: 644–652.

Morrish, D.W., Shaw, A.R.E., Seehofer, J., Bhardwaj, D. and Paras, M.T. (1991) Preparation of fibroblast-free cytotrophoblast cultures utilising differential expression of the CD9 antigen. *In Vitro Cellular and Developmental Biology* **27A**: 303–306.

Morrison-Graham, K. and Takahashi, Y. (1993) Steel factor and c-*kit* receptor: from mutants to a growth factor system. *BioEssays* **15**: 77–83.

Morriss, G.M. (1975) Placental evolution and embryonic nutrition. In: *Comparative Placentation*, Ed. Steven, D.H., Academic Press, London, pp. 87–107.

Mosher, W.D. (1985) Reproductive impairments in the United States 1965–1982. *Demography* **22**: 415–430.

Moss, L., Prakobphol, A., Wiedmann, T.-W., Fisher, S.J. and Damsky, C.H. (1994) Glycosylation of human trophoblast integrins is stage and cell-type specific. *Glycobiology* **4**: 567–575.

Motro, B., Van der Kooy, D., Rossant, J., Reith, A. and Bernstein, N.K. (1991) Contiguous patterns of c-*kit* and steel expression: analysis of mutations at the *W* and *Sl* loci. *Development* **113**: 1207–1221.

Mueller, S.C. and Chen, W.T. (1991) Cellular invasion into matrix beads: localization of β_1 integrins and fibronectin to the invadopodia. *Journal of Cell Science* **99**: 213–226.

Mülhauser, J., Crescimano, C., Kaufmann, P., Höfler, H., Zaccheo, D. and Castellucci, M. (1993) Differentiation and proliferation patterns in human trophoblast revealed by c-*erb*B-2 oncogene product and EGF-R. *Journal of Histochemistry and Cytochemistry* **41**: 165–173.

Müller, R., Tremblay, J.M., Adamson, E.D. and Verma, I.M. (1983) Tissue and cell type–specific expression of two human c-*onc* genes. *Nature* **304**: 454–456.

Multhaupt, H.A.B., Mazar, A., Cines, D.B., Warhol, M.J. and McCrae, K.R. (1994) Expression of urokinase receptors by human trophoblast: a histochemical and ultrastructural analysis. *Laboratory Investigation* **71**: 392–400.

Murphy, C.R., Rogers, P.A.W., Hosie, M.J., Leeton, J. and Beaton, L. (1992) Tight junctions of human uterine epithelial cells change during the menstrual cycle: a morphometric study. *Acta Anatomica* **144**: 36–38.

Murphy, S.M., Bergman, M. and Morgun, D.O. (1993) Deletion of the SH3 domain of *src* interferes with regulation by the phosphorylated carboxyl-terminal tyrosine. *Molecular and Cellular Biology* **13**: 5290–5300.

Murray, B.A. and Jensen, J.J. (1992) Evidence for heterophilic adhesion of embryonic retinal cells and neuroblastoma cells to substratum-adsorbed NCAM. *Journal Cell Biology* **117**: 1311–1320.

Mutter, G.L., Stewart, C.L., Chaponot, M.L. and Pomponio, R.J. (1993) Oppositely imprinted genes H19 and insulin-like growth factor 2 are coexpressed in human androgenetic trophoblast. *American Journal of Human Genetics* **53**: 1096–1102.

Mwenda, J.M., Maher, P.M., Melling, G.C., Lyden, T.W. and Johnson, P.M. (1994) A murine monoclonal antibody (RV3-27) raised against isolated human placental endogenous retroviral particles and reactive with syncytiotrophoblast. *Journal of Reproductive Immunology* **26**: 75–95.

Mylona, P., Kielty, C.M., Hoyland, J.A. and Aplin, J.D. (1995) Expression of type VI collagen mRNAs in human endometrium during the menstrual cycle and first trimester of pregnancy. *Journal of Reproduction and Fertility* – in press.

Nagler, A., Lanier, L.L., Cwirla, S. and Phillips, J.H. (1989) Comparative studies of human FcRIII-positive and negative natural killer cells. *Journal of Immunology* **143**: 3183–3191.

Nakarai, T., Robertson, M.J., Streuli, M., Wu, Z., Ciardelli, T.L., Smith, K.A. and Ritz, J. (1994) Interleukin 2 receptor γ chain expression on resting and activated lymphoid cells. *Journal of Experimental Medicine* **180**: 241–251.

Naume, B., Johnsen, A.-C., Espevik, T. and Sundan, A. (1993) Gene expression and secretion of cytokines and cytokine receptors from highly purified CD56$^+$ natural killer cells stimulated with interleukin-2, interleukin-7 and interleukin-12. *European Journal of Immunology* **23**: 1831–1838.

Navot, D., Karstaedt, A., Drews, M.R., Scott, R.T., Bergh, P.A., Garrisi, G.J., Guzman, I. and Hofmann, G.E. (1994) Age-related decline in female fertility is not due to diminished capacity of the uterus to sustain embryo implantation? *Fertility and Sterility* **61**: 97–101.

Nelson, D.M., Enders, A.C. and King, B.F. (1978a) Cytological events involved in protein synthesis in cellular and syncytial trophoblast of human placenta: an electronmicroscope autoradiographic study of [³H]leucine incorporation. *Journal of Cell Biology* **76**: 400–417.

Nelson, D.M., Enders, A.C. and King, B.F. (1978b) Cytological events involved in glycoprotein synthesis in cellular and syncytial trophoblast of human placenta: an electron microscope autoradiographic study of [³H]galactose incorporation. *Journal of Cell Biology* **76**: 418–429.

Nelson, J.A., Leong, J.-A. and Levy, J.A. (1978) Normal human placentas contain RNA-directed DNA polymerase activity like that in viruses. *Proceedings of the National Academy of Sciences USA* **75**: 6263–6267.

Nelson, J.A., Levy, J.A. and Leong, J.C. (1981) Human placentas contain a specific inhibitor of RNA-directed DNA polymerase. *Proceedings of the National Academy of Sciences USA* **78**: 1670–1674.

Nickoloff, B.J., Mitra, R.S., Green, J., Zheng, X.G., Shimizu, Y., Thompson, C. and Turka, L.A. (1993) Accessory cell function of keratinocytes for superantigens: dependence on lymphocyte function-associated antigen-1/intercellular adhesion molecule-1 interaction. *Journal of Immunology* **150**: 2148–2159.

Nicosia, R.F., Nicosia, S.V. and Smith, M. (1994) Vascular endothelial growth factor, platelet-derived growth factor, and insulin-like growth factor-1 promote rat aortic angiogenesis *in vitro*. *American Journal of Pathology* **145**: 1023–1029.

Nilsen-Hamilton, M. (1990) *Growth Factors and Development*. Current Topics in Developmental Biology 24, Academic Press San Diego.

Nishikawa, K., Saito, S., Morii, T., Hamada, K., Ako, H., Narita, N., Ichijo, M., Kurahayashi, M. and Sugamura, K. (1991) Accumulation of CD16⁻ CD56⁺ natural killer cells with high affinity interleukin 2 receptors in human early pregnancy decidua. *International Immunology* **3**: 743–750.

Nishikawa, S., Kusakabe, M., Yoshinaga, K., Ogawa, M., Hayashi, S.I., Kunisada, T., Sakakura, T. and Nishikawa, S.O. (1991) *In utero* manipulation of coat colour formation by a monoclonal anti c-*kit* antibody: two distinct waves of c-*kit* dependency during melanocyte development. *EMBO Journal* **10**: 3287–3294.

Nishino, E., Matsuzaki, N., Masuhiro, K. et al. (1990) Trophoblast-derived IL-6 regulates human chorionic gonadotropin release through IL-6 receptor on human trophoblasts. *Journal of Clinical Endocrinological Methods* **21**: 436–441.

Norment, A.M. and Littman, D.R. (1988) A second subunit of CD8 is expressed in human T cells. *EMBO Journal* **7**: 3433–3439.

O'Brien, R.L. and Born, W. (1991) Heat shock proteins as antigens for γδ T cells. *Seminars in Immunology* **3**: 81–87.

O'Connell, C.D. and Cohen, M. (1984) The long terminal repeat sequences of a novel human endogenous retrovirus. *Science* **226**: 1204–1206.

O'Connell, C., O'Brien, S., Nash, W.G. and Cohen, M. (1984) ERV3, a full-length human endogenous provirus: chromosomal localisation and evolutionary relationships. *Virology* **138**: 225–235.

Odum, N., Ledbetter, J.A., Martin, P., Geraghty, D., Tsu, T., Hansen, J.A. and Gladstone, P. (1991) Homotypic aggregation of human cell lines by HLA Class II-, Class Ia- and HLA-G-specific monoclonal antibodies. *European Journal of Immunology* **21**: 2121–2131.

Ogawa, O., McNoe, L.A., Eccles, M.R., Morison, I.M. and Reeve, A.E. (1993) Human insulin-like growth factor type I and type II receptors are not imprinted. *Human Molecular Genetics* **2**: 2163–2165.

Oglesby, T.J., Allen, C.J., Liszewski, M.K., White, D.J. and Atkinson, J.P. (1992) Membrane cofactor protein (CD46) protects cells from complement-mediated attack by an intrinsic mechanism. *Journal of Experimental Medicine* **175**: 1547–1551.

Oksenberg, J.R., Mor-Yosef, S., Persitz, E., Schenker, Y., Mozes, E. and Brautbar, C. (1986) Antigen-presenting cells in human decidual tissue. *American Journal of Reproductive Immunology* **11**: 82–88.

Ombelet, W., Vandermerwe, J.V. and Van Assche, F.A. (1988) Advanced extrauterine pregnancy: description of 38 cases with literature survey. *Obstetrical and Gynecological Survey* **43**: 386–397.

Ono, M. (1986) Molecular cloning and long terminal repeat sequences of human endogenous retrovirus genes related to types A and B retrovirus genes. *Journal of Virology* **58**: 937–944.

Ortenzi , C., Miceli, C., Bradshaw, R.A. and Luporini, P. (1990) Identification and initial characterization of an autocrine pheromone receptor in the protozoan ciliate *Euplotes raikovi*. *Journal of Cell Biology* **111**: 607–614.

Osborn, L. (1990) Leucocyte adhesion to endothelium in inflammation. *Cell* **62**: 3–6.

Ossowski, L. (1988) *In vivo* invasion of modified chorioallantoic membrane by tumor cells: the role of cell surface-bound urokinase. *Journal of Cell Biology* **107**: 2437–2445.

Osteen, K.G., Hill, G.A., Hargrove, J.T. and Gorstein, F. (1989) Development of a method to isolate and culture highly purified populations of stromal and epithelial cells from human endometrial biopsy specimens. *Fertility and Sterility* **52**. 965–972.

Osteen, K.G., Rodgers, W.H., Gaire, M., Hargrove, J.T., Gorstein, F. and Matrisian, L.M. (1994) Stromal-epithelial interaction mediates steroidal regulation of metalloproteinase expression in human endometrium. *Proceedings of the National Academy of Sciences USA* **91**: 10129–10133.

Oudejans, C.B.M., Krimpenfort, P., Ploegh, H.L. and Meijer, C.J.L.M. (1989) Lack of expression of HLA-B27 gene in transgenic mouse trophoblast. *Journal of Experimental Medicine* **169**: 447–456.

Owens, R.J., Tanner, C.C., Mulligan, M.J., Srinivas, R.V. and Compans, R.W. (1990) Oligopeptide inhibitors of HIV-induced syncytium formation. *AIDS Research and Human Retroviruses* **6**: 1289–1296.

Pace, D., Morrison, L. and Bulmer, J.N. (1989) Proliferative activity in endometrial stromal granulocytes throughout the menstrual cycle and early pregnancy. *Journal of Clinical Pathology* **42**: 35–39.

Pace, D., Longfellow, M. and Bulmer, J.N. (1991) Characterization of intraepithelial lymphocytes in human endometrium. *Journal of Reproduction and Fertility* **91**: 165–174.

Page, H. (1989) Estimation of the prevalence and incidence of infertility in a population: a pilot study. *Fertility and Sterility* **51**: 571–577.

Pal, N., Wadey, R.B., Buckle, B., Yeomans, E., Pritchard, J. and Cowell, K. (1990) Preferential loss of maternal alleles in sporadic Wilms' tumour. *Oncogene* **5**: 1665–1668.

Pampfer, S., Daiter, E., Barad, D. and Pollard, J.W. (1992) Expression of the colony-stimulating factor-1 receptor (c-*fms* proto-oncogene product) in the human uterus and placenta. *Biology of Reproduction* **46**: 48–57.

Panayotou, G., End, P., Aumailley, M., Timpl, R. and Engel, J. (1989) Domains of laminin with growth-factor activity. *Cell* **56**: 93–101.

Paneth, N. and Susser, M. (1995) Early origin of coronary heart disease (the 'Barker hypothesis'). *British Medical Journal* **310**: 411–412.

Parem, S. (1979) C-type virus expression in the placenta. *Current Topics in Pathology* **66**: 175–189.

Parham, P. (1994a) The rise and fall of great class I genes. *Seminars in Immunology* **6**: 373–382.

Parham, P. (1994b) Evolution of class I HLA antigen presenting molecules. In: *Immunology of Human Papillomaviruses*, Ed. Stanley, M.A., Plenum Press, New York, pp. 161–172.

Parham, P. (1994c) Chewing the fat. *Nature* **372**: 615–616.

Parham, P. (1995) Antigen presentation by class I major histocompatibility complex molecules: a context for thinking about HLA-G. *American Journal of Reproductive Immunology* **34**: 10–19.

Paria, B.C., Huet-Hudson, Y.M. and Dey, S.K. (1993) Blastocyst's state of activity determines the 'window' of implantation in the receptive mouse uterus. *Proceedings of the National Academy of Sciences USA* **90**: 10159–10162.

Parker, C.M., Cepek, K.L., Russell, G.J., Shaw, S.K., Posnett, D.N., Schwarting, R. and Brenner, M.B. (1992) A family of β_7 integrins on human mucosal lymphocytes. *Proceedings of the National Academy of Sciences USA* **89**: 1924–1928.

Parr, E.L., Young, L.H.Y., Parr, B.P. and Young, J.D.-E. (1990) Granulated metrial gland cells of pregnant mouse uterus are natural killer-like cells that contain perforin and serine esterases. *Journal of Immunology* **145**: 2365–2372.

Patterson, P.H. (1994) Leukemia inhibitory factor, a cytokine at the interface between neurobiology and immunology. *Proceedings of the National Academy of Sciences USA* **91**: 7833–7835.

Paulesu, L., Bocci, V., King, A. and Loke, Y.W. (1991a) Immunocytochemical localization of interferons in human trophoblast populations. *Journal of Biological Regulators and Homeostatic Agents* **5**: 81–85.

Paulesu, L., King, A., Loke, Y.W., Cintorino, M., Bellizzi, E. and Boraschi, D. (1991b) Immunohistochemical localization of IL-1α and IL-1β in normal human placenta. *Lymphokine and Cytokine Research* **10**: 443–448.

Paulesu, L., Romagnoli, R., Cintorino, M., Ricci, M.G. and Garotta, G. (1994) First trimester human trophoblast expresses both interferon-γ and interferon-γ-receptor. *Journal of Reproductive Immunology* **27**: 37–48.

Peles, E., Bacus, S.S., Koski, R.A., Lu, H.S., Wen, D., Ogden, S.G., Levy, R.B. and Yarden, Y. (1992) Isolation of the *neu*/HER-2 stimulatory ligand: a 44kd glycoprotein that induces differentiation of mammary tumour cells. *Cell* **69**: 205–216.

Perrot-Applanat, M., Deng, M., Fernandez, H., Lelaidier, C., Meduri, G. and Bouchard, P. (1994) Immunohistochemical localization of estradiol and progesterone receptors in human uterus throughout pregnancy: expression in endometrial blood vessels. *Journal of Clinical Endocrinology and Metabolism* **78**: 216–224.

Perussia, B. (1991) Lymphokine-activated killer cells, natural killer cells and cytokines. *Current Opinion in Immunology* **3**: 49–55.

Pesheva, P., Probstmeier, R. and Skubitz, A.P.N. (1994) Tenascin-R (J1 160/180) inhibits fibronectin-mediated cell adhesion: functional relatedness to tenascin-C. *Journal of Cell Science* **107**: 2323–2333.

Peyman, J.A. and Hammond, G.L. (1992) Localization of IFN-γ receptors in first trimester placenta to trophoblasts but lack of stimulation of HLA-DR, -DRB, or invariant chain mRNA expression by IFN-γ. *Journal of Immunology* **149**: 2675–2680.

Peyman, J.A., Nelson, P.J. and Hammond, G.L. (1992) HLA-DR genes are silenced in human trophoblasts and stimulation of signal transduction pathways does not circumvent interferon-γ unresponsiveness. *Transplantation Proceedings* **24**: 470–471.

Pfeifer-Ohlsson, S., Goustin, A.S., Rydnert, J., Bjersing, L., Wahlström, T., Stehelin, D. and Ohlsson, R. (1984) Spatial and temporal pattern of cellular *myc* oncogene expression in developing human placenta: implications for embryonic cell proliferation. *Cell* **38**: 585–596.

Phillips, J.H., Hori, T., Nagler, A., Bhat, N., Spits, H. and Lanier, L.L. (1992) Ontogeny of human natural killer (NK) cells: fetal NK cells mediate cytolytic function and express cytoplasmic CD3ε proteins. *Journal of Experimental Medicine* **175**: 1055–1066.

Picillo, U., Marcialis, R.M., Longobardo, A., LaPolombara, R., Faeta, G., Migliaresi, S. and Tirri, G. (1992) Pregnancy and antiphospholipid antibodies. *Annals of Rheumatic Diseases* **51**: 1103.

Pijnenborg, R. (1994) Trophoblast invasion. *Reproductive Medicine Review* **3**: 53–73.

Pijnenborg, R., Dixon, G., Robertson, W.B. and Brosens, I. (1980) Trophoblastic invasion of human decidua from 8 to 18 weeks of pregnancy. *Placenta* **1**: 3–19.

Pijnenborg, R., Robertson, W.B., Brosens, I. and Dixon, G. (1981) Trophoblast invasion and the establishment of haemochorial placentation in man and laboratory animals. *Placenta* **2**: 71–91.

Pijnenborg, R., Bland, J.M., Robertson, W.B. and Brosens, I. (1983) Uteroplacental arterial changes related to interstitial trophoblast migration in early human pregnancy. *Placenta* **4**: 397–414.

Polakova, K., Karpatova, M. and Russ, G. (1993) Dissociation of β2-microglobulin is responsible for selective reduction of HLA class I antigenicity following acid treatment of cells. *Molecular Immunology* **30**: 1223–1230.

Pollard, J.W. (1991) Lymphohematopoietic cytokines in the female reproductive tract. *Current Opinion in Immunology* **3**: 772–777.

Polotskaya, A., Zhao, Y., Lilly, M.L. and Kraft, A.S. (1993) A critical role for the cytoplasmic domain of the granulocyte-macrophage colony-stimulating factor α receptor in mediating cell growth. *Cell Growth and Differentiation* **4**: 523–531.

Pook, M.A., Woodcock, V., Tassabehji, M., Duncan Campbell, R., Summers, C.W., Taylor, M. and Strachan, T. (1991) Characterisation of an expressible nonclassical class I HLA gene. *Human Immunology* **32**: 102–109.

Porter, S. and Gilkes, C.B. (1993) Genomic imprinting: a proposed explanation for the different behaviours of testicular and ovarian germ cell tumours. *Medical Hypotheses* **41**: 37–41.

Postlethwait, J.H. and Hopson, J.L. (1992) *The Nature of Life.* McGraw-Hill, New York, pp. 378–424.

Potts, J.R. and Campbell, I.D. (1994) Fibronectin structure and cell assembly. *Current Opinion in Cell Biology* **6**: 648–655.

Press, M.F., Udove, J.A. and Greene, G.L. (1988) Progesterone receptor distribution in the human endometrium. *American Journal of Pathology* **131**: 112–124.

Press, M.F., Cordon-Cardo, C. and Slamon, D.J. (1990) Expression of the HER-2/*neu* proto-oncogene in normal human adult and fetal tissues. *Oncogene* **5**: 953–962.

Probstmeier, R., Kuhn, K. and Schachner, M. (1989) Binding properties of the neural cell adhesion molecule to different components of the extracellular matrix. *Journal of Neurochemistry* **53**: 1794–1801.

Purcell, D.F.J., McKenzie, I.F.C., Lublin, D.M., Johnson, P.M., Atkinson, J.P., Oglesby, T.J. and Deacon, N.J. (1990) The human cell surface glycoproteins HuLy-m5, membrane cofactor protein (MCP) of the complement system, and trophoblast-leucocyte common (TLX) antigen are CD46. *Immunology* **70**: 155–161.

Queenan, J.T., Kao, L.C., Arboleda, C.A., Ulloa-Aguirre, A., Golos, T.G., Clines, D.B. and Strauss, J.F. (1987) Regulation of urokinase-type plasminogen activator production by cultured human trophoblasts. *Journal of Biological Chemistry* **262**: 10903–10906.

Rabinowich, H., Sedlmayr, P., Herberman, R.B. and Whiteside, T.L. (1993) Response of human NK cells to IL-6 alterations of the cell surface phenotype, adhesion to fibronectin and laminin, and tumor necrosis factor-α/β secretion. *Journal of Immunology* **150**: 4844–4855.

Rachmilewitz, J., Gileadi, O., Eldar-Geva, T., Schneider, T., De Groot, N. and Hochberg, A. (1992) Transcription of the H19 gene in differentiating cytotrophoblasts from human placenta. *Molecular Reproduction and Development* **32**: 196–202.

Rainer, S., Johnson, L.A., Dobry, C.J., Ping, A.J., Grundy, P.E. and Feinberg, A.P. (1993) Relaxation of imprinted genes in human cancer. *Nature* **362**: 747–749.

Raines, E.W., Bowen-Pope, D.F. and Ross, R. (1990) Platelet-derived growth factor. In: *Peptide Growth Factors and Their Receptors: I*, Eds. Sporn, M.B. and Roberts, A.B., Springer-Verlag, Berlin, pp. 173–262.

Ramsey, E.M. and Donner, M.W. (1980) *Placental Vasculature and Circulation*. Georg Thieme, Stuttgart, pp. 12–13.

Ramsey, E.M., Houston, M.L. and Harris, J.W.S. (1976) Interactions of the trophoblast and maternal tissues in closely related primate species. *American Journal of Obstetrics and Gynecology* **124**: 647–652.

Randall, S., Buckley, C.H. and Fox, H. (1987) Placentation in the Fallopian tube. *International Society of Gynecology and Pathology* **6**: 132–139.

Rast, J.P. and Litman, G.W. (1994) T-cell receptor gene homologs are present in the most primitive jawed vertebrates. *Proceedings of the National Academy of Sciences USA* **91**: 9248–9252.

Rathjen, P.D., Toth, S., Willis, A., Heath, J.K. and Smith, A.G. (1990) Differentiation inhibition activity is produced in matrix associated and diffusible forms that are generated by alternate promotor usage. *Cell* **62**: 1105–1114.

Ratner, S. (1992) Motility of IL-2 stimulated lymphocytes in neutral and acidified extracellular matrix. *Cellular Immunology* **139**: 399–410.

Raulet, D.H. (1992) A sense of something missing. *Nature* **358**: 21–22.

Ravetch, J.V. and Margulies, D.H. (1994) New tricks for old molecules. *Nature* **372**: 323–324.

Ravn, V., Stubbe Teglbjaerg, C., Mandel, U. and Dabelsteen, E. (1992a) The distribution of type-2 chain histo-blood group antigens in normal cycling human endometrium. *Cell and Tissue Research* **270**: 425–433.

Ravn, V., Stubbe Teglbjaerg, C., Visfeldt, J., Brock, J.E., Sorensen, H. and Dabelsteen, E. (1992b) Mucin-type carbohydrates (type 3 chain antigens) in normal cycling human endometrium. *International Journal of Gynecological Pathology* **11**: 38–46.

Ravn, V., Stubbe Teglbjaerg, C., Mandel, U. and Dabelsteen, E. (1993) The distribution of type I chain ABH and related histo-blood group antigens in normal cycling human endometrium. *International Journal of Gynecological Pathology* **12**: 70–79.

Ravn, V., Mandel, U., Svenstrup, B. and Dabelsteen, E. (1994a) Expression of type-2 histo-blood group carbohydrate antigens (Le^x, Le^y, and H) in normal and malignant human endometrium. *Virchows Archiv A: Pathological Anatomy and Histopathology* **424**: 411–419.

Ravn, V., Mandel, U., Svenstrup, B. and Dabelsteen, E. (1994b) Type–1 chain histo-blood group antigens (Le^a, monosialosyl-Le^b, disialosyl-Le^a, Le^b, and H) in normal and malignant human endometrium. *Virchows Archiv A: Pathological Anatomy and Histopathology* **424**: 495–502.

Rebut–Bonneton, C., Bontemy-Roulier, S. and Evain-Brion, D. (1993) Modulation of pp60^{c-src} activity and cellular localisation during differentiation of human trophoblast cells in culture. *Journal of Cell Science* **105**: 204–210.

Reed, M.L. and Leff, S.E. (1994) Maternal imprinting of human SNRPN, a gene deleted in Prader-Willi syndrome. *Nature Genetics* **6**: 163–167.

Regan, L. (1992) Recurrent early pregnancy failure. *Current Opinion in Obstetrics and Gynecology* **4**: 220–228.

Regan, L., Braude, P.R. and Trembath, P.L. (1989) Influence of past reproductive performance on risk of spontaneous abortion. *British Medical Journal* **299**: 541–545.

Regan, L., Braude, P.R. and Hill, D.P. (1991) A prospective study of the incidence, time of appearance and significance of anti-paternal lymphocytotoxic antibodies in human pregnancy. *Human Reproduction* **6**: 294–298.

Repaske, R., Steele, P.E., O'Neill, R.R., Rabson, A.B. and Martin, M.A. (1985) Nucleotide sequence of a full-length human endogenous retroviral segment. *Journal of Virology* **54**: 764–772.

Rettenmier, C.W., Sacca, R., Furman, W.L., Roussel, M.F., Holt, J.T., Nienhuis, A.W., Stanley, E.R. and Sherr, C.J. (1986) Expression of the human c-*fms* proto-oncogene product (colony-stimulating factor-1 receptor) on peripheral blood mononuclear cells and choriocarcinoma cell lines. *Journal of Clinical Investigation* **77**: 1740–1746.

Rinaldo, C.R. (1994) Modulation of major histocompatibility complex antigen expression by viral infection. *American Journal of Pathology* **144**: 637–650.

Rippmann, F., Taylor, W.R., Rothbard, J.B. and Green, N.M. (1991) A hypothetical model for the peptide binding domain of hsp 70 based on the peptide binding domain of HLA. *EMBO Journal* **10**: 1053–1059.

Ritson, A. and Bulmer, J.N. (1987a) Extraction of leucocytes from human decidua. A comparison of dispersal techniques. *Journal of Immunological Methods* **104**: 231–236.

Ritson, A. and Bulmer, J.N. (1987b) Endometrial granulocytes in human decidua react with a natural-killer (NK) cell marker, NKH-1. *Immunology* **62**: 329–331.

Roberts, A.B. and Sporn, M.B. (1990) The transforming growth factor-βs. In: *Peptide Growth Factors and Their Receptors: I*, Eds. Sporn, M.B. and Roberts, A.B., Springer-Verlag, Berlin, pp. 419–472.

Roberts, R.M. (1989) Conceptus interferons and maternal recognition of pregnancy. *Biology of Reproduction* **40**: 449–452.

Roberts, R.M., Leaman, D.W., Hernandez-Ledezma, J.J. and Cosby, N.C. (1993) Trophoblast interferons: expression during development and gene organization.

In: *Trophoblast Cells: Pathways for Maternal Embryonic Communication*, Eds Soares, M.J., Handwerger, S. and Talamantes, F., Serono Symposium, Springer Verlag, Berlin, pp. 206–221.

Roberts, W.M., Look, A.T., Roussel, M.F. and Sherr, C.J. (1988) Tandem linkage of human CSF-1 receptor (c-*fms*) and PDGF receptor genes. *Cell* **55**: 655–661.

Roberts, W.M., Shapiro, L.H., Ashmun, R.A. and Look, A.T. (1992) Transcription of the human colony-stimulating factor-1 receptor gene is regulated by separate tissue-specific promoters. *Blood* **79**: 586–593.

Robertson, S.A., Seamark, R.F., Guilbert, L.J. and Wegmann, T.G. (1994) The role of cytokines in gestation. *Critical Reviews in Immunology* **14**: 239–292.

Robertson, W.B. (1987) Pathology of the pregnant uterus. In: *Obstetrical and Gynaecological Pathology*, Ed. Fox, H., Churchill Livingstone, Edinburgh, pp.1149–1176.

Robillard, P.-Y., Hulsey, T.C., Alexander, G.R., Kennan, A., de Caines, F. and Papiernik, E. (1993) Paternity patterns and risk of pre-eclampsia in the last pregnancy in multipara. *Journal of Reproductive Immunology* **24**: 1–12.

Robillard, P.-Y., Hulsey, T.C., Perianin, J., Janky, E., Miri, E.H. and Papiernik, E. (1994) Association of pregnancy-induced hypertension with duration of sexual cohabitation before conception. *Lancet* **344**: 973–975.

Rodesch, F., Simon, P., Donner, C. and Jauniaux, E. (1992) Oxygen measurements in endometrial and trophoblastic tissues during early pregnancy. *Obstetrics and Gynecology* **80**: 283–285.

Rogers, P. (1993) Uterine receptivity. In: *Handbook of In Vitro Fertilization*, Eds. Trounson, A. and Gardner, D.K., CRC Press, Boca Raton, pp. 263–285.

Ross, R. (1989) Platelet-derived growth factor. *Lancet* **i**: 1179–1182.

Roth, C., Kourilsky, P. and Ojcius, D.M. (1994) Ly-49-independent inhibition of natural killer cell-mediated cytotoxicity by a soluble major histocompatibility complex class I molecule. *European Journal of Immunology* **24**: 2110–2114.

Roubey, R.A.S. (1994) Autoantibodies to phospholipid-binding plasma proteins: a new view of lupus anticoagulants and other ''antiphospholipid'' autoantibodies. *Blood* **84**: 2854–2867.

Ruoslahti, E. and Pierschbacher, M.D. (1987) New perspectives in cell adhesion: RGD and integrins. *Science* **238**: 491–497.

Russell, S.M. Sparrow, R.L., McKenzie, I.F.C. and Purcell, D.F.C. (1992) Tissue specific and allelic expression of the complement regulator CD46 is controlled by alternative splicing. *European Journal of Immunology* **22**: 1513–1518.

Rutanen, M. (1993) Cytokines in reproduction. *Annals of Medicine* **25**: 343–347.

Sage, E.H. and Bornstein, P. (1991) Extracellular proteins that modulate cell–matrix interactions: SPARC, tenascin, and thrombospondin. *Journal of Biological Chemistry* **266**: 14831–14834.

Saito, S., Nishikawa, K., Morii, T., Narita, N., Enomoto, M. and Ichijo, M. (1992) Expression of activation antigens CD69, HLA-DR, interleukin-2 receptor-alpha (IL-2Rα) and IL-2Rβ on T cells of human decidua at an early stage of pregnancy. *Immunology* **75**: 710–712.

Saito, S., Morii, T., Enomoto, M., Sakakura, S., Nishikawa, K., Narita, N. and Ichijo, M. (1993a) The effect of interleukin 2 and transforming growth factor-β2 (TGF-β2) on the proliferation and natural killer activity of decidual CD16⁻ CD56^bright natural killer cells. *Cellular Immunology* **152**: 605–613.

Saito, S., Motoyoshi, K., Saito, M., Kato, Y., Enomoto, M., Nishikawa, K., Morii, T. and Ichijo, M. (1993b) Localization and production of human macrophage colony-stimulating factor (hM-CSF) in human placental and decidual tissues. *Lymphokine and Cytokine Research* **12**: 101–107.

Saito, S., Nishikawa, K., Morii, T., Enomoto, M., Narita, N., Motoyoshi, K. and Ichijo, M. (1993c) Cytokine production by CD16⁻ CD56^bright natural killer cells in the human early pregnancy decidua. *International Immunology* **5**: 559–563.

Saito, S., Saito, M., Enomoto, M., Ito, A., Motoyoshi, K., Nakagawa, T. and Ichijo, M. (1993d) Human macrophage colony-stimulating factor induces the differentiation of trophoblast. *Growth Factors* **9**: 11–19.

Saito, S., Kasahara, T., Sakakura, S., Enomoto, M., Umekage, H., Harada, N., Morii, T., Nishikawa, K., Narita, N. and Ichijo, M. (1994a) Interleukin-8 production by natural killer cells in the human early pregnancy decidua. *Biochemical and Biophysical Research Communications* **20**: 378–383.

Saito, S., Nishikawa, K., Morii, T., Narita, N., Enomoto, M., Ito, A. and Ichijo, M. (1994b) A study of CD45RO, CD45RA and CD29 antigen expression on human decidual T cells in an early stage of pregnancy. *Immunology Letters* **40**: 193–197.

Sakakibara, H., Taga, M., Saji, M., Kida, H. and Minaguchi, H. (1994) Gene expression of epidermal growth factor in human endometrium during decidualisation. *Journal of Clinical Endocrinology* **79**: 223–226.

Saksela, O. and Rifkin, D.B. (1988) Cell-associated plasminogen activation: regulation and physiological functions. *Annual Review of Cell Biology* **4**: 93–126.

Salcedo, M., Momburg, F., Hämmerling, G.J. and Ljunggren, H.-G. (1994) Resistance to natural killer cell lysis conferred by TAP1/2 genes in human antigen-processing mutant cells. *Journal of Immunology* **152**: 1702–1708.

Sánchez, M.J., Muench, M.O., Roncarolo, M.G., Lanier, L.L. and Phillips, J.H. (1994) Identification of a common T/natural killer cell progenitor in human fetal thymus. *Journal of Experimental Medicine* **180**: 569–576.

Sanders, S.K., Giblin, P.A. and Kavathas, P. (1991) Cell-cell adhesion mediated by CD8 and HLA-G, a nonclassical major histocompatibility complex class I molecule on cytotrophoblasts. *Journal of Experimental Medicine* **174**: 737–740.

Santis, A.G., López-Cabrera, M., Hamann, J., Strauss, M. and Sánchez-Madrid, F. (1994) Structure of the gene coding for the human early lymphocyte activation antigen CD69: a C-type lectin receptor evolutionarily related with the gene families of natural killer cell-specific receptors. *European Journal of Immunology* **24**: 1692–1697.

Sargent, I.L. (1993) Maternal and fetal immune responses during pregnancy. *Experimental and Clinical Immunogenetics* **10**: 85–102.

Sargent, I.L., Arenas, J. and Redman, C.W.G. (1987) Maternal cell-mediated sensitisation to paternal HLA may occur, but is not a regular event in normal human pregnancy. *Journal of Reproductive Immunology* **10**: 111–120.

Sargent, I.L., Wilkins, T. and Redman, C.W.G. (1988) Maternal immune responses to the fetus in early pregnancy and recurrent miscarriage. *Lancet* **ii**: 1099–1104.

Sastry, S.K. and Horwitz, A.F. (1993) Integrin cytoplasmic domains: mediators of cytoskeletal linkages and extra- and intracellular initiated transmembrane signaling. *Current Opinion in Cell Biology* **5**: 819–831.

Sato, N. and Miyajima, A. (1994) Multimeric cytokine receptors: common versus specific functions. *Current Opinion in Cell Biology* **6**: 174–179.

Satyaswaroop, P.G., Bressler, S., de la Penna, M.M. and Gurpide, E. (1979) Isolation and culture of human endometrial glands. *Journal of Clinical Endocrinology and Metabolism* **48**: 639–641.

Schaller, M.D. and Parsons, J.T. (1994) Focal adhesion kinase: an integrin-linked protein tyrosine kinase. *Trends in Cell Biology* **3**: 258–262.

Schatz, F., Gordon, R.E., Laufer, N. and Gurpide, E. (1990) Culture of human endometrial cells under polarizing conditions. *Differentiation* **42**: 184–190.

Scherer, M.T., Ignatowicz, L., Winslow, G.M., Kappler, J.W. and Marrack, P. (1993) Superantigens: bacterial and viral proteins that manipulate the immune system. *Annual Review of Cell Biology* **9**: 101–128.

Schild, H., Mavaddat, N., Litzenberger, C., Ehrich, E.W., Davis, M.M., Bluestone, J.A., Matis, L., Draper, R.K. and Chien, Y.-H. (1994) The nature of major histocompatibility complex recognition by γδ T cells. *Cell* **76**: 29–37.

Schmidt, C.M. and Orr, H.T. (1991) A physical linkage map of HLA-A, -G, -7.5p and -F. *Human Immunology* **31**: 180–185.

Schmidt, C.M. and Orr, H.T. (1993) Maternal/fetal interactions: the role of the MHC class I molecule HLA-G. *Critical Reviews in Immunology* **13**: 207–224.

Schmidt, C.M., Ehlenfeldt, R.G.F., Athanasiou, M.C., Duvick, L.A., Heinrichs, H., David, C.S. and Orr, H.T. (1993) Extraembryonic expression of the human MHC class I gene HLA-G in transgenic mice. *Journal of Immunology* **151**: 2633–2645.

Schmidt, C., Bladt, F., Goedecke, S., Brinkmann, V., Zschiesche, W., Sharpe, M., Gherardi, E. and Birchmeier, C. (1995) Scatter factor/hepatocyte growth factor is essential for liver development. *Nature* **373**: 699–702.

Schofield, P.N. (ed.) (1992). *The Insulin-like Growth Factors: Structure and Biological Functions,*. Oxford University Press, Oxford.

Schofield, V.L., Schlumpberger, J.M., West, L.A. and Weissman, I.L. (1982) Protochordate allorecognition is controlled by a MHC-like gene system. *Nature* **295**: 499–502.

Schroeder, W.T., Chao, L.-Y., Dao, D.D., Strong, L., Pathak, S., Riccardi, V., Lewis, W.H. and Saunders, G.F. (1987) Non-random loss of maternal chromosome 11 alleles in Wilms' tumors. *American Journal of Human Genetics* **40**: 413–420.

Schultz, R.M., Silberman, S., Persky, B., Bajkowski, A.S. and Carmichael, D.F. (1988) Inhibition by human recombinant tissue inhibitor of metalloproteinases of human amnion invasion and lung colonization by murine B16-F10 melanoma cells. *Cancer Research* **48**: 5539–5545.

Schwarz, R.E. and Hiserodt, J.C. (1988) The expression and functional involvement of laminin-like molecules in non-MHC restricted cytotoxicity by human Leu-19[+]/CD3[−] natural killer lymphocytes. *Journal of Immunology* **141**: 3318–3323.

Scott, P.A.E. and Bicknell, R. (1993) The isolation and culture of microvascular endothelium. *Journal of Cell Science* **105**: 269–273.

Seftor, R.E.B., Seftor, E.A., Gehlsen, K.R., Stetler-Stevenson, W.G., Brown, P.D., Ruoslahti, E. and Hendrix, M.J.C. (1992) Role of the $\alpha_v\beta_3$ integrin in human melanoma cell invasion. *Proceedings of the National Academy of Sciences USA* **89**: 1557–1561.

Selick, C.E., Horowitz, G.M., Gratch, M., Scott, R.T., Novot, D. and Hofmann, G.E. (1994) Immunohistochemical localization of transforming growth factor-β in human implantation sites. *Journal of Clinical Endocrinology and Metabolism* **78**: 592–596.

Seman, G., Levy, B.M., Panigel, M. and Dmochowski, L. (1975) Type-C virus particles in placenta of the cottontop marmoset (*Sanguinus oedipus*). *Journal of the National Cancer Institute* **54**: 251–252.

Seppälä, M., Riitinen, L. and Julkunen, M. (1988) Structural studies, localization in tissue and clinical aspects of human endometrial protein. *Journal of Reproduction and Fertility* **36**: 127–131.

Seppälä, M., Koistinen, R. and Rutanen, E.-M. (1994) Uterine endocrinology and paracrinology: insulin-like growth factor binding protein-1 and placental protein 14 revisited. *Human Reproduction* **9**: 917–925.

Serhal, P.F. and Craft, I. (1987) Immune basis for pre-eclampsia: evidence from oocyte recipients. *Lancet* **ii**: 744.

Serle, E., Aplin, J.D., Li, T.-C., Warren, M.A., Graham, R.A., Seif, M.W. and Cooke, I.D. (1994) Endometrial differentiation in the peri-implantation phase of women with recurrent miscarriage: a morphological and immunohistochemical study. *Fertility and Sterility* **62**: 989–996.

Sharkey, A.M., Charnock-Jones, D.S., Brown, K.D. and Smith, S.K. (1992) Expression of mRNA for kit ligand in human placenta: localisation by *in-situ* hybridisation and identification of alternatively spliced variants. *Molecular Endocrinology* **6**: 1235–1241.

Sharkey, A.M., Charnock-Jones, D.S., Boocock, C.A., Brown, K.D. and Smith, S.K. (1993) Expression of mRNA for vascular endothelial growth factor in human placenta. *Journal of Reproduction and Fertility* **99**: 609–615.

Sharkey, A.M., Jokhi, P.P., King, A., Loke, Y.W., Brown, K.D. and Smith, S.K. (1994) Expression of c-*kit* and kit ligand at the human materno-fetal interface. *Cytokine* **6**: 195–205.

Sharman, G.B. (1976) Evolution of viviparity in mammals. In: *The Evolution of Reproduction*, Eds. Austin, C.R. and Short, R.V., Cambridge University Press, Cambridge, pp. 32–70.

Sherr, C.J. (1990) Colony-stimulating factor-1 receptor. *Blood* **75**: 1–12.

Sheth, K.V., Roca, G.L., Al-Sedairy, S.T., Parhar, R.S., Hamilton, C.J.C.M. and Al Abdul Jabbar, F. (1991) Prediction of successful embryo implantation by measuring interleukin-1-α and immunosuppressive factor(s) in preimplantation embryo culture fluid. *Fertility and Sterility* **55**: 952–957.

Shi, W.-L., Wang, J.-D., Fu, Y. and Zhu, P.-D. (1993a) Estrogen and progesterone receptors in human decidua after RU486 treatment. *Fertility and Sterility* **60**: 69–74.

Shi, W.-L., Wang, J.-D., Fu, Y., Xu, L.-K. and Zhu, P.-D. (1993b) The effect of RU 486 on progesterone receptor in villous and extravillous trophoblast. *Human Reproduction* **8**: 953–958.

Shimizu, Y. and Shaw, S. (1991) Lymphocyte interactions with extracellular matrix. *FASEB Journal* **5**: 2292–2299.

Shimizu, Y., Van Seventer, G.A., Horgan, K.J. and Shaw, S. (1990) Costimulation of proliferative responses of resting CD4[+] T cells by the interaction of VLA-4 and VLA-5 with fibronectin or VLA-6 with laminin. *Journal of Immunology* **145**: 59–67.

Shinkai, Y., Rathbun, G., Lam, K.-P., Oltz, E.M., Stewart, V., Mendelsohn, M., Charron, J., Stall, M. and Alt, F.W. (1992) RAG-2-deficient mice lack mature lymphocytes owing to inability to initiate V(D)J rearrangement. *Cell* **68**: 855–867.

Shirakawa, F., Tanaka, Y., Eto, S., Suzuki, H., Yodoi, J. and Yamashita, U. (1986) Effect of interleukin-1 on the expression of interleukin-2 receptor (Tac antigen) on human natural killer cells and natural killer-like cells (YT cells). *Journal of Immunology* **137**: 551–556.

Shorter, S.C., Jackson, M.C., Sargent, I.L., Redman, C.W.G. and Starkey, P.M. (1990) Purification of human cytotrophoblast from term amniochorion by flow cytometry. *Placenta* **11**: 505–513.

Shorter, S.C., Starkey, P.M., Ferry, B.L., Clover, L.M., Sargent, I.L. and Redman, C.W.G. (1993) Antigenic heterogeneity of human cytotrophoblast and evidence for the transient expression of MHC class I antigens distinct from HLA-G. *Placenta* **14**: 571–582.

Shukla, H., Swaroop, A., Srivastava, R. and Weissman, S.M. (1990) The mRNA of a human class I gene HLA G/HLA 6.0 exhibits a restricted pattern of expression. *Nucleic Acids Research* **18**: 2189.

Sima, P. and Vetvicka, V. (1993) Evolution of immune reactions. *Critical Reviews in Immunology* **13**: 83–114.

Simón, C., Piquette, G., Frances, A. and Polan, M.L. (1993) Localization of interleukin-1 type I receptor and interleukin-1β in human endometrium throughout the menstrual cycle. *Journal of Clinical Endocrinology and Metabolism* **77**: 549–555.

Simón, C., Frances, A., Piquette, G.N., Danasouri, I.E., Zurawski, G., Dang, W. and Polan, M.L. (1994a) Embryonic implantation in mice is blocked by interleukin-1 receptor antagonist. *Endocrinology* **134**: 521–528.

Simón, C., Frances, A., Piquette, G., Hendrickson, M., Milki, A. and Polan, M.L. (1994b) Interleukin-1 system in the materno-trophoblast unit in human implantation: immunohistochemical evidence for autocrine/paracrine function. *Journal of Clinical Endocrinology and Metabolism* **78**: 847–854.

Simon, P., Decoster, C., Brocas, H., Schwers, J. and Vassart, G. (1986) Absence of human chorionic somatomatrophin during pregnancy associated with two types of gene deletion. *Human Genetics* **74**: 235–238.

Sims, J.E., Gayle, M.A., Slack, J.L., Alderson, M.R., Bird, T.A., Giri, J.G., Colotta, F., Re, F., Mantovani, A., Shanebeck, K., Grabstein, K.E. and Dower, S.K. (1993) Interleukin-1 signaling occurs exclusively via the type I receptor. *Proceedings of the National Academy of Sciences USA* **90**: 6155–6159.

Singer, D.S. and Maguire, J.E. (1990) Regulation of the expression of class I MHC genes. *Critical Reviews in Immunology* **10**: 235–257.

Singleton, T.P. and Strickler, J.G. (1992) Clinical and pathologic significance of the c-*erb*B-2 (HER-2/*neu*) oncogene. *Pathology Annals* **27**: 165–190.

Slukvin, I.I., Chernyshov, V.P., Merkulova, A.A., Vodyanik, M.A. and Kalinovsky, A.K. (1994) Differential expression of adhesion and homing molecules by human decidual and peripheral blood lymphocytes in early pregnancy. *Cellular Immunology* **158**: 29–45.

Smith, H.R.C., Karlhofer, F.M. and Yokoyama, W.M. (1994) Ly-49 multigene family expressed by IL-2-activated NK cells. *Journal of Immunology* **153**: 1068–1079.

Smith, L.C. and Davidson, E.H. (1992) The echinoid immune system and the phylogenetic occurrence of immune mechanisms in deuterostomes. *Immunology Today* **13**: 356–362.

Smith, L.C. and Hildemann, W.H. (1986) Allograft rejection, autograft fusion and inflammatory responses to injury in *Callyspongia diffusa* (Porifera; Demospongia). *Proceedings of the Royal Society of London, Series B* **226**: 445–464.

Snijders, M.P.M.L., de Goeij, A.F.P.M., Debets-Te Baerts, M.J.C., Rousch, M.J.M., Koudstaal, J. and Bosman, F.T. (1992) Immunocytochemical analysis of eostrogen receptors and progesterone receptors in the human uterus throughout the menstrual cycle and after the menopause. *Journal of Reproduction and Fertility* **94**: 363–371.

Somersalo, K. and Saksela, E. (1991) Fibronectin facilitates the migration of human natural killer cells. *European Journal of Immunology* **21**: 35–42.

Sone, S., Utsugi, T., Nii, A. and Ogura, T. (1988) Differential effects of recombinant interferons α, β, and γ on induction of human lymphokine (IL-2)-activated killer activity. *Journal of the National Cancer Institute* **80**: 425–431.

Sonnenberg, A., Linders, C.J.T., Daams, J.H. and Kennel, S.J. (1990) The $\alpha_6\beta_1$ (VLA-6) and $\alpha_6\beta_4$ protein complexes: tissue distribution and biochemical properties. *Journal of Cell Science* **96**: 207–217.

Soubiran, P., Zapitelli, J.-P. and Schaffer, L. (1987) IL-2-like material is present in human placenta and amnion. *Journal of Reproductive Immunology* **12**: 225–234.

Spits, H., Yssel, H., Paliard, X., Kastelein, R., Figdor, C. and de Vries, J.E. (1988) IL-4 inhibits IL-2-mediated induction of human lymphokine-activated killer cells, but not the generation of antigen-specific cytotoxic T lymphocytes in mixed leukocyte cultures. *Journal of Immunology* **141**: 29–36.

Spriggs, M.K. (1994) Cytokine and cytokine receptor genes 'captured' by viruses. *Current Opinions in Immunology* **6**: 526–529.

Springer, T.A. (1990) Adhesion receptors of the immune system. *Nature* **346**: 425–434.

Stanley, E., Lieschke, G.J., Grail, D., Metcalf, D., Hodgson, G., Gall, J.A.M., Maher, D.W., Cebon, J., Sinickas, V. and Dunn, A.R. (1994) Granulocyte/macrophage colony-stimulating factor-deficient mice show no major perturbation of hematopoiesis but develop a characteristic pulmonary pathology. *Proceedings of the National Academy of Sciences USA* **91**: 5592–5596.

Starkey, P.M. (1991) Expression on cells of early human pregnancy decidua of the p75, IL-2 and p145, IL-4 receptor proteins. *Immunology* **73**: 64–70.

Starkey, P.M., Sargent, I.L. and Redman, C.W.G. (1988) Cell populations in human early pregnancy decidua: characterisation and isolation of large granular lymphocytes by flow cytometry. *Immunology* **65**: 129–134.

Starkey, P.M., Clover, L.M. and Rees, M.C.P. (1991) Variation during the menstrual cycle of immune cell populations in human endometrium. *European Journal of Obstetrics and Gynecology* **39**: 203–207.

Steel, S.A., Pearce, J.M., McParland, P. and Chamberlain, G.V.P. (1990) Early Doppler ultrasound screening in prediction of hypertensive disorders of pregnancy. *Lancet* **335**: 1548–1551.

Stetler-Stevenson, W.G., Liotta, L.A. and Kleiner, D.E. (1993) Extracellular matrix. VI. Role of matrix metalloproteinases in tumor invasion and metastasis. *FASEB Journal* **7**: 1434–1441.

Stewart, C.L., Kaspar, P., Brunet, L.J., Bhatt, H., Gadi, I., Köntgen, F. and Abbondanzo, S.J. (1992) Blastocyst implantation depends on maternal expression of leukaemia inhibitory factor. *Nature* **359**: 76–79.

Stewart, F., Lennard, S.H. and Allen, W.R. (1995) Mechanisms controlling formation of the equine chorionic girdle. *Biology of Reproduction*, Monograph Series 1. In press.

Stewart, I.J. (1987) Differentiation of granulated metrial gland cells in ovariectomized mice given ovarian hormones. *Journal of Endocrinology* **112**: 23–26.

Stewart, I.J. (1994) Granulated metrial gland cells: not part of the natural killer cell lineage? *Journal of Reproductive Immunology* **26**: 1–15.

Stewart, I.J. and Mukhtar, D.D.Y. (1988) The killing of mouse trophoblast cells by granulated metrial gland cells *in vitro*. *Placenta* **9**: 417–425.

Storkus, W.J. and Dawson, J.R. (1991) Target structures involved in natural killing (NK): characteristics, distribution and candidate molecules. *Critical Reviews in Immunology* **10**: 393–416.

Story, C.M., Mikulska, J.E. and Simister, N.E. (1994) A major histocompatibility complex class I-like Fc receptor cloned from human placenta: possible role in transfer of immunoglobulin G from mother to fetus. *Journal of Experimental Medicine* **180**: 2377–2381.

Streuli, C.H., Schmidhauser, C., Kobrin, M., Bissell, M.J. and Derynck, R. (1993) Extracellular matrix regulates expression of the TGF-β1 gene. *Journal of Cell Biology* **120**: 253–260.

Strobino, B.R., Fox, H.E., Kline, Z., Susser, M. and Warburton, D. (1986) Characteristics of women with recurrent spontaneous abortions and women with favourable reproductive histories. *American Journal of Public Health* **76**: 986–991.

Stromberg, K. and Huot, R.I. (1981) Preferential expression of endogenous type C viral antigen in rhesus placenta during ontogenesis. *Virology* **112**: 365–369.

Stroynowski, I. and Lindahl, K.F.L. (1994) Antigen presentation by non-classical class I molecules. *Current Opinion in Immunology* **6**: 38–44.

Su, H.C., Orange, J.S., Fast, L.D., Chan, A.T., Simpson, S.J., Terhorst, C. and Biron, C.A. (1994) IL-2-dependent NK cell responses discovered in virus-infected β₂-microglobulin-deficient mice. *Journal of Immunology* **153**: 5674–5681.

Sugama, Y., Tiruppathi, C., Janakidevi, K., Andersen, T.T., Fenton, J.W. and Malik, A.B. (1992) Thrombin-induced expression of endothelial P-selectin and intercellular adhesion molecule. I. A mechanism for stabilizing neutrophil adhesion. *Journal of Cell Biology* **119**: 935–944.

Suni, J., Närävnen, A., Wahlstrom, T., Lehtovirta, P. and Vaheri, A. (1984a) Monoclonal antibody to human T-cell leukemia virus p19 defines polypeptide antigen in human choriocarcinoma cells and syncytiotrophoblasts of first trimester placentas. *International Journal of Cancer* **33**: 293–298.

Suni, J., Närävnen, A., Washlstrom, T., Aho, M., Pakkanen, R., Vaheri, A., Copeland, T., Cohen, M. and Oroszian, S. (1984b) Human placental syncytiotrophoblast *Mr* 75 000 polypeptide defined by antibodies to a synthetic peptide based on a cloned human endogenous retroviral DNA sequence. *Proceedings of the National Academy of Sciences USA* **81**: 6197–6201.

Suzuki, N., Suzuki, T. and Engleman, E.G. (1991) Evidence for the involvement of CD56 molecules in alloantigen-specific recognition by human natural killer cells. *Journal of Experimental Medicine* **173**: 1451–1461.

Szulman, A.E. and Surti, U. (1978) The syndromes of hydatidiform mole. I. Cytogenetic and morphologic correlations. *American Journal of Obstetrics and Gynecology* **131**: 665–671.

Tabarelli, S., Tang, B. and Gurpide, E. (1992) *In vitro* decidualization of human endometrial stromal cells. *Journal of Steroid Biochemistry and Molecular Biology* **42**: 337–344.

Tabibzadeh, S. (1990) Proliferative activity of lymphoid cells in human endometrium throughout the menstrual cycle. *Journal of Clinical Endocrinology and Metabolism* **70**: 437–443.

Tabibzadeh, S.S. and Satyaswaroop, P.G. (1988) Differential expression of HLA-DR, HLA-DP and HLA-DQ antigenic determinants of the major histocompatibility complex in human endometrium. *American Journal of Reproductive Immunology* **18**: 124–130.

Tabibzadeh, S.S., Gerber, M.A. and Satyaswaroop, P.G. (1986) Induction of HLA-DR antigen expression in human endometrial epithelial cells *in vitro* by recombinant γ-interferon. *American Journal of Pathology* **125**: 90–96.

Taga, T. and Kishimoto, T. (1995) Signaling mechanisms through cytokine receptors that share signal transducing receptor components. *Current Opinion in Immunology* **7**: 17–23.

Takagi, N. (1991) Abnormal X-chromosome dosage compensation as a possible cause of early developmental failure in mice. *Development, Growth and Differentiation* **33**: 429–435.

Takagi, N. and Sasaki, M. (1975) Preferential inactivation of the paternally derived X chromosome in the extraembryonic membranes of the mouse. *Nature* **256**: 640–642.

Tamaki, J., Arimura, Y., Koda, T., Fujimoto, S., Fujino, T., Wakisaka, A. and Kakinuma, M. (1993) Heterogeneity of HLA-G genes identified by polymerase chain reaction/single strand conformational polymorphism (PCR/SSCP). *Microbiology and Immunology* **37**: 633–640.

Tao, Y.-X. and Cao, Y.-Q. (1993) Modulation of interferon secretion by concanavalin A and interleukin-2 in first trimester placental explants *in vitro*. *Journal of Reproductive Immunology* **24**: 201–212.

Tartaglia, L.A. and Goeddel, D.V. (1992) Two TNF receptors. *Immunology Today* **13**: 151–153.

Tauber, A.I. (1994) The immune self: theory or metaphor? *Immunology Today* **15**: 134–136.

Taverne, J. (1993) Transgenic mice in the study of cytokine function. *International Journal of Experimental Pathology* **74**: 525–546.

Tedesco, F., Narchi, G., Radillo, O., Meri, S., Ferrone, S. and Betterle, C. (1993) Susceptibility of human trophoblast to killing by human complement and the role of the complement regulatory proteins. *Journal of Immunology* **151**: 1562–1570.

Testa, J.E. and Quigley, J.P. (1988) Protease receptors on cell surfaces: new mechanistic formulas applied to an old problem. *Journal of the National Cancer Institute* **80**: 712–713.

Theide, H.A. (1960) Studies of the human trophoblast in tissue culture. I. Cultural methods and histochemical staining. *American Journal of Obstetrics and Gynecology* **79**: 636–647.

Thiry, L., Sprecher-Goldberger, S., Bossens, M. and Neuray, F. (1978) Cell-mediated immune response to simian oncornovirus antigens in pregnant women. *Journal of the National Cancer Institute* **60**: 527–532.

Thiry, L., Loke, Y.W., Whyte, A., Hard, R.C., Sprecher-Goldberger, S. and Buekens, P. (1981) Heterologous antiserum to human syncytiotrophoblast membrane is cytotoxic to retrovirus-producing cells and to some cancer cell lines. *American Journal of Reproductive Immunology* **1**: 240–245.

Thornton, J.C. and Onwude, J.L. (1991) Pre-eclampsia: discordance among identical twins. *British Medical Journal* **303**: 1241–1242.

Thrailkill, K.M., Golander, A., Underwood, L.E. and Handwerger, S. (1988) Insulin-like growth factor 1 stimulates the synthesis and release of prolactin from human decidual cells. *Endocrinology* **123**: 2930–2934.

Torry, D.S. and Cooper, G.M. (1991) Proto-oncogenes in development and cancer. *American Journal of Reproductive Immunology* **25**: 129–132.

Tortosa, C.G., Vargas, M.L., Camara, M., Aleman, P., Montes, M.J., Ruiz, C. and Olivares, E.G. (1993) Expression of adhesion molecules by endothelial cells of early human decidua. *Virchows Archiv A: Pathological Anatomy and Histopathology* **423**: 287–290.

Trinchieri, G. (1989) Biology of natural killer cells. *Advances in Immunology* **47**: 187–376.

Trinchieri, G. (1994) Recognition of major histocompatibility complex class I antigens by natural killer cells. *Journal of Experimental Medicine* **180**: 417–421.

Trinchieri, G. and Perussia, B. (1985) Immune interferon: a pleiotropic cytokine with multiple effects. *Immunology Today* **6**: 131–136.

Turner, M.L. (1992) Cell adhesion molecules: a unifying approach to topographic biology. *Biological Reviews* **67**: 359–377.

Turpeenniemi-Hujanen, T., Rönnberg, L., Kauppila, A. and Puistola, U. (1992) Laminin in the human embryo implantation: analogy to the invasion by malignant cells. *Fertility and Sterility* **58**: 105–113.

Tycko, B. (1994) Genomic imprinting: mechanism and role in human pathology. *American Journal of Pathology* **144**: 431–443.

Uehara, Y., Minowa, O., Mori, C., Shiota, K., Kuno, J., Noda, T. and Kitamura, N. (1995) Placental defect and embryonic lethality in mice lacking hepatocyte growth factor/scatter factor. *Nature* **373**: 702–705.

Ulbrecht, M., Rehberger, B., Strobel, I., Messer, G., Kind, P., Degitz, K., Bieber, T. and Weiss, E.H. (1994) HLA-G: expression in human keratinocytes *in vitro* and in human skin *in vivo*. *European Journal of Immunology* **24**: 176–180.

Vairo, G. and Hamilton, J.A. (1991) Signalling through CSF receptors. *Immunology Today* **12**: 362–369.

Van de Velde, H., von Hoegen, I., Luo, W., Parnes, J.R. and Thielemans, K. (1991) The B-cell surface protein CD72/Lyb-2 is the ligand for CD5. *Nature* **351**: 662–665.

Vanderpuye, O.A., Beville, C.M. and McIntyre, J.A. (1994) Characterisation of co-factor activity for factor I: cleavage of complement C4 in human syncytiotrophoblast microvilli. *Placenta* **15**: 157–170.

van der Ven, K. and Ober, C. (1994) HLA-G polymorphisms in African Americans. *Journal of Immunology* **153**: 5628–5633.

van der Ven, K., Verp, M.S. and Ober, C. (1994) Missense mutations in the α2 domain of the human leukocyte antigen (HLA)-G gene in neonates with idiopathic intrauterine growth retardation (IUGR). Abstract (no. 031) from 41st Meeting of Society for Gynecologic Investigation, Chicago.

Van Eijkeren, M.A., Peters, P.J. and Geuze, H.J. (1991) Polarized expression of major histocompatibility complex class I molecules in human endometrial and endocervical epithelial cells. *European Journal of Immunology* **21**: 3049–3052.

Varmusa, S. and Mann, M. (1994) Genomic imprinting: defusing the ovarian time bomb. *Trends in Genetics* **10**: 118–123.

Vassalli, P. (1992) The pathophysiology of tumor necrosis factors. *Annual Review of Immunology* **10**: 411–452.

Vegeto, E., Shahbaz, M.M., Wen, D.X., Goldman, M.E., O'Malley, B.W. and McDonnell, D.P. (1993) Human progesterone receptor A form is a cell- and promoter-specific repressor of human progesterone receptor B function. *Molecular Endocrinology* **7**: 1244–1255.

Vernon, M.L., McMahon, J.M. and Hackett, J.J. (1974) Additional evidence of C particles in human placentas. *Journal of the National Cancer Institute* **52**: 987–989.

Vestweber, D. (1992) Selectins: cell surface lectins which mediate the binding of leukocytes to endothelial cells. *Seminars in Cell Biology* **3**: 211–220.

Vicovac, L., Papic, N. and Aplin, J.D. (1993) Tissue interactions in first trimester trophoblast-decidua co-cultures. *Trophoblast Research* **7**: 223–236.

Vicovac, L., Jones, C.J.P. and Aplin, J.D. (1995) Trophoblast differentiation during formation of anchoring villi in a model of the early human placenta *in vitro*. *Placenta* **16**: 41–56.

Vilcek, J. (1990) Interferons. In: *Peptide Growth Factors and Their Receptors II*, Eds. Sporn, M.B. and Roberts, A.B., Springer-Verlag, Berlin, pp. 4–38.

Vilcek, J. and Lee, T.H. (1991) Tumor necrosis factor: new insights into the molecular mechanisms of its multiple actions. *Journal of Biological Chemistry* **266**: 7313–7316.

Vince, G.S., Starkey, P.M., Jackson, M.C., Sargent, I.L. and Redman, C.W.G. (1990) Flow cytometric characterisation of cell populations in human pregnancy decidua and isolation of decidual macrophages. *Journal of Immunological Methods* **132**: 181–189.

Vince, G., Shorter, S., Starkey, P., Humphreys, J., Clover, L., Wilkins, T., Sargent, I. and Redman, C. (1992) Localization of tumour necrosis factor production in cells at the materno/fetal interface in human pregnancy. *Clinical and Experimental Immunology* **88**: 174–180.

Viselli, S.M., Stanek, E.M., Mukherjee, P., Hymer, W.C. and Mastro, A.M. (1991) Prolactin-induced mitogenesis of lymphocytes from ovarietomized rats. *Endocrinology* **129**: 983–990.

Visvader, J. and Verma, I.M. (1989) Differential transcription of exon 1 of the human c-*fms* gene in placental trophoblasts and monocytes. *Molecular and Cellular Biology* **9**: 1336–1341.

von Numers, C. (1953) On the specific granular cells (globular leukocytes) of the human endometrium. *Acta Pathologica Microbiologica et Immunologica Scandinavica* **33**: 250–256.

Wada, T., Quian, X. and Greene, M.I. (1990) Intermolecular association of the p185neu protein and EGF receptor modulates EGF receptor function. *Cell* **61**: 1339–1347.

Wahl, S.M., Allen, J.B., Weeks, B.S., Wong, H.L. and Klotman, P.E. (1993) Transforming growth factor β enhances integrin expression and type IV collagenase secretion in human monocytes. *Proceedings of the National Academy of Sciences USA* **90**: 4577–4581.

Waites, G.T. and Bell, S.C. (1989) Immunohistological localization of human pregnancy-associated endometrial α2-globulin (α2-PEG), a glycosylated β-lactoglobulin homologue, in the decidua and placenta during pregnancy. *Journal of Reproduction and Fertility* **87**: 291–300.

Wallenburg, H.C.S. and Visser, W. (1994) Pregnancy-induced hypertensive disorders. *Current Opinion in Obstetrics and Gynecology* **6**: 19–29.

Walsh, C.M., Matloubian, M., Liu, C.-C., Ueda, R., Kurahara, C.G., Christensen, J.L., Huang, M.T.F., Young, J.D.-E., Ahmed, R. and Clark, W.R. (1994) Immune function in mice lacking the perforin gene. *Proceedings of the National Academy of Sciences USA* **91**: 10854–10858.

Walsh, F.S. and Doherty, P. (1991) Structure and function of the gene for neural cell adhesion molecule. *Seminars in Neuroscience* **3**: 271–284.

Walsh, L.A., Tone, M., Thiru, S. and Waldmann, H. (1992) The CD59 antigen – a multifunctional molecule. *Tissue Antigens* **40**: 213–220.

Wang, B., Biron, C., She, J., Higgins, K., Sunshine, M.-J., Lacy, E., Lonberg, N. and Terhorst, C. (1994) A block in both early T lymphocyte and natural killer cell development in transgenic mice with high-copy numbers of the human CD3E gene. *Proceedings of the National Academy of Sciences USA* **91**: 9402–9406.

Wang, J.-D., Fu, Y., Shi, W.-L., Zhu, P.-D., Cheng, J., Qiao, G.-M., Wang, Y.-Q. and Greene, G.L. (1992) Immunohistochemical localisation of progesterone receptor in human decidua or early pregnancy. *Human Reproduction* **7**: 123–127.

Wang, Z.-Q., Fung, M.R., Barlow, D.P. and Wagner, E.F. (1994) Regulation of embryonic growth and lysosomal targeting by the imprinted Igf2/Mpr gene. *Nature* **372**: 464–467.

Watkins, D.I., Chen, Z.W., Hughes, A.L., Evans, M.G., Tedder, T.F. and Letvin, N.L. (1990) Evolution of the MHC class I genes of a New World primate from ancestral homologues of human non-classical genes. *Nature* **346**: 60–63.

Watkins, D.I., Garber, T.L., Chen, Z.W., Toukatly, G., Hughes, A.L. and Letvin, N.L. (1991) Unusually limited nucleotide sequence variation of the expressed major histocompatibility complex class I genes of a New World primate species (*Sanguinus oedipus*). *Immunogenetics* **33**: 79–89.

Watt, F.M., Kubler, M.-D., Hotchin, N.A., Nicholson, L.J. and Adams, J.C. (1993) Regulation of keratinocyte terminal differentiation by integrin-extracellular matrix interactions. *Journal of Cell Science* **106**: 175–182.

Wegmann, T.G. (1990) The cytokine basis for cross-talk between the maternal immune and reproductive systems. *Current Opinion in Immunology* **2**: 765–769.

Wegmann, T.G. (1992) Lymphohematopoietic cytokines in the placenta: their role in reproduction. In: *Immunology of Pregnancy*, Ed. Chaouat, G., CRC Press, Boca Raton, pp.143–150.

Wei, X. and Orr, H.T. (1990) Differential expression of HLA-E, HLA-F, and HLA-G transcripts in human tissue. *Human Immunology* **29**: 131–142.

Weill, P. (1921) Etudes sur les leukocytes. I. Les cellules granuleuses des muqueuses intestinale et uterine. *Archives d'Anatomie Microscopique* **17**: 77–82.

Weiner, H.L. (1994) Oral tolerance. *Proceedings of the National Academy of Sciences USA* **91**: 10762–10765.

Weintraub, B.C., Jackson, M.R. and Hedrick, S.M. (1994) γδ T cells can recognize nonclassical MHC in the absence of conventional antigenic peptides. *Journal of Immunology* **153**: 3051–3058.

Weissman, I.L., Saito, Y. and Rinkevich, B. (1990) Allorecognition histocompatibility in a protochordate species: is the relationship to MHC somatic or structural? *Immunological Reviews* **113**: 227–241.

Welsh, R.M. and Vargas-Cortez, M. (1992) Natural killer cells in viral infection. In: *The Natural Killer Cell*, Eds. Lewis, C.E. and McGee, J.O'D., IRL Press, Oxford, pp. 108–150.

Werb, Z., Tremble, P.M., Behrendtsen, O., Crowley, E. and Damsky, C.H. (1989) Signal transduction through the fibronectin receptor induces collagenase and stromelysin gene expression. *Journal of Cell Biology* **109**: 877–889.

West, J.D., Frels, W.I. and Chapman, V.M. (1977) Preferential expression of the maternally derived X chromosome in the mouse yolk sac. *Cell* **12**: 873–882.

Wewer, U.M., Faber, M., Liotta, L.A. and Albrechtsen, R. (1985) Immunochemical and ultrastructural assessment of the nature of the pericellular basement membrane of human decidual cells. *Laboratory Investigation* **53**: 624–633.

Whaley, A.E., Meka, C.S., Harbison, L.A., Hunt, J.S. and Imakawa, K. (1994) Identification and cellular localization of unique interferon mRNA from human placenta. *Journal of Biological Chemistry* **269**: 10864–10868.

White, S. and Kimber, S.J. (1994) Changes in α(1-2) fucosyltransferase activity in the murine endometrial epithelium during the estrous cycle, early pregnancy, and after ovariectomy and hormone replacement. *Biology of Reproduction* **50**: 73–81.

Whyte, A. and Loke, Y.W. (1979) Antigens of the human trophoblast plasma membrane. *Clininical and Experimental Immunology* **37**: 359–366.

Wigglesworth, J.S. (1989) Aetiology of fetal undergrowth. In: *Fetal Growth*, Eds. Sharp, F., Fraser, R.B. and Milner, R.D.G., Royal College of Obstetricians and Gynaecologists, London, pp. 185–195.

Wilcox, A.J., Weinberg, C.R., O'Connor, J.F., Baird, D.D., Schlatterer, J.P., Canfield, R.E., Armstrong, E.G. and Nisula, B.C. (1988) Incidence of early loss of pregnancy. *New England Journal of Medicine* **319**: 189–194.

Williams, J. and Kieffer, N. (1994) Adhesion molecules in cellular interactions. *Trends in Cell Biology* **4**: 102–104.

Wooding, F.B.P. (1992) The synepitheliochorial placenta of ruminants: binucleate cell fusions and hormone production. *Placenta* **13**: 101–113.

Wordinger, R.J., Jackson, F.L. and Morrill, A. (1988) Implantation, deciduoma formation and live births in mast cell-deficient mice *(W/Wv)*. *Journal of Reproduction and Fertility* **77**: 471–476.

Wu, W.-X., Brooks, J., Millar, M.R., Ledger, W.L., Glasier, A.F. and McNeilly, A.S. (1993) Immunolocalization of oestrogen and progesterone receptors in the human decidua in relation to prolactin production. *Human Reproduction* **8**: 1129–1135.

Yabe, T., McSherry, C., Bach, F.H., Fisch, P., Schall, R.P., Sondel, P.M. and Houchins, J.P. (1993) A multigene family on human chromosome 12 encodes natural killer-cell lectins. *Immunogenetics* **37**: 455–460.

Yagel, S., Parhar, R.S., Jeffry, J.J. and Lala, P.K. (1988) Normal non-metastatic human trophoblast cells share *in vitro* invasive properties of malignant cells. *Journal of Cell Physiology* **136**: 455–462.

Yagel, S., Casper, R.F., Powell, W., Parhar, R.S. and Lala, P.K. (1989a) Characterisation of pure human first-trimester cytotrophoblast cells in long-term culture: growth pattern, markers and hormone production. *American Journal of Obstetrics and Gynecology* **160**: 938–945.

Yagel, S., Lala, P.K., Powell, W.A. and Casper, R.F. (1989b) Interleukin-1 stimulates human chorionic gonadotropin secretion by first trimester human trophoblast. *Journal of Clinical Endocrinology and Metabolism* **68**: 992–995.

Yamada, A., Nikaido, Y., Nojima, S.F., Schlossman, S.F. and Morimoto, C. (1991) Activation of human CD4 T lymphocytes. *Journal of Immunology* **146**: 53–56.

Yamada, K.M. (1989) Fibronectins: structure, functions and receptors. *Current Opinion in Cell Biology* **1**: 956–963.

Yamamoto, T., Ikawa, S., Akiyama, T., Semba, K., Nomura, N., Miyajima, N., Saito, T. and Toyoshima, K. (1986) Similarity of protein encoded by the human c-*erb*B-2 gene to epidermal growth factor receptor. *Nature* **319**: 230–234.

Yarden, Y., Escobedo, J.A., Kuang, W.J., Yang-Feng, T.L., Daniel, T.O., Tremble, P.M., Chen, E.Y., Ando, M.E., Harkins, R.N., Francke, U., Fried, V.A., Ulrich, A. and Williams, L.T. (1986) Structure of the receptor for platelet-derived growth factor helps define a family of closely related growth factor receptors. *Nature* **323**: 226–232.

Yaron, Y., Peyser, M.R., Botcham, A., David, M.P., Amit, A. and Lessing, J.B. (1994) Endometrial receptivity in the light of modern assisted reproductive technologies. *Fertility and Sterility* **62**: 225–232.

Yawata, H., Yasukawa, K., Natsuka, S., Murakami, M., Yamasaki, K., Hibi, M., Taga, T. and Kishimoto, T. (1993) Structure–function analysis of human IL-6 receptor: dissociation of amino acid residues required for IL-6 binding and for IL-6 signal transduction through gp130. *EMBO Journal* **12**: 3341–3351.

Yeh, C.C., Bulmer, J.N., Hsi, B., Tian, W., Rittershaw, C. and Ip, S.H. (1990) Monoclonal antibodies to T cell receptor γδ complex react with human endometrial glandular epithelium. *Placenta* **11**: 253–261.

Yelavarthi, K.K. and Hunt, J.S. (1993) Analysis of p60 and p80 tumor necrosis factor-α receptor messenger RNA and protein in human placentas. *American Journal of Pathology* **143**: 1131–1141.

Yelavarthi, K.K., Fishback, J.L. and Hunt, J.S. (1991) Analysis of HLA-G mRNA in human placental and extraplacental membrane cells by in-situ hybridization. *Journal of Immunology* **146**: 2847–2854.

Yelavarthi, K.K., Schmidt, C.M., Ehlenfeldt, R.G., Orr, H.T. and Hunt, J.S. (1993) Cellular distribution of HLA-G mRNA in transgenic mouse placentas. *Journal of Immunology* **151**: 3638–3645.

Yokoyama, W.M. (1995) Natural killer cell receptors. *Current Opinion in Immunology* **7**: 110–120.

Yokoyama, W.M. and Seaman, W.E. (1993) The Ly-49 and NKR-P1 gene families encoding lectin-like receptors on natural killer cells: the NK gene complex. *Annual Review of Immunology* **11**: 613–635.

Yokoyama, W.M., Jacobs, L.B., Kanagawa, O., Shevach, E.M. and Cohen, D.I. (1989) A murine lymphocyte antigen belongs to a supergene family of type II integral membrane proteins. *Journal of Immunology* **143**: 1379–1386.

Yokoyama, W.M., Kehn, P.J., Cohen, D.I. and Shevach, E.M. (1990) Chromosomal location of the Ly-49 (A1, YE1/48) multigene family: genetic association with the NK1.1 antigen. *Journal of Immunology* **145**: 2353–2358.

Yu, D., Hamada, J.-I., Zhang, H., Nicolson, G.L. and Hung, M.-C. (1992) Mechanisms of c-*erb*B2/*neu* oncogene-induced metastasis and repression of metastatic properties by adenovirus 5EIA gene products. *Oncogene* **7**: 2263–2270.

Yui, J., Garcia-Lloret, M., Brown, A.J., Berdan, R.C., Morrish, D.W., Wegmann, T.G. and Guilbert, L.J. (1994) Functional long-term cultures of human term trophoblasts purified by column-elimination of CD9 expressing cells. *Placenta* **15**: 231–246.

Zarcone, D., Cemiti, G., Tenca, C., Arancia, G., Malorni, W., Iosi, F. and Grossi, C.E. (1992) Human NK cell adhesion molecules (CAMs). In: *NK Cell Mediated Cytotoxicity: Receptors, Signalling and Mechanisms*, Eds. Lotzová, E. and Herberman, R.B., CRC Press, Boca Raton, pp. 77–82.

Zdravkovic, M., Aboagye-Mathiesen, G., Zachar, V., Toth, F.D., Dalsgard, A.M., Hager, H. and Ebbesen, P. (1994) Immunosuppressive effects of human placental trophoblast interferon-β on lymphocytes *in vitro*. *Placenta* **15**: 591–600.

Zemmour, J. and Parham, P. (1992) Distinctive polymorphism at the HLA-C locus: implications for the expression of HLA-C. *Journal of Experimental Medicine* **176**: 937–950.

Zhang, Y. and Tycko, B. (1992) Monoallelic expression of the human H19 gene. *Nature Genetics* **1**: 40–44.

Zhou, Y., Damsky, C.H., Chio, K., Roberts, J.M. and Fisher, S.J. (1993) Preeclampsia is associated with abnormal expression of adhesion molecules by invasive cytotrophoblast. *Journal of Clinical Investigation* **91**: 950–960.

Zhu, H.H., Huang, J.R., Mazela, J., Elias, J. and Tseng, L. (1992) Progestin stimulates the biosynthesis of fibronectin and accumulation of fibronectin mRNA in human endometrial stromal cells. *Human Reproduction* **7**: 141–146.

Zini, J.-M., Murray, S.C., Graham, C.H., Lala, P.K., Barnathan, E.S., Mazar, A., Henkin, J., Cines, D.B. and McCrae, K.R. (1992) Characterization of urokinase receptor expression by human placental trophoblasts. *Blood* **79**: 2917–2929.

Zolti, M., Ben-Rafael, Z., Meirom, R., Shemesh, M., Bider, D., Mashiach, S. and Apte, R. (1991) Cytokine involvement in oocytes and early embryos. *Fertility and Sterility* **56**: 265–272.

Zuccotti, M. and Monk, M. (1995) Methylation of the mouse *Xist* gene in sperm and eggs correlates with imprinted *Xist* expression and paternal X-inactivation. *Nature Genetics* **9**: 316–320.

Index